PRAISES FOR
AWAKEN YOUR H

"This book is an eye-opener! Just when we [illegible] had seen it all with books like Lynne McTaggart's *The Field* and Rupert Sheldrake's *Seven Experiments That Could Change the World*, along comes the exciting and scientifically-backed account of people like John Wong, who defied the odds and went against conventional medical wisdom to emerge triumphant in a face-off with death. A must-read for those who wish to keep in good health and maintain their vitality, youth and vigor by simply changing the way they see the world around them. This book has reminded me that all of life, including my body, is a spectacular miracle. I highly recommend this book!"
– **DR MEL GILL**, author of the international bestseller *The Meta Secret*

"John proved himself to be a miracle maker when my mom was admitted to the hospital on the brink of death. Through his healing touch, my mom made a miraculous recovery that left the managing doctors dumbfounded. John is truly a healer and I am thankful and extremely blessed to have been touched and influenced by his amazing work."
– **DR VINCENT TAN** MBBS, MRCS, MMED (Surgery), Founder of Wizard Warrior Training

"When my father was warded in the hospital for a heart attack, I called John and asked him what I could do on my part to help my father. John shared that I could help my father by praying for his life energy to increase. Fortunately, I heeded John's advice and my father's condition did indeed improve. I strongly believe that having faith in prayers gave my family and me the extra boost that we needed. John's sharing on how we should pray from the heart continues to make a difference in our lives."
– **SHAN LIM**, author of *How Do Ordinary People Achieve Extraordinary Dreams*

"Thanks a lot, John. You've been of much help to me. Whatever you told me that day is still strongly imprinted on my mind. And I didn't even need to write it down! I knew we were connected when you understood what I was going through even without me having to tell you about it!"
– **JANE**, healer, oracle and tarot cards reader with an autistic son

"I was inspired by John's courage to overcome his illness. He made me believe that I have the strength and ability to battle my illness myself. This belief was the beginning of my process to recovery and it gave me hope that I would fully recover."
– **STACEY LIM**, teacher, recovered from transverse myelitis

"I, too, was inspired by the way John overcame his illness and his struggle to get well. I realized then that our belief system is one of the key forces in life. With belief, we have the hope and courage to face any obstacles that come our way. I now view any obstacles as challenges that we will eventually overcome."
– **MARK**, husband of Stacey Lim who suffered from transverse myelitis

"Now, I know how my mind and spirit are connected to my illness. And, since I own my body and my sickness, I can overcome it. I have the confidence again to improve further."
– **LUKE**, suffers from hereditary neurofibromatosis

"During my time with John, I have learned the following about him: he is very passionate about his work, he is quite an inspirational person, his enthusiasm rubs off on others around him, and he is very committed to helping people use their mental state to help manage their physical one. This book is one demonstration of his commitment in this area of treatment."
– **ASSISTANT PROFESSOR CHARLES GULLO**, Ph.D (Duke/NUS Graduate Medical School, Singapore), author of *Cancer Made Simple*

"John is a walking miracle. I am so inspired by his story, in particular his determination to live on, that I feel that everything in life is possible; only if you want it bad enough."
– **SHERYN YEO**, author of *How Do Ordinary People Achieve Extraordinary Dreams*

"It has transformed me and altered my views on my existing condition of terminal nose cancer and Parkinson's disease. By keeping a strong faith, I have already become healthier. And compared to how I had suffered previously, the severe cramps that I used to face on a regular basis have reduced dramatically. I aim to recover and go back to work in the near future."
– **DARRYL**, optometrist, suffers from nose cancer and Parkinson's disease

"During our time of need, you and your friends encouraged us greatly, and after the passing of our son Nicholas, we were able to accept this devastating turn with much needed fortitude. As Dr Daisaku Ikeda once said, "Winter always turns to spring." With that in mind, we have been sincerely practicing our faith as we have since learned that connecting to our higher selves is the key to overcoming life's sufferings. Thanks to you and your group of dear friends for all your help."
– **PHILLIP CHONG & SERENE CHONG**, parents of Nicholas Chong (deceased)

"Having been John's close friend since we were 18, I know that we share a common dream of becoming scientists who can make a difference. As we pursued our dreams, I witnessed John taking very hard knocks along the way. The first time he was lying in hospital, I thought that, like before, he would be up and about in no time. As reality unfolded, we were told that this unknown affliction would be permanent as damaged nerves do not regenerate. This was definitely the toughest battle that John had to ever face on his own. It was a despairingly helpless situation, and an agonizing one for his loved ones.

From rock bottom, John miraculously picked himself back up and put himself together piece by piece, muscle by muscle, step by step. It was a phenomenal recovery over a

very painfully long period. Today, John stands before us, having done what was thought to be the unimaginable and the impossible. John truly has a unique personality and I cannot begin to express my pride in him and how honored I am that he is my friend and living proof of what nerves of steel really means. In my eyes, he is the Ironman."
– **DR CHRISTOPHER YANG**, research fellow, Immunology Programme, Department of Microbiology, National University of Singapore

"I first met John Wong back in 2002 when Adam Khoo held his first Patterns of Excellence Program (based on Neuro-Linguistic Programming strategies). I did not meet John again until very recently. And I did not realize that the dynamic young man before me had, in the intervening years, suffered sudden paralysis and blindness to the extent that even specialists in neurosurgery were baffled at his affliction and could not really help him. So, it is truly remarkable and indeed a miracle that John Wong has not only fully recovered, but that this highly intelligent, caring and compassionate young man has now formulated strategies to help others who have been similarly afflicted. However, based on my own studies and research into the teachings of Dr Rudolf Steiner (founder of Anthroposophical medicine and nutrition), Dr Deepak Chopra (Mind/Body Connection), Neuro-Linguistic Programming and orthomolecular psychiatry/treatments, and the amazing curative powers of natural foods (to heal both mind and body), I am not at all surprised that, with God's grace and guidance, John has healed himself and is now well on his mission to help others heal."
– **BETTY L. KHOO-KINGSLEY**, eco-educator and environmentalist, author of *Cancer Cured & Prevented Naturally*

"The human body is a masterpiece of God's creation that has its own ability to heal when the conditions are favorable. John, through his own experience, has shown how one can overcome a crisis to heal oneself and help heal others. This book is a wonderful reflection of this ability and gift that God has endowed in everyone."
– **DR CHUA TECK-MEAN**, researcher, Energy Medicine

"My mother's friend, Donna, was in critical stage after she collapsed with a pain in her stomach. John taught her family on how to awaken her when all the doctors had given up hope. She has regained consciousness and is now resting at home. Thank you, John!"

– **ISAAC KK LOONG**, inventor, architect

Hi Meron,

Stillness is
your Inner Liberation.
Leads to Happiness.

29.2.12

AWAKEN YOUR HEALING POWER

a molecular biologist's journey in reversing **paralysis** and **blindness** through Transcendental Connection®

JOHN WONG CW

Candid Creation Publishing

First published March 2011

Reprinted May 2011, September 2011

AWAKEN YOUR HEALING POWER

A molecular biologist's journey in reversing paralysis and blindness through Transcendental Connection®

Author:	John Wong CW
Publisher:	Phoon Kok Hwa
Copyeditor:	Louise Lim
Layout:	Zoe Toh
Cover design:	Jacquelyn Chen
Cover photography:	Lim Kok Wee
Published by:	Candid Creation Publishing LLP
	524, Kampong Bahru Road, #03-00
	Singapore 099455
Website:	www.SingaporeBookPublisher.com
Email:	enquiry@SingaporeBookPublisher.com
ISBN:	978-981-08-7869-6

National Library Board, Singapore Cataloguing-in-Publication Data

Wong, John C. W., 1974-

Awaken your healing power : a molecular biologist's journey in reversing paralysis and blindness through Transcendental Connection / John Wong C.W. – Singapore : Candid Creation Pub., 2011.

p. cm.

Includes bibliographical references.

ISBN : 978-981-08-7869-6 (pbk.)

1. Wong, John C. W., 1974- 2. Quadriplegics – Singapore – Biography. 3. Molecular biologists – Singapore – Biography.

4. Spiritual healing. 5. Spiritual healing – Buddhism. 6. Self-actualization (Psychology) I. Title.

RC406.Q33

362.1968420092 -- dc22 OCN707456601

To my Father and Mother,
who have loved me and taught me to seek
and improve myself in many ways.

Disclaimer

The purpose of this book is to educate. It is sold with the understanding that the publisher and author shall have neither liability nor responsibility for any injury caused or alleged to be caused directly or indirectly by the information contained in this book. While every effort has been made to ensure its accuracy, the book's contents should not be construed as medical advice. Each person's health needs are unique. To obtain recommendations appropriate to your particular situation, please consult a qualified health care provider.

Author's view and interpretations expressed in this book does not represent any institutions which he worked in or collaborated. They are solely the views established by the author.

CONTENTS

Foreword		xiii
Message		xv
Preface		xvii
PART I –		
HOW I HEALED MYSELF		1
Chapter One	Uncovering the Blueprint for Disease	3
Chapter Two	A Disease Waiting to Happen	14
Chapter Three	The Manifestation of My Disease	26
Chapter Four	The Toll of My Disease	37
Chapter Five	The Key to Healing Lies Within	48
Chapter Six	My Road to Recovery	65
PART II –		
UNDERSTANDING HEALING BY TRANSCENDENTAL CONNECTION		89
Chapter Seven	3,000 Realms in a Single Living Moment	91
Chapter Eight	Five Mutual Elements	100

Part III –
HOW OTHERS HAVE HEALED THEMSELVES 129
Chapter Nine Passing the Light On 131

Epilogue 148
Annex: Tips for Recovery 153
Acknowledgements 157
Bibliography 159

FOREWORD

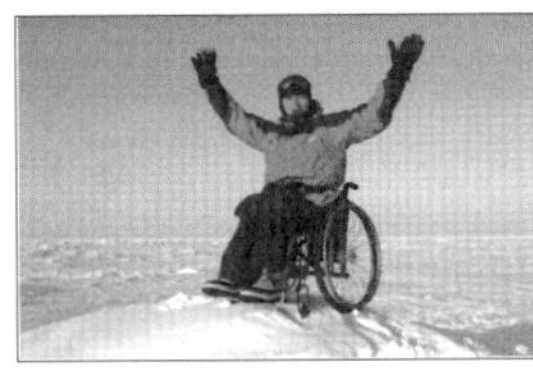

Our journey in life is never without problems, setbacks and failures. What really matters is being able to turn such setbacks into comebacks. This book is a celebration of the triumphs of John Wong. Through great determination and perseverance, he has overcome a debilitating neurological disease. As a survivor, he has turned his experiences into a passion to help others who are afflicted by illnesses affecting their brains, spinal cords, and/or their peripheral nerves.

Neurological disease is debilitating and affects every aspect of the sufferer's life. Even more devastating is the fact that there is often no cure at all. And the chronic nature of neurological disease poses a huge burden on patients and their families. Unlike other causes, such as cancer, heart disease and kidney failure, neurological diseases do not receive much support from the community. As Chairman of the National Neurological Foundation, we are very grateful to John for dedicating part of the proceeds from the sale of his book to support the Foundation's work of helping those afflicted and their families.

I congratulate you, John, for your efforts in documenting your journey. Your fighting spirit and passion to help others serve as a great inspiration to us all.

Dr William Tan
International Inspirational Speaker
www.willpower.com.sg

MESSAGE

It is with great pleasure and privilege that I've been asked to write this message for the remarkable account of John's personal journey into his illness, recovery and beyond.

I first met John several years ago as his managing physician in hospital. An intelligent and successful man, he had just been struck by a devastating illness, resulting in profound disability. He sustained widespread demyelinating polyneuropathy – a disorder that affects many nerves in the body, including nerves to the eyes (resulting in significant visual impairment), to all the limbs (resulting in weakness and sensory loss), and to the bowel and bladder (resulting in incontinence).

This left him unable to do virtually any of the activities of daily life, including eating, bathing, getting dressed, going to the toilet, getting up and walking.

The pattern of his illness was unusual and he was diagnosed at different stages to be suffering from conditions such as Guillain-Barré Syndrome and Chronic Inflammatory Demyelinating Polyneuropathy (CIDP). He underwent many tests, saw many doctors, and received many forms of treatment, including intravenous steroids and immunoglobulins, and chemotherapy.

Despite all these, his recovery progress continued to be slow and painful. Not surprisingly, he become extremely depressed and was in much despair.

However, despite all this adversity, the desire in his heart to recover remained strong. Drawing from a wide range of sources, including his faith, spirituality, complementary medicine, specific diets and a never-say-die attitude, recovery was slow but sure. He started to see again, regained control of his strength and senses, and successfully integrated back into society.

Today, John looks forward to a life full of promise and hope.

There are lessons for us all to draw from in this autobiography, particularly the unwavering strength of the human spirit that triumphs over adversity.

Happy and meaningful reading!

Dr Ng Yee Sien
Head, Department of Rehabilitation Medicine, Singapore General Hospital

** This message has been contributed in the author's personal capacity and does not reflect the views of other physicians or the institutions that he works in.*

PREFACE

At school, I majored in molecular genetics and biotechnology. Upon graduating, I embarked on a career in the life sciences industry, where I delved deeper into the dynamics of how the body works for the next fifteen years. Such was the depth that I had acquired in this specific field that I was one of the pioneering few who introduced a ground-breaking piece of new technology – tandem mass spectrometry – into South East Asia while I was working for one of the largest US-based multinational biotech corporations.

At that time, I was supposedly at the peak of my career – one that ironically involved a deep understanding of human physiology – when my own body unexpectedly failed me and life as I had known it then, came to a standstill.

In 2005, I was struck by a peculiar illness that led to my paralysis from my neck down. Most of my internal organs were also badly affected and some were malfunctioning. As if that was not enough for me to bear, I even lost my ability to see. Yet, I somehow managed to defy the better judgment of most doctors who thought that I was a lost cause and miraculously recovered from my paralysis and blindness.

Today, my doctors are not only bowled over by the fact that I am able to walk, run and dance, but are even more amazed that I have returned to my normal life and am actually living more vivaciously than ever, in the healing workshops, charitable drives and even amateur opera performances that I participate in.

Although these trials have been long and arduous, they have been necessary. My paralysis was just one of many chapters in my life that I had to experience, on top of a failed marriage, which shook the foundations of my world. Prior to all these tribulations, it seemed to me that I had been fast asleep from the truth that had been residing within me all the while. Looking back, it appeared that I had needed to experience repeated pains and failures in life for me to 'wake up' from my stupor, until I had arrived at a new and necessarily deeper understanding in life. While some might refer to this awakening as enlightenment, salvation or even being touched by God, I choose to call it a Transcendental Connection.

In the course of this book, I will be referring to a Transcendental Connection as our awakening to who we are and the profound mutual connection we have to the divine power or universal consciousness. Based on my personal experience of a Transcendental Connection, I will share how it has led to my miraculous healing and how it has allowed me to be a vehicle for further healing in others, as I continue to tread this lifelong path of self-awakening.

Not to be mistaken as a phenomenon that leans towards a specific religion, this Transcendental Connection is one that transcends all religions to encompass the bigger picture of one's spirituality. As such, you will be able to relate to the message in this book regardless of your religious beliefs.

Having said that, I need to clarify that I am Buddhist by faith. Owing to what I have been exposed to, I will be making some references to the principles of Buddhism within the pages of this book, although I will also briefly highlight insights from other faiths, as well as my own insights, about Transcendental Connection.

With due respect to all religions, I perceive myself to be spiritually-inclined in general. I embrace and respect all religions and believe that they inherently impart the same beautiful truth, albeit expressed in different ways due to the varying languages, cultures and historical contexts that shaped them. Essentially, I believe that there is only one spiritual Source, but that it is manifested in many ways and has been represented through different voices. To me, there is only one Source and it resides everywhere, in any form. And, if we look within, we will realize that we are one with the Source. Similar to how Jesus and Buddha were awakened to the truth without the need for a teacher, I acknowledge that there are many ways for us to reach God, or the Source, within us. These great teachers have always asked us to strive to look inward and see our connection to our Source as a personal journey that all of us need to embark on alone.

As you read on, I urge you to keep an open mind. It took me five long years after I had recovered from my paralysis before I felt ready to pen this book and share with a wider audience my experiences. Through my story, I hope to extend to you the conviction that we are capable of things that we never thought possible when we are finally connected to our Source. Based on my insights, I will share with you how you can reach optimal health, or even gain wealth and find love for that matter, and how you will be able to assist others in doing so too. I will also share how health, wealth and love are able to bring about happiness, albeit fleeting, but it is an inner liberation that results in true bliss.

In this book, I will also talk about how seeking perfection in others can have a limiting effect on our ability to change our lives. For when we place someone else on a pedestal, or think that others are perfect and have all the answers, we unknowingly hand our power to them and think of ourselves as imperfect, lowly, inadequate, unworthy, flawed and even sinful. In doing so, we subconsciously dissociate our own entity from our Source. By extending to you the belief that we are in fact all one and that all of us have an equal standing in the eyes of the universe, we no longer need to seek healing from someone or something that is outside of us, since true healing can only begin from within us.

I hope this book will help you broaden your awareness about yourself and your life. As you read on, I will even shed light on how and why miracles happen when there is a Transcendental Connection, from a scientific point of view. However, it must be said that some things in life cannot be explained by science, or at least not yet.

Even though I am healed from my paralysis and blindness, I recognize that I am not 'The Healer' per se. To me, Mother Nature or the Source is responsible for my miraculous healing and I am simply a messenger who is here to share the healing that I and others of different faiths have gratefully experienced.

Remember that I am not here to teach, but to share. I used to think that those who reach out to others must first be able to lead a perfect life but I have since learnt that this is a self-limiting belief. In fact, history has always pointed otherwise; great spiritual teachers like Buddha, Jesus, Muhammad, Lao Tzu and Gandhi fell hard and had to humble themselves before they could share their newfound wisdom with the world and before the world was ready to listen to them. These teachers never once professed to be perfect and even suggested that we too – though we are imperfect people – can be like them.

Today, I know that I do not have to be rich to share. I also do not have to be perfect before I can share what I have learnt with others. In fact, life is never about being rich or perfect. Rather, life is a journey where we continually work to overcome our own weaknesses, scale greater heights and impart our lessons learnt to others.

No matter what message you derive from the words in this book, there is no denying that this book has power because words have power. Similarly, consciousness has power and your actions after reading this book will have power. This power stays with you and it has always been in and with you. You are always connected whether you are aware of it or not – transcendentally connected.

PART I
How I Healed Myself

The ultimate measure of a man is not
the greatness of his deeds or words.
But rather, how he reacts to his life daily.

Chapter One
Uncovering the Blueprint for Disease

My childhood

If health is indeed wealth, then being struck by a disease is akin to having a thief take all our wealth away from us. Like a thief, a disease sneaks around unnoticed and robs a person of good night's sleep. But quite unlike a thief who walks away with one's valued possessions overnight, a disease seldom strikes quickly nor is its full impact always apparent from the start. Diseases can lie dormant in the body for months, years or even decades before they eventually rear their ugly head.

As such, the full account of my disease cannot be told from the very fateful day when all hell broke loose. Instead, the story of my disease must be traced back to its roots in my childhood...

I come from a poor family, where my parents had to struggle to make ends meet. With no education, my father, the sole breadwinner, earned a meager income that could barely meet the basic needs of the family. Such was the situation at home when I was a child that we often fretted over where our next meal would come from and even required the aid of relatives and friends from time to time to get by.

"Diseases can lie dormant in the body for months, years or even decades before they eventually rear their ugly head."

When I was five and our family's livelihood was a constant source of worry, the atmosphere at home was mostly quite grim. To make matters worse, my mother's growing discontent and frustration often erupted into frequent heated quarrels with my father.

In times like those, it did not help that my father was admittedly the kindest and most honest man that my mother had ever met. During those quarrels, she never failed to reproach my father for being the honest and trusting man that he was, and as a result of it, had often wound up being conned in whatever little business undertakings he had attempted.

Brought up in an environment where love was found wanting, I became a font of deep-seated anger. By the age of six, I began to hold so little regard for a man who provided so poorly for his family that I spoke less to my father and grew increasingly estranged towards him over the years to come.

But in spite of my resentment towards my father, what angered me most as a child were my mother's incessant remarks about how poor our family was and how stupid my siblings and I were. Even though my mother is now a completely changed woman, her remarks back then contributed much to my agony as a child.

"Their children are so smart and you are so stupid!" my mother would often grunt at me under the watchful eyes of relatives or friends. As much as I would try to appear nonchalant, I actually felt indignant and downright humiliated inside. On various occasions, my mother would even make it a point to remind me that, "My parents were poor and now we are also poor and uneducated! We will never be able to amount to anything in life!"

Although she probably did not think much about what she was saying, the degree of hurt inflicted on me was nonetheless damaging. I had to face such insensitive remarks on more occasions than I would like to remember and, as a young and impressionable child, the pain that they caused me became deeply etched in my memory, like a bad taste that lingered in the mouth.

Yet, I did not truly believe a word that she uttered.

Firstly, I did not think that I was stupid. Secondly, even though we were undeniably poor, I did not believe that we had achieved nothing. I could not resign myself, as she had, to the belief that any hope for progress was futile.

So, the more frequently and with the greater amount of conviction she professed her contempt for the family and me, the more I found myself resisting her absurd beliefs and, eventually, her. And the more I resisted, the greater the anger that raged silently within me.

I am not stupid! I would constantly affirm, like a mantra. I will become someone, someday!

Deep inside, I wanted nothing more than to prove my mother wrong. I wanted to prove to my mother that her son was not stupid and that her family would amount to something, someday. Even at a young age, I knew intuitively that I had to break out of this vicious cycle of poverty. Instead of resigning to a lifetime of poverty just because my parents were poor, I held a deep and strong conviction that I wanted very much to become someone, someday. So, while most children would say that they want to become a doctor, fireman or dancer, when asked what it is that they want to do when they grow up, I would say, "The chairman of a big company!"

> ... as a young and impressionable child, thc pain that thcy causcd me became deeply etched in my memory, like a bad taste that lingered in the mouth.

But how do I do that?

Trapped in an environment that was mired in constant negativity, I was completely at my wits end. With no answers to my questions, I found myself mentally and emotionally entangled in a web where I strived to be better to prove my mother wrong, while struggling with the seething anger inside me that intensified each time she lashed out at the family.

My anger towards my parents, my upbringing, the environment and even the world turned me bitter and angry. And over time, I developed a streak of rebelliousness that often got me into hot soup.

On one particular occasion, I had accompanied my mother to the local town council office, where she had to pay our monthly rental and utilities bill. While she was waiting in line to make her payment, I stood by a big pond outside of the office, where a handful of children were squatting, with their backs facing me, admiring and feeding the fishes swimming there. Out of sheer boredom, I strode over and kicked as many children as I could into the pond.

"Trapped in an environment that was mired in constant negativity, I was completely at my wits end."

Ploop! Ploop! Ploop! I looked on with satisfaction as, one by one, the children plunged helplessly into the water and their panic-stricken parents scrambled frantically to hoist them out.

Needless to say, I received a harsh beating from my mother over that. But that incident was just one of many where I got beaten by my mother for badly misbehaving. It reached the point where, on another occasion, the police were called in as I had been hit by my mother till I bled.

I had not been conducting myself well at home, and I was certainly no better at school. My unruly behavior persisted throughout primary school. Nicknamed 'The Little Volcano' by a teacher whom I am fondly in touch with till today, I was an angry and highly strung boy who picked fights with his peers almost every other week. In school, I became a notorious figure and it did not help matters when I won most fights that I fought. Deep inside, I secretly harbored the thought of becoming a king and even conquering the world!

Still, I was not altogether bad. Just as there are two sides of a coin, each of us possesses a polarity of traits that is both good and bad. As angry and rebellious as I was then, I caught glimpses of my compassionate side when it was not otherwise eclipsed by my defiant streak. One particular instance that best exemplifies my surprising occasional empathy for others took place when I was seven.

One day, one of the blocks in my neighborhood was engulfed by a big fire. As a young boy, I watched helplessly as the residents fled their homes and the fire consumed what was left of a very old block. With little that I could do to help, I turned instinctively towards my mother to ask her if I could pray for the victims of the fire. Seeing my earnest desire to help in what little way I could, my mother just smiled approvingly. By that time, I was no stranger to Buddhist chanting as my mother had just been introduced to Buddhist chanting and practices. With her consent, I dropped to my knees at once and started to chant for hours on end, on my own accord.

Little did I know then, that the next time that I would be taking the initiative to chant again would be many years later. And little did I know that this desire to pray would also become one of my saving graces later in life...

Mind over matter

"... a disease is the confluence of internal and external factors, such as one's genetic makeup, environment and thoughts."

A "dis-ease", as the word suggests, can be loosely defined as the lack of ease. While most of us would immediately associate this lack of ease with some problem solely in the body, this lack of ease may be extended to the mind.

Not to be perceived as separate and distinct entities, the mind and body are, in fact, facets of a higher intelligence that is still being researched on, at this very moment. This connection between the mind and the body suggests that there is a conduit between the mental and physical being of a person. So, when one is happy, endorphins are released into the body. Conversely, when one is under stress, stress hormones are then secreted into the body.

In the realm of science, many schools of thought hold divided views on the same subject. But it is widely accepted that each of us embodies an amalgamation of traits and characters inherited from our parents at the genetic level. While nature plays an essential role in molding our inherent characters and traits, we are also influenced by environmental factors on a mental and habitual level, conditioning us to behave and respond in a certain ways.

And similar to how our character is necessarily molded by a convergence of internal and external factors, a disease is the confluence of internal and external factors, such as one's genetic makeup, environment and thoughts.

In fact, recent studies in epigenetic and genetic dynamics have proven that our adopted thinking patterns, diet, behavior, and even the vibration of light, electromagnetic spectrum, and also sound wave, are capable of altering our DNA.[1] Such changes affect our resultant genetic blueprint and our blood biochemistry, which in turn, have an influence on our physiological health in the long run. As such, the internal causes of a disease can be traced to one, if not a pool of, abnormal genes that are waiting upon an external cause, such as an intense level of mental or environmental stress, to be triggered.

Since we can most certainly exert some control over the external factors in our life, we necessarily have the means to alter our own DNA and, hence, reverse any disease.

With this understanding, our mind can be our best friend or our worst enemy. It is a faculty that can help make or break us. With regards to our body, our mind certainly holds the master key to our physiological well being.

The power of the subconscious

Our mind comprises of a conscious mind and a subconscious mind that speaks two discrete languages. While the language of the conscious mind is fluent in articulating rational thoughts that receive, process, and analyze information, the language of the subconscious mind delves into a reservoir of emotions, thoughts and salient memories that sits at the outer realm of our conscious awareness. While the conscious mind has a tendency to forget, the subconscious mind, which is believed by researchers to be running our daily life about ninety

> "... the subconscious mind... is an enduring memory powerhouse that stores our salient memories or silent beliefs based on experiences and information that have been previously processed by the conscious mind."

percent of the time, is an enduring memory powerhouse that stores our salient memories or silent beliefs based on experiences and information that have been previously processed by the conscious mind.

For example, when we learn to drive or scuba dive for the first time, we are using our conscious mind to acquire the necessary skills and knowledge. But once we have mastered them, these skills and knowledge then become consequently recorded in our subconscious mind.

To be able to function normally in our daily lives, both our conscious and subconscious minds come into equal play, so that there is no saying one is better than the other. However, some scientists suggested that our subconscious mind has a far more powerful processing ability at 40 million bits per second, as compared to our conscious mind which processes information at a mere 40 bits per second.[2] So, once information is mastered at the conscious level, our subconscious mind, which also serves as a highly effective and intelligent processor, will instinctively respond to these tasks when stimulated.

Using the example cited earlier, we are using our conscious mind when we are learning to drive as we have to first think before we act. But once we have learnt how to drive, we are actually tapping into our subconscious mind when our reflexes respond seemingly on autopilot (when, for instance, we instinctively put our foot down on the brake the moment the vehicle in front of us comes to a sudden stop). Without the need to navigate through the conscious path in our minds first, we steer through our journey *mindlessly* as it is one that we are already familiar with. In another word, we live mostly on some form of playback or reflex!

But driving is one thing; it is an entirely different ballgame altogether when the subconscious mind is similarly responsible for a person's behavior.

Today, researchers have revealed that children below the age of eight, with an undeveloped conscious mind, have a high susceptibility to absorbing a myriad of information from the world around them and consequently have this very same information programmed at their subconscious level.

Even though we might have been too young to truly know right from wrong then, we would have subconsciously made some important judgments or adopted some beliefs during our early years. Unknowingly, these thoughts would tend to form our inner beliefs and behavioral tendencies later in life.

Regardless of whether our judgments were sound or whether our beliefs were relevant, they would have already become so grounded in our subconscious mind as a child that they would unknowingly still influence us as we react to situations when we have grown up. Because of such conditioning, it is not easy to alter one's subconscious mind or behavior unless one is very conscious of the need for change on a fundamental level.

"And such is the power of the subconscious mind that the person we are today is the result of our conditioning in the past."

Such is the power of the subconscious mind that all that we are, or have ever been, is imprinted like a seal on a piece of paper. And such is the power of the subconscious mind that the person we are today is the result of our conditioning in the past.

As a child, my world inevitably revolved around my family. Brought up in an environment where negativity constantly loomed like a dark cloud overhead, I believe I must have subconsciously registered that the world is a full of conflict and lack. Coupled with my mother's bitter attitude towards her life and her family, I held a belief that this world is also full of regret and anger. And since I perceived my world to be no more than a nasty, brutish struggle resulting in the survival of the fittest, I subconsciously developed a pressing desire to win and my competitive drive soon became second nature.

Academically, I was not the best but I was quite content with being amongst the top ten students in class. However, I did strive to be the best at sports in school. At home, my desire to win was so apparent that my family and relatives gave me the nickname 'Number One'!

Throughout those formative years – which I later found had a profound bearing on my later life – I continued to tread a belief system which viewed the world as a harsh place filled with either winners or losers. Never once did I forget the sense of humiliation that accompanied my mother's belittling comments and never did a day pass when I did not yearn to prove to my mother that I was capable of greater achievements. Coupled with my parents' constant complaints about how they had been ill-treated at work as a result of their lack of education, I was all the more determined to excel in life.

Perhaps it was a very early warning sign of what was to befall me in my adulthood, but when I was eleven, I started to experience a bout of vomiting, backaches and a series of headaches that was so bad that it interfered with my ability to walk at times. Because of these symptoms, I had to be hospitalized as the doctors needed to place me under observation and ran a chain of tests on me. But after two long months in the hospital, the doctors were unable to determine the cause of my symptoms and I was eventually discharged.

Through word of mouth, my mother had learnt of a very famous Chinese acupuncturist and decided to bring me to see him. After conducting a brief examination of me, the Chinese acupuncturist told my mother, "It's just a migraine!" And, by the end of the first acupuncture session, most of my symptoms were alleviated. Much to the relief of my mother and myself, I seemed to have completely recovered after a course of ten sessions.

As I reflect on the past, I find this brief episode to have been a tell tale sign of what was about to become something more severe and devastating. Just like how Western medicine – even at its best and with the best of intentions – was not able to heal me when I was just eleven, it was to prove equally inadequate when I was eventually paralyzed in my adulthood. At both times, it was my encounter with with traditional and holistic medicine and healing that made a difference to my health.

So, even in my childhood, there were undoubtedly signs that pointed at the poor state of my health. And since mind and body are inseparable, I believe that my poor psyche, or rather my angst-filled state and limiting self-belief, as a child had already had a profound physiological effect on my body. And this, in my opinion, had in turn altered my genetic makeup and affected the quality of my body's tissues right up to my adulthood.

---

[1] *John Cloud, "Why Your DNA Isn't Your Destiny," TIME 18 Jan. 2010: 49-53.*

[2] *Bruce Lipton, The Biology of Belief: Unleashing the Power of Consciousness, Matter and Miracles (USA: Sounds True, 2008) Disc 3 Track 2. Audio book.*

Chapter Two
A Disease Waiting to Happen

The need to rise above expectations

If my childhood were the breeding years for my disease, then my years as a teenager most likely contributed to the further proliferation of my physical degeneration.

During my teenage years, my habitual need to compete and rebel did not change or lessen. Even though my mother showed more compassion in her words and deeds, perhaps owing to the fact that she had found some peace though daily Buddhist practice, anger habitually continued to besiege me on the inside.

By then, my anger was no longer directed towards my parents, but towards our continued state of lack, which had not changed over the years. And it most certainly did not help matters when there was not enough money to go round at home and I was always to be seen wearing the same set of clothes when I was out with my friends.

"John, why are you always wearing the same polo shirt? Don't you have another polo shirt to wear?" my friends would ask innocently, as I felt my face burn in embarrassment. Although they meant no insult, I did not like to be reminded that my family was poor.

As an angry and rebellious teenager, I was easily led astray and joined a gang, where frequent fights only reinforced my underlying desire to compete and win. Instead of focusing my attention on my studies, I began to take on part-time jobs so that I had the money to join my peers at activities such as disco skating and making merry on the streets. Such was my indifference towards schooling and the authorities that I had already made a name for myself by getting into a fight with some boys on the first day at my secondary school.

With little direction and guidance in life, I spent most of my time and energy preoccupied with girls, my looks and being seen with the right crowd at school. Over time, my lack of interest in my studies became apparent in my poor grades.

During the first two years of my secondary education, I managed to scrape by in my examinations. But my seeming stroke of good luck waned in Secondary Three when I failed every single subject. Instead of marginally passing my subjects, as I had done for my first two years in secondary school, I scored a mere 30 marks out of a total of 100 marks for subjects like English and Mathematics.

As I stared with disbelief at the grades on my results slip, I felt a wave of unease sweep through my body.

I will have to repeat my third year if I do not pass in the final examinations! I remember thinking to myself with fear.

For the first time in my life, I faced the real possibility that my mother had actually been right all this while. For the first time in my life, I became acquainted with the word 'failure' – a word that I had thought never existed in my vocabulary, until then. And for the first time in my life, I truly felt threatened by the prospect that I would wind up never amounting to anything in life.

The mere thought of it sent shudders down my spine. The mere thought of the humiliation that accompanied a failure in my final examinations was too daunting for someone like me to bear.

For once, the competitive streak within me served me well. There and then, I felt propelled by a sudden impetus to work hard at my studies.

I have had enough fun. I cannot bear the thought of repeating a year at school. I will have to start studying! Determined to reverse the situation, I made a commitment to turn over a new leaf and study hard.

> "The mere thought of the humiliation that accompanied a failure in my final examinations was too daunting for someone like me to bear."

Such was my resolution that I made a drastic overhaul to my lifestyle. No longer was I gallivanting on the streets with my friends and no longer was I a fellow accomplice in senseless gang fights.

With only four months to the final examinations, I began to toil day and night at my books. During that semester, I literally lived, ate and breathed on the knowledge offered in my books. Not wanting to waste even a second, I even studied in the bus on my way to school, as well as on my journey back home. And, I would even study in the toilet.

Just to play it safe, I also began to adopt the habit of praying daily. From someone who would not want to pray, as the mere thought of it seemed too boring and monotonous, I transformed completely into a person who would pray for hours each day. In my prayers, I never asked to be the best, but only held the hope that I would pass my final examinations.

Lo and behold, my hard work and perseverance praying eventually paid off. Not only did I pass my examinations as a whole, I had passed each and every one of my subjects with flying colors! But what was most astounding, not only to the principal, the teachers, my peers and even myself, was that I had obtained the highest marks for all but one subject, in the entire level!

Just like that, the indescribable low that I had experienced when I failed my mid-year examinations translated into an unimaginable high after the final examinations. Just like that, I had morphed from a zero into a hero overnight. What had started out as a desperate attempt to avert the fate of repeating my third year had become by far the most invaluable lesson in my life at that point. For the first time, I learnt that studying can be a very gratifying process. And for the first time, it dawned on me that I was actually capable of outdoing others in my studies.

"Through this unexpected brush with success, I found myself overwhelmed with a sense of liberation that I had never encountered before."

Through this unexpected brush with success, I found myself overwhelmed with a sense of liberation that I had never encountered before. Although I was giddy with disbelief, I was also bursting with a happiness that was simply beyond words. To me, my surprisingly good grades were not only an affirmation that I was capable of reaping good results when I placed my heart and mind into achieving something, but most importantly, it confirmed my belief that I was not stupid after all.

"See, I told you that I can be better than others!" I exclaimed with beaming pride, as I held my results slip out to my mother when I returned home that day.

I have finally proved you wrong! I thought to myself triumphantly.

Even though I appeared to be too happy by my newfound feeling of accomplishment to be bothered by my mother's response, I did quietly observe my mother's reaction and do still recall that she did not breathe a single word. It was as if she too found the news quite hard to believe. A woman who was not too expressive or fond of words, my mother just stood still in silence. However, a reticent smile on her lips revealed much more than could possibly be conveyed with words. To me, that smile was simply priceless.

With this brand new insight into my academic capabilities, I became a radically changed person. Instead of neglecting my studies, I began to approach it with renewed vigor. Apart from showing a keen interest in the subjects in school, I started to pour over any book that I could land my hands on. It was as if I had an unquenchable thirst for knowledge and, to satisfy it, I started to read widely and voraciously on a wide range of topics that spanned everything from medicine to philosophy, physics to the arts.

As one of the top students in school, I enjoyed being in the limelight. Apart from having teachers shower their attention on me, peers whom I had started coaching in school began to look up to me as a worthy role model. For my GCE 'O' Levels at the end of my final year, I scored 'A's for all my subjects, except English, for which I had obtained a 'B'. Just like that, a once subversive gangster in Secondary One had become one of the top students in school upon graduation.

When expectations face limitations

After I graduated from secondary school, I embarked on a three-year course in biotechnology at a local polytechnic, with the goal to pursue my PhD and become a scientist subsequently. With high hopes of becoming the best in class, I continued to immerse myself in books day in and day out. If I was not studying for school, I would be reading other books, in the bus and in toilet.

Such was the degree of curiosity that I held towards the world and what made it go round that I found myself constantly generating a stream of endless questions. *Who are we? Why are we here? Why are some people so successful, while others are not? What is the meaning of life? How do we have control of our life? How do I become happy? Why do people think and behave this way?* And the list went on.

With all these questions circling in my head, I ploughed through volumes of books in search for the answers. When there appeared to be no answer, I would become even more intrigued and determined to get to the bottom of it. And when I did chance upon an answer to a question, a new set of questions emerged. It was a situation perhaps best described by Socrates when he said, "The more I learn, the less I know."

"It was as if my mind had taken on a life of its own and there was no 'stop' button to put an end to those mental conversations."

At the back of my mind, I began to feel that I was growing overly obsessed with my never-ending questions about life. On hindsight, I felt that I was not able to cope with my new-found intellectual state and the constant influx of information. Even in the quiet of the night, the silence was disturbed by the internal chatter. It was as if my mind had taken on a life of its own and there was no 'stop' button to put an end to those mental conversations. I would think long and hard into the night and, as hard as I tried to shake those thoughts from my mind and catch some sleep, I simply could not. As most nights were spent tossing and turning in bed, I started to dread each night as it approached.

As physically drained and mentally frustrated as I was then, I did not share my problem with anyone as I saw it as a sign of weakness. Instead, I pushed myself to press on, as if through mere perseverance and mind power, my problems would go away.

However, as my insomnia dragged on for days, weeks and even months on end, my physical and mental reserve took such a severe beating that my body finally succumbed under the weight of the pressure upon it. Perhaps owing to a prolonged lack of sleep, which I later discovered is essential for the regeneration of our body (see section on Wood element in Chapter Eight), as well as the high levels of mental stress that I was under, stemming from my competitive need to be the best in my studies, my body began to show signs of protest.

What started out as a harmless rash in the first year of my polytechnic studies, in 1991, intensified to become more severe by the time I was in the second year. By then, the rash had spread to most parts of my body. As if it was not bad enough that the rash looked unpleasant to the eye, it would flare into an extreme itch and sharp pain whenever water came into contact with my body. The pain was often so excruciating that bathing became a chore and I cringed at the mere thought of it each time. There was even a time when the itch was so torturing that an ambulance had to be sent for to take me to hospital. Eventually, I stopped bathing altogether but that resulted in a foul body odor. Over time, I also developed a stiff neck. Not only was I unable to turn my head freely, it eventually became an annoying twitch that would act up every few minutes.

As a result of my bad rash, constant twitching and body odor, I developed such a poor sense of self esteem that I started to distance myself from my friends. Physically and mentally worn out, my studies began to go downhill, much against my will. Within the span of a year, I had dropped from being one of the top students in school, to one of the students with the lowest grades.

Sensing the distress I felt, my mother brought me to consult a psychiatrist. After a few sessions, the psychiatrist concluded that I had a higher than average intelligence. And, despite being merely seventeen, I displayed the mentality and maturity of someone in their forties.

However, because of my strange physical condition and declining grades, some of my lecturers started to see me in a different light and some of my classmates would openly tease me. As if a regression in my grades was not already a big blow to my esteem, the comments that others made about me added to my mental and emotional stress. On top of feeling frustrated and even angry that all these things were happening to me, I felt misunderstood and hurt. However, I chose to keep my grievances to myself.

But little did I know that these signs were just the first of many other symptoms to follow. The more I tried to suppress my emotions and pretended that everything was alright, the more acute my condition grew.

It did not take long before I started to encounter a series of mini strokes, or ischemic strokes[3] as it is termed medically, in late 1992, when I was still in my second year of tertiary studies. These mini strokes struck me regularly, around twice a year, and each time they struck, I found myself unable to move or speak for hours. Stricken, my body would quiver uncontrollably and I would be on the verge of passing out. My face would turn pale and my entire body would become numb and cold, almost as if I was dead.

"The more I tried to suppress my emotions and pretended that everything was alright, the more acute my condition grew."

Being the headstrong and stubborn person that I was, I refused to fully acknowledge and accept my condition. Even though my doctor told me that I was suffering from a manic depression and prescribed me some anti-depressants, I refused to take them out of spite.

Above all else, I still harbored the goal of becoming the best in my studies. As much as I was irritated with myself for letting my grades suffer in the first place, I urged myself to overcome all odds and pushed myself to study as much and as hard as I could. Looking back, I now realize that I was not managing the exceedingly high expectations I had placed upon myself well, and I had upset the much needed balance that all of us require in our lives to stay healthy.

> "I wanted so much to break loose from this impaired shell but felt like I was locked behind a glass window that offered no way out."

The final straw eventually came when the mounting pressure from my expectations became too much for me to bear in my third and final year of studies. It was as if I had reached my breaking point and something within me just snapped. I felt desensitized from my surroundings and the people around me. I would stare into space like a zombie and my ability to absorb new information seemed blocked by a trance-like veil that numbed my senses.

Despite what was happening to me on the outside, I was still sound inside. I felt like I was trapped in a foreign body that I had absolutely no control of. I wanted so much to break loose from this impaired shell but felt like I was locked behind a glass window that offered no way out. Even though my heart and mind were willing, my body was not. With only one more semester to go, I made a decision to quit my studies.

Why is my life filled with so many obstacles? I would wonder to myself, as I pondered the meaninglessness of the days that followed, when I shut myself at home and watched cartoons all day. But at the back of my mind, I knew that I would never give up on myself.

With this resolve to recover, I went back to the same doctor during one of my regular checkups and told him, "Doctor, I want to recover."

"But what if you can never recover?" the doctor replied with brutal frankness. "What if you can never recover and your parents have to take care of you for the rest of your life?"

Upon hearing such a curt response, I resolved to never step into his clinic again. *How could I seek treatment from someone who does not even believe that I can recover?*

Instinctively, I knew that I could not put the fate of my recovery in his hands. As the bald-headed doctor went on with his speech on how I should accept my condition, I had already convinced myself to pick up the broken pieces, regain my health and eventually prove him wrong.

The calm before the storm

Not knowing how she could help me, my mother then decided to call upon a fellow Buddhist friend to come by and give me encouragement. Once a drug addict who had gone through a trying phase of depression himself, this friend shared how the power of prayers had helped him to overcome the adversities he had faced in life.

When I told him that it was hard for me to pray as I was not even able to concentrate, he said something that resonated with me deeply even till today.

"Pray with your heart, John. Not with your mind."

With no one and nowhere to turn to for help, and with the encouragement of this friend, I decided to turn to the divine again for intervention. From that day onwards, I struggled to filter out thoughts and feelings of hopelessness, anguish, fear and anxiety, as I filled my heart with earnest prayer.

Instead of being at the mercy of my inner demons for once, I sought a place in my heart where my deepest desires, hopes and dreams resided. From this place in my heart, I prayed for divine strength to recover and manifest a better me.

> "Pray with your heart, John. Not with your mind."

Six months after I had dropped out of school, I returned to my third year of studies with the support of my family and some close friends who had journeyed in faith with me during that period. This time around, I was no longer gripped with the notion of being the best student, but was merely content with graduating.

I want to live my life with no regrets. It's okay even if I fail, so long as I have given my best. Although I had not fully recovered, there were signs of improvement in my health and that was good enough to keep me going.

In spite of the problems I was facing, I also committed to helping others. Perhaps by lighting the path of others, my own path would be lit as well. By sharing my story on how I was never going to give up on myself, I encouraged others to similarly walk out of their state of depression and their obsession with their personal problems, and this courage also rubbed off positively on me.

Even though I was in a better place physically, it was still a struggle for me to go to school and sit through all the lessons. As I was unable to take in all the information at school, I decided to pick five, out of twenty chapters per subject to study for the examinations and pray that those very same chapters would be tested. Although it was admittedly not a good study practice, it was all that I could manage then.

Miraculously, all the chapters that I had picked to study were tested in the examinations! This did not merely happen for one subject, but all the subjects that I had taken. Call it a stroke of good luck if you will, but I believe that such an occurrence was the result of the good fortune that I had reaped from helping others even when I was most in need of help myself.

Upon graduation, I was enlisted to serve my national service. Due to my condition then, I was assigned to conduct research work at the Defense Research Laboratory at the National University of Singapore. During that period, my health gradually picked up and life as I had known it, was back to being normal again.

By the age of eighteen, I married a wonderful lady out of an act of rebelliousness against our parents' wishes. Due to the differences in our life directions then, we gradually drifted apart. And it was not long before we eventually parted ways mutually and peacefully. Despite our amicable separation, I was filled with regret and remorse. Deep inside, I berated myself for the rash decision to get married as a teenager. In fact, I was so ashamed of myself that I found it hard to divulge to others that I was a divorcee as I was afraid that others would see me as a failure in life.

Having weathered such an extreme physical, emotional and mental ordeal as a teenager, one would think that I had learnt a painful lesson and would never be caught repeating the same mistakes as an adult. But who would have guessed that fate had planned it otherwise...

[3] *An ischemic stroke attack is a temporary neurological dysfunction (that persists for less than 24 hours) as a result of a change in the blood supply level to an area in the brain.*

Chapter Three
The Manifestation of My Disease

The beginning of my decline

I joined the workforce in 1997, while I was still studying. At that time, I was doing very well at my job. But after I had completed my varsity education by 2000, I took on a technical sales position in another multinational company that had just set up its first business unit in the region. As I was thought to be rather young and lacking in experience, many of my colleagues in the industry thought that I would struggle to cope with the demands of the job and bow out of the highly competitive corporate setting in no time.

But little did they know that I was someone who thrived on competition.

> "Like most young adults, I was transfixed on carving the perfect future for myself and my focus then was to acquire more wealth and have greater personal growth."

Instead of calling it quits, I performed better than expected in my job. As the department had started from scratch and grew to become one of the most dominant players in Singapore and within the region, I watched as the headcount of my own division expanded. At that time, I was the sole person in charge of spearheading the growth of the division's business organically. With the continued expansion of the business, my team was at the receiving end of top regional awards and industry recognitions that could not have made the morale of the team any higher.

By then, I was earning a comfortable income and had a beautiful girlfriend whom I loved and planned to settle down with. Like most young adults, I was transfixed on carving the perfect future for myself and my focus then was to acquire more wealth and have greater personal growth. I dreamt of living in a larger private property, driving a larger posh car and leading the high life. Blinded by what this world had to offer, I looked towards the possession of material things as a source of happiness.

"... I once again found myself plagued by a familiar level of unnerving physical and mental stress..."

Riding on a career high, I was motivated to accomplish bigger and better things. To make progress in the corporate rat race, I understood that compromises had to be made. And I did. In my bid to keep up with the growing business and escalating expectations, I started to work practically every single day of the week. Each day, I worked until the wee hours of the morning, leaving myself just a couple of hours to sleep before the first stream of daylight broke and I woke up to get ready to report to work again.

As if my lack of sleep was not disturbing enough, my constant need to travel abroad for work meant that my body had to frequently adjust to a new environment and sometimes the time difference of the countries that I visited. Coupled with a rich diet of poultry and alcohol – so necessary while entertaining clients – my body was overloaded in more ways than one (see section on Earth element in Chapter Eight).

Almost like a mirror that reflected my woes as a teenager, I once again found myself plagued by a familiar level of unnerving physical and mental stress, which I still refused to acknowledge as a problem. Unable to cope with the mounting physical stress that my body and mind was subjected to, I became very irritable and critical of people and things around me. Even the most trivial matters rubbed me the wrong way and caused me to lose my temper at my family, my girlfriend, close friends and even strangers.

Thinking back, I probably knew as much that worse was to come, but I had simply chosen to ignore my worst fears.

The first signs

As much as I had chosen to play down on the impact that my career and an unhealthy lifestyle had on me, there was simply no fooling Mother Nature.

In late December 2004, my company organized a Christmas lunch at the office, where everyone could bring their families. Spirits were high and everyone, young and old alike, was in a festive mood. The day could not have been more perfect but I was not to know, however, that fate had charted a different course for me.

That afternoon, I remembered running alongside my colleagues' children in one of the games, when I found that I could not keep up with the pace. Within moments, I realized that I could no longer command my legs to run. It was as if the act of running was too rigorous for my mind and body to perform. It felt as though my legs had become so rooted to the ground that try as I might, I simply could not summon my legs to build into the fluid momentum of a run. But if it was any consolation at all, I could still walk.

For the rest of the afternoon, I was left feeling slightly perturbed, but I was quick to recover from the incident and wasted no time in dismissing any negative thoughts that followed.

It is probably some muscle ache. I shall sleep it off. I thought to myself naively.

But this was clearly not one of the problems that one could sleep off. Instead, my legs began to turn sporadically weaker over the next few days and many a time, I would even collapse under the weight of my body when my legs gave way. On a few occasions, I fell onto the bathroom floor while I was shampooing my hair with my eyes closed.

This persisted for days before my body displayed further signs of a downward spiral. By then, I would slip in and out of consciousness for seconds or even minutes, without any prior warning. It was as if I had been given a strong dose of sleeping gas and my body had no choice but to succumb to its influence. I also began to lose control of my arms intermittently. But being the stubborn person that I was, I continued to go about my daily affairs, caring little about the seriousness of my predicament.

It was not until I had several nasty encounters on the road, where I would unknowingly fall asleep whilst driving along the expressway or when the grip of my hands had slipped off the steering wheel, that I realized for the first time that my condition could probably endanger the lives of others, as well as mine. It was only then that I decided that I needed some sort of medical attention.

At the private clinic, the neurologist conducted an examination on the reflexes of my limbs. He placed wires on my limbs and tested for nerve electrical impulses. Without saying more to me, the neurologist simply scribbled his observations on a piece of paper and told me to seek treatment at Singapore General Hospital (SGH) immediately. It was with such a sense of urgency that the neurologist referred me to another hospital, yet I was still blissfully ignorant of the severity of my condition.

Perhaps I was being hopelessly optimistic, but I guess now that I was mostly in self-denial. Just like how I had not conceded defeat in life and had competed to become the very best, I would not yield to a failing body. Not again, at least. Furthermore, I had not even caught a cold for a long time, which led me to believe that my body was strong and well.

It's just a minor viral infection. I thought to myself reassuringly. *I will recover in no time and get back to work and carry on with my life!*

Resistance

My journey to SGH was harrowing to say the least. My legs were threatening to give way against the pedals and my hands felt like rubber as I tried to grip the steering wheel and navigate. It was amazing that I even arrived at my destination unscathed.

Upon admittance to SGH, I was rerouted to Alexandra Hospital. There, my condition immediately took a dive. I could not stand upright, let alone walk. I was immediately warded and specifically instructed to stay in my room while a series of observations and tests were underway. At that time, I called my family to inform them of what had happened, but kept my friends in the dark.

Still reluctant to admit the gravity of my condition and adamant about returning to my work and normal life, I decided to sneak out of the hospital when night fell. At that point, I was confident that through sheer willpower, I could command my body to be well. Using the wall as a source of support, I groped along its surface as I slowly staggered towards the car park. What should have been a breeze became a task that was immeasurably taxing for me.

When I finally made it to the car park, after a very long while, I felt what little strength was left in me ebb away rapidly. My legs seemed strangely detached from my body and, at the same time, the rest of my body seemed to have dissolved into nothingness. Almost instantaneously, I dropped like a rag doll as I collapsed onto the hard, coarse tarmac. My head hit the ground with a thud and blood began to gush out of a deep wound on my forehead.

> At that point, I was confident that through sheer willpower, I could command my body to be well.

Although my body could not obey my wishes, my perception remained acute and I was conscious of the horror of what had just happened. As I lay motionless on the floor, I was aware that I had lost most, if not all the control of my limbs. As I stared towards the night sky, I allowed the severity of my condition to set in a little.

What do I do now? I could be lying here for the whole night! So, I started to shout for help.

Slowly, a crowd started to form around me. But much to my chagrin, they just stood by inquisitively, watching me. From where I was lying, I could see them just staring, whispering amongst themselves and gesturing towards me. At the back of their minds, they must have been wondering why I was not getting up as I looked perfectly fine on the outside. So, there I was, feeling buried alive and frustrated as I just stared helplessly at those bystanders. To make matters worse, my bowel went into a massive cramp and I started to purge. Just like that, I began to defecate uncontrollably in front of an audience of bystanders. Smeared with blood and surrounded by my defecation while tossing and turning, I had never felt more pathetic and humiliated.

What is happening to me? I wondered quizzically as I lay captive in a body that was no longer recognizable to me – a body that was no longer connected to my mind. Everything was falling apart so quickly that I was unable to comprehend the reality of what was happening. I was flabbergasted!

The more I tried to wriggle my body to get up, the messier I got. After a long time, three policemen and a male nurse finally arrived at the scene and hauled me back into the hospital. By then, my clothes and my body were mostly soaked with feces and blood. I was not a pleasant sight and it was also almost impossible to breathe with the bad stench that I was emitting! Back at the ward, I received a scolding from one of the senior staff nurses who threatened to tie up my limbs should I harbor any more thoughts of leaving the hospital. By then, my girlfriend had arrived and she stood vigil over me till the next morning.

The very next day, I quickly became the subject of a series of tests. Medical staff would come in unannounced, observe and probe me, and then leave without a word. I began to feel less like a patient and more like some curious scientific specimen on a laboratory table

Do they not interact with their patients? Are they simply too stressed to care for their patients and put in a sympathetic word? I wondered to myself critically.

At one point, a junior doctor, accompanied by a senior doctor, was instructed to practice puncturing a needle into my spine in order to extract samples of my cerebrospinal fluid for further testing. According to the senior doctor, they were testing for antibodies in my nerve tissues and the protein content in my cerebrospinal fluid.

Since the spinal cord is a spongy conduit at the back which houses all the nerves necessary for all sensory experiences, motor transmissions and communication throughout the body, one can only imagine the pain and discomfort when a sharp needle is pierced right into the spine, even when administered by a pair of experienced hands. So, imagine the extent of my pain and agony when this junior doctor tried unsuccessfully, on more than one attempt, to insert the needle into my spinal cord. Each time she inserted the needle into my spine, my body clenched in fear and my teeth grit in anguish. The pain was so unimaginably acute and excruciating that I would never ever wish it upon anyone.

My family and girlfriend were by my side throughout the procedure. And even though their faces registered shock and disbelief, I remained optimistic that I would be back on my feet in no time. In fact, my mind was preoccupied with work the whole time I was hospitalized. I kept telling the nurses that I was a busy man with a lot at stake at work and that I needed to bring in a laptop to work from the hospital. But of course, the nurses never acceded to my request.

After a few days of waiting, the doctors finally rallied round with a prognosis to offer my family and me. They explained that they could not arrive at a conclusive diagnosis. However, they suspected that I was suffering from Guillain-Barré Syndrome (GBS). They added that GBS could not be cured but a kind of specialized chemotherapy or a high dosage of steroids could be of use to minimize the deterioration. Triggered by numerous suspected factors, like the flu, vaccinations, food poisoning, toxins and even allergens, amongst others, GBS has many variants and rare sub-variants and can affect any part of one's body or organs. Based on what little was known about this rare condition, GBS could potentially have a mild, debilitating or even deadly effect on a person's body. As my condition was merely a suspicion on the doctor's part, I remained very positive about a full recovery. Without the need for medication, I was placed under observation for possible improvements.

Even with this new insight into my condition, I remained insistent about returning to work. Looking back, I was perhaps being an impossible workaholic, but I was also probably trying to cling onto anything that would make my life feel like it had gone back to normal.

Since there was no cure per se and there was simply no way for me to get back to work unless I was discharged from the hospital, I decided to put on a healthy and normal front before the doctors and nurses, to trick them into believing that I had recovered after all. So, during the next two weeks of physiotherapy and rehabilitation, I harnessed all my will power and strength to move about normally. On top of that, I would also appear to be upbeat and cheerful. Based on what little acquired knowledge I had about medicine and biology, I did my best to mimic a satisfactory reflex response when tests were being conducted, so that the physician was fully convinced that my condition was turning around. I was able to stand up for a short while and also started to walk in a wobbly fashion for up to 5 faint steps. Coupled with several sessions of physiotherapy that recorded improvement in my progress, as well as much persuasion on my part, I was finally allowed to be discharged by reluctant doctors.

When I was finally discharged in the second week of January 2005, my family was constantly there to attend to my needs. Like a toddler, I was learning to walk steadily again and my family took turns to keep a close watch on me. In the hopes of recovering faster, I started to go for acupuncture. But the car trips to the acupuncturist soon proved to be too horrifically punishing and physically taxing for me.

For some reason I could not grasp, my head would throb with an unbearable pain each time I travelled to the acupuncturist. My head would be spinning so badly that I felt almost detached from my body. By the time I had arrived at my destination, I would be feeling out of breath. On top of that, a nauseating wave would leave me grappling with a violent cramp in my stomach. Such trips were so bad that I even cried at the mere thought of travelling in a car and begged my family not to drag me for treatments anymore.

By then, the disturbing reality of my condition finally hit home. As I watched my body crumble into pieces and my life thrown out of synchrony, there was simply no denying that something was inherently wrong with me. Although I was still lucid, my body had become an impenetrable wall that stood between me and a lifestyle that I was once familiar with. I could barely make it out the door and my work had come to a halt. My condition challenged my sense of self and it disrupted the very core of who I was and what I would normally have been capable of performing on my own. My limbs almost lost all its functions. I no longer had the strength and control to climb the stairs, stand for more than 1 minute without assistance, use the laptop, make a phone call, handle the chopsticks, bathe myself and brush my teeth.

But in spite of an uneasy sense of foreboding, my spirit remained unbowed and I started to pray more fervently. During times of such extreme vulnerability, my perspective on life shifted and I felt compelled to journey inwards. I would reflect upon what I had done in my life.

Why is this happening to me? Is this the result of something I did? Did I do something wrong? Why am I being punished this way?

Amid all the uncertainties that surrounded me, I remained steadfast in my prayers, as I hoped for a recovery.

Although the process was grindingly slow and laborious, I was soon able to walk without much of a struggle. Following that, I was able to get up from a chair by myself and could at least stand for a full minute. The doctors grew increasingly optimistic about my ability to recover and deep in my heart, I firmly believed it too. During the span of a month, I made such tremendous leaps in my recovery that many people who had learnt about my story, rallied round and encouraged me to share how my faith had healed me.

"During times of such extreme vulnerability, my perspective on life shifted and I felt compelled to journey inwards. I would reflect upon what I had done in my life."

But the sense of relief that accompanied my short bout of recovery was unfortunately short-lived. Just when my road to recovery seemed to be all set in stone, my health took a sudden and sharp turn for the worst in the weeks to come.

Chapter Four
The Toll of My Disease

My body was no longer mine

In the first week of February 2005, I started to have bizarre, and oftentimes unsettling, visions. Throughout the course of the day, I would see objects morphing into other things. Such was the peculiarity of the phenomenon that I would see pots transformed into oranges and baskets into crabs. On some occasions, I even saw shadows pass me by out of the corner of my eyes. Once, a plant even morphed into an alien and came walking towards me. It was as though my perception of things had become distorted and my reality had been entangled in some twilight zone where shapes and forms were subjective.

How could this be happening?

Considering how outlandish these sightings were, I had trouble coming to terms with them and I decided not to breathe a word about them. Besides, my academic background in biochemistry gave me reason to believe that those disconcerting visions were the result of some temporary disturbances at a physiological level in my brain.

But by the second week of February, my health continued to go downhill. Physical activities that previously did not require much effort on my part became increasingly laborious to perform. Firstly, I grew easily lethargic and breathless as I literally felt my energy being drained by the minute. My fingers started to become weak and I slowly lost the ability to even clasp a spoon at mealtimes. Next, my speech became affected. Sentences became chopped into fragments of words and my voice reduced to a somewhat inaudible slur. Within days, I had lost every inch of control over my limbs as they became increasingly frail and numb to my senses. By then, things had completely spiraled out of control and I found myself unable to engage my body normally. Eventually, I could not even turn around in bed, not to mention hauling myself out of it.

When my body refused to comply with the desires of my mind, my parents took on the arduous duty of attending to my daily needs at home. But as my mother and father were already at an advanced age (late fifties and early sixties), and not in the most optimal of health, dealing with all of my physical needs proved to be immeasurably taxing for them.

Although my parents never did grunt a word of complaint, I could read the expression of unspoken struggle on their faces whenever they tried to sit me up in bed. During that time, my father had a serious problem with both knees – he could easily dislocate either knee if he strained them or moved them in the wrong way. My mother also had a numbing pain in all the joints of her hands due to her constant contact with cleaning chemicals and water while washing dishes and cups during all those years as an office cleaner. Upon seeing the tremendous strain that they were under, my heart sank with a deep sense of guilt and remorse. Plagued by deteriorating health, I was not only carrying the burden of a failing body, but also the pressing weight of anger and frustration that I held at my helplessness. This persisted for days before I next consulted a medical professional.

On the morning of Valentine's Day (14 February) 2005, I had a scheduled appointment to return to SGH for a routine checkup. As I was unable to get out of bed, my family called for an ambulance to send me to the hospital. So, what really should have been an easy and effortless trip to the hospital became a dramatic affair where I had to be supported by an elaborate machine and towed down some steps as there was no elevator serving the floor where I lived. And what really should have been a routine checkup that might last a couple of hours at most, dragged on to become a long, much dreaded and miserable stay in the hospital.

"What happened to you?" my senior neurologist shrieked as she jumped to her feet and slammed her hands on her table in shocked disbelief when she saw me. Instead of reflecting a recovery that was in full swing, as she clearly had expected, my nerve conduction test recorded a sharp decline in my condition.

Much to my dismay, my neurologist ordered me to be hospitalized at once. At that point, my spirits were low as I thought that I would be as fit as a fiddle by February and able to take my girlfriend out for a celebration on Valentine's Day. I thought I would be able to resume my regular life and no longer be a source of worry for my family and girlfriend. But I could not have been more wrong.

In spite of the disappointment I felt in being admitted to hospital once again, I continued to hope that I would be discharged within weeks or even days, as had been the case during my previous bout of ill health. But as fate would have it, this stay in the hospital became the longest and most treacherous chapter of my life.

Fear was my dominant state of mind

This time around, the sudden relapse in my disease left me completely paralyzed from the neck down. Such was my inability to control my body that I was not even able to sit on a wheelchair as I would just slide down onto the floor like a limp ribbon. As such, I had to be confined to the bed at all times. During the first two weeks of my hospitalization at SGH, I was so physically drained that I was reduced to a semi-conscious state most of the time, barely aware of my surroundings. Soon, I lost the sensation of touch. I could not even feel the touch of my love ones. My body had gone completely numb.

The sensory interactions that governed my world had vanished.

By the second week, I was more conscious of what was happening around me. But this awareness also jolted me to an appalling realization that my body was treading the path to perdition. At first, swallowing became increasingly difficult, as I would choke on the food ingested. Subsequently, eating became a chore altogether and I had completely lost my ability to produce a sound. Within an alarmingly short span of time, most of my organs started to malfunction one by one.

I could not even expel my urine or feces. As a result of this problem, my bladder began to swell and my bowel became bloated. Due to the large amount of gas trapped within my body that I did not have the means to release, my insides became subject to bruising aches and violent pains. Whenever the nurses tried to adjust my body on the bed, I felt sudden spells of excruciating pain, as though my organs were being punched and stabbed! What made the pain more insufferable was that the nurses adjusted me a few times each a day and I was too weak to even protest each time. As there was no way that they could read my mind, the nurses were puzzled at why my face expressed fear whenever they approached me. On their part, they must have thought that I had lost my mind. To me, life was a living hell every day.

But the worst was yet to come. Within a month of my hospitalization, my vision faded, leaving me in a grey, clouded and dim world where I could hardly see a thing. As though losing my sight on top of all the other faculties of my body was not hard enough to bear, I was constantly irritated by sharp pains, like sudden pulses of electrical current, behind my eye, causing me extreme discomfort throughout the day.

Just like that, all the basic functions of my nervous system and muscular system had come apart one by one, resulting in a body that was totally impaired. Within what seemed to be the blink of an eye, my body had crumbled under the devastation of a disease that had left it an empty shell and one that no longer seemed to be mine.

I had heard of other conditions like cancer, stroke and other common ailments to befall others, but I had never expected that I would be subject to such a severe condition that would result in such a fast, painful and extreme deterioration of my body.

> "My body was like a time bomb that could go off at any time."

As time passedAs time passed, my spirit was getting weaker and my life hung precariously in the balance. My weight dropped by 25 kilograms or more, and my heartbeat and blood pressure levels were still extremely erratic and oftentimes threatening to my life. My body was like a time bomb that could go off at any time. Every now and then, doctors and nurses would swing by to monitor my situation and watch out for any signs of impending danger.

Countless tests were conducted on me during those first few weeks in hospital. And as the doctors were not offering my family and me much information about my condition, I could not help but try to put together the pieces of the puzzle by eavesdropping on their conversations.

Although my poor eyesight meant that I could not read their body language, the tone of their voices communicated the gravity of my situation. Through the bits of information that I gleaned from the hushed conversations that I managed to overhear, my worst fears were confirmed. Not only was my condition getting from bad to worse, but they were also clueless as to why this was happening to me! So there I was, unable to move or see and encapsulated in a dark chamber of helplessness all by myself.

How could it be that the doctors do not know what is happening to me even after so many weeks of study and tests? I thought to myself in dismay.

My thoughts soon ran further and wilder, fueled by my intense anxiety. By then, the severity of my condition really hit home hard and it occurred to me that my life had seemingly arrived at a dead end. What little glimmer of hope that I had clung onto was overshadowed by a wave of crippling fear that was impossible to defy.

What will happen to me if I am permanently trapped in this hellish state for the rest of my life?

“... the severity of my condition really hit home hard and it occurred to me that my life had seemingly arrived at a dead end.”

As the days went by, my fear intensified exponentially. Apart from being overwhelmed by an underlying fear that I would never be able to recover and get up on my feet again, there were also the daily fears that I had to confront as a result of the callous treatment I received at times. For example, I needed to be bathed by the nurses. Whilst lying on the bathing bed, the nurses would shower water onto my body and head. Unknown to them, I often wound up choking and gasping for air as the water channeled into my mouth. Unable to protest, I actually thought I would drown while bathing. As a result of that, bathing became such a punishing act for me that I began to develop a fear of something as simple as bathing.

Dying seemed to be the answer

As my spirit and my body slipped away, there was only one thing that I could still control in my life – my mind. My wondering mind was also a breeding ground for my pain and misery during this period. But try as I might to muster the will to fight this disease, I realized that the sheer brutality of this disease was enough to humble even the most conceited man and bring down the resilience of even the strongest-willed individual. At that time, I realized that sheer will power was not the be all and end all to everything in life. Positive thinking was also futile as the physical pain and trauma of what I was going through could not be ignored. Reduced to such a state of desolation, sheer will power and positive thinking would not bring me back on my feet and no amount of motivation would be able to move me.

As weeks slipped into months, I felt denied of the basic dignity that every human being is entitled to. On days when I could still gather the strength to mumble, I had to plea, cry and scream for nurses or even strangers to adjust my sore and frail body. On other occasions, I had to beg with tears in my eyes for the nurses to feed me with water and food gently. Unable to fend for myself, I was at the mercy of nurses to bath, feed and move me about. Oftentimes, I felt like a piece of dead poultry, as nurses man-handled my then lifeless body. As much as I dreaded the feeling of being dependent on others, I knew that I was not in a position to choose, but had to simply resign myself to such a sorry and even forlorn plight. For a go-getter like me, my inability to change anything about my life was a horrific reality that was simply too cruel for me to grasp and accept. I remember thinking to myself how horrible and painful it was to still be alive!

"I realized that sheer will power was not the be all and end all to everything in life. Positive thinking was also futile as the physical pain and trauma of what I was going through could not be ignored."

Not a day passed when I was not embroiled in constant pain, dark and fear. Time seemed to have stood still and every moment seemed like an eternity. Gone were the days when I thrived on targets and goals. Instead, I could no longer make out any purpose in life. Trapped in a body that had left me immobile, there was absolutely nothing I could do but to journey into the realms of my tortured mind.

In the silence of the night, I would recall those good old days when I was healthy and up and about. I thought about the challenges that I used to face in life and knew that despite all those odds, nothing could possibly compare to what I was experiencing then. And what made it worse was that no one could tell me when or even whether this suffering would eventually come to an end.

During my stay in the hospital, I had relatives and friends who came by to visit me. While most of them tried to support me in my time of distress, others were less empathetic. So, while the majority conveyed words of encouragement to my family and me, others were quick to pass vile remarks with unsettling claims that I must have sinned terribly in my life.

Why me? I would plead in desperation. *What have I done to deserve this? Did I swallow a toxin? Did I catch a virus from some country that I visited? Did someone perform black magic on me?*

My mind constantly swarmed with endless questions as I tried to make sense of the seemingly senseless. I thought that if I could get to the root of the problem, I would be able to work something out with the doctors to cure me. When I was left with no satisfactory answers, I started to question if I had indeed sinned terribly in my present or past lives and this was the consequence of

> "For a go-getter like me, my inability to change anything about my life was a horrific reality that was simply too cruel for me to grasp and accept."

my karma. Guilt multiplied inside my mind, torturing me no end.

What is this guilt going to do to me besides this?

At the mercy of an unresponsive body, I felt isolated from all things and inevitably the world around me. It seemed to me like I was in my own world – a world that prohibited me from any contact or interaction with the outside world that I was once a part of. I was like a captive held in a prison cell that offered not even a glimpse of light. Every morning, I woke up barely able to see a thing. And what little I could see appeared dim. Consumed with so much sadness and fear, I would scream at the top of my lungs until I eventually lost my voice. Still, no one answered my calls of desperation. No one came to my rescue. No one could.

> At the mercy of an unresponsive body, I felt isolated from all things and incvitably thc world around me.

Even though I was burning with desire to connect with the outside world, my family and my girlfriend, the compulsion only drove me to further frustration as I was not even able to feel the encouraging touch of a loved one! Without being able to feel my mouth or my tongue, I found it testing to even acknowledge my own physical existence. I felt robbed of my sense of self and it seemed as though the very core of my identity had been cruelly taken from me. Immured within the tomb of my failing body, I felt like a ghost or a spirit that had faded into an existence where the line between life and death blurred.

As grueling as it was for me, the patient, to endure this ordeal, my loved ones did not have it any easier. If it was any solace at all, my family and my girlfriend came by to visit me every day. My mother, unable to contain her emotions, often cried hysterically in the initial months when she visited me. Although I could not see my mother's face clearly, I could hear the anxiety and helplessness in her bitter sobs. My father, on the other hand, was less expressive of his emotions. But come rain or shine, my father would visit me at half past six every morning before he headed to work.

"Son, I am here." My father would tap me gently on my shoulder before retreating to a corner of the room and praying for a whole hour for me. Although my vision had been compromised, my heart finally saw him for the good man that he was. My father's virtues, which I had chosen to turn a blind eye to for years, became all of a sudden apparent to me.

Even though he was equally stricken with fear, he kept his worries to himself and silently supported me during those trying times in ways that he knew best. Through my father's simple, yet steadfast, acts of love for me, my longstanding resentment towards him evaporated and was instead replaced by a newfound respect. For the first time in my life, I truly allowed myself to experience my father's love for me and I felt like a newborn child once again in the embrace of his arms.

But who would have thought that their love for me was actually emotionally punishing for me. The more selflessly they cared for me, the greater it brought to light my failures as a son. In the midst of all that love, I could not help but feel like a complete disappointment and a heavy burden to my parents.

What if my parents have to take care of me for as long as they live? What if I can never repay their love for me?

I found it impossible to define myself within the parameters of my seemingly vague and burdensome existence and cried myself to sleep on most nights. On days when the physical discomfort and emotional anguish became too unbearable, I contemplated death as the answer to all my sufferings. On days when I felt so alone and seemed to be on the brink of death, I courted the idea of ending my life prematurely. But even that eluded me.

“Such was my level of incompetence as a human being that I could not even exercise my freedom to choose death over life.”

I could neither lift a finger to silt my own throat, nor bite my tongue and hope to bleed to death. Such was my level of incompetence as a human being that I could not even exercise my freedom to choose death over life. It had never crossed my mind till then, that dying could actually become a privilege. I was certain that this was what hell was like.

At that point, I was ready to surrender whatever remained of my life when a series of events took place that made me rethink my outlook towards life and its value.

Chapter Five
The Key to Healing Lies Within

My near-death experience

In life, I have come to realize that we learn the most when we face the greatest adversity. Oftentimes, we require a life-changing event to shake us, as if by our shoulders, before we experience a shift in our perception and have a true glimpse of the value of life.

After spending a total of three months in the hospital, I was so physically, emotionally and mentally drained that I was truly at the end of my tenterhooks. On top of the gnawing pain that I suffered as the weight of my rib cage constantly pressed on my lungs, I had to deal with other frequent but intermittent problems, such as a pounding headache, floating dizziness, a constant pulse of pain behind my eye that burned my brain, and difficulty in inhaling. Above the constant torment of the pain was the nagging thought that I was a downright burden to my family and was probably better off dead. In fact, I felt certain that I was losing the battle against my disease and was ready to surrender my life, when the unthinkable took place.

One evening in early March 2005, I was all by myself in the quiet of my ward. As usual, I was immersed in a deep pain that left me physically depleted. Then, the pain seemed to fade into the background and an overwhelming sense of tiredness came upon me slowly but surely and I found myself slipping out of consciousness.

As surreal as it seemed, my recollection of what was to follow was surprisingly vivid.

At first, my breathing became much easier. In fact, it was almost effortless. But I began to feel a sense of foreboding as my eyes slowly closed. All of a sudden, I found myself engulfed by some indescribable universal force as I felt myself falling deeper and deeper into an abyss. I realized that I was, in fact, no longer breathing. Somehow, I knew that I had become detached from my immobile body and I began to panic. As my consciousness continued to fade and I continued gliding silently down a dark, silent abyss, almost as if on a soft, invisible cushion, I was shaken by the realization that I was going to die, and perhaps was even in the process of dying right now.

Not like this... not in this manner. I begged desperately. *Help me please, benevolent universe!*

Suddenly, I no longer wanted to die. Instead, I tried to paddle my way upwards. However, I continued to fall and, as it became increasingly quiet and peaceful as I fell deeper, I knew that my life would eventually come to an end. At that instant, the succession of events in my life flashed before me and I realized that I was looking at myself from a new and totally different plane and dimension. All that had happened to me during my past lifetimes became apparent to me in just a few short seconds. Events that had spanned decades took mere seconds to replay before my very eyes, as if time itself had become subjective.

> "... I found myself engulfed by some indescribable universal force as I felt myself falling deeper and deeper into an abyss."

Intuitively, I knew that I was waiting for my higher consciousness or my ultimate true self to sum up the totality of my existence. For the first time, I was privileged enough to understand that

> "This emerging true self would be the sole truth of our real identity."

> "... my near-death experience was one of the most fearful, yet most beautiful, humbling and profound experiences ever."

at death, we would be judged by our emerging true self alone. This emerging true self would be the sole truth of our real identity. As it had emerged from within me while I was slowly departing this world, I discovered that my true self is in fact also part of the universe and universal consciousness.

I became part of the Divine Consciousness, yet I was still aware of my own identity on earth. I must confess that no words in the world can accurately describe the way I felt at that moment. In that instant, I finally realized that I was connected to the universe and that the universe is, in fact, in me. Suddenly, the silence of space was filled by the resonance of Buddhist chanting and I was swept off my feet by what seemed to be a rising carpet that was preventing me from falling deeper.

As fleeting as it was, my near-death experience was one of the most fearful, yet most beautiful, humbling and profound experiences ever. At that moment, I became aware that I was one with the vastness of the universe. At that moment, I came to the realization that I was merely a physical manifestation of the ebb and flow of the universe. I understood that our physical being and consciousness are synchronized in the same space, yet this space is also multi-dimensional in its content and activity. Each of us is like a drop of water, part of the cosmic ocean of space and time. When the drop of water returns to the ocean, the drop becomes one with the ocean. And just as the drop is the ocean, the ocean is made up of many drops. Essentially, we are all one, regardless of our form.

I understood that God, or what some call the Source, the higher self or even the Mystic Law, is actually the universal and cosmic consciousness pulsating in everything and everywhere around us. And just as how the Old Testament suggested that God had made each and every one of us in his image, we are also the consciousness of this universe (Genesis 1:27). This was, at once, both very profound and very simple.

I recognized that the universe exists within us, but also outside of us. Time, space, matter and energy make up this cosmic oceanic space and we are, in turn, made of these elements. We are one within the never-ending momentum of cause and effect operating in this vast cosmic space.

Although many books have cited similar experiences, for me, encountering the depth of this profoundness first hand surpassed all the head knowledge that I could possibly have gleaned from mere words in a book.

It truly was a moment of epiphany. I had come face to face with death but had been held back in the nick of time. And, everything in life suddenly became crystal clear to me, as if I had been given true insight by a higher intelligence.

> “I understood that God, or what some call the Source, the higher self or even the Mystic Law, is actually the universal and cosmic consciousness pulsating in everything and everywhere around us.”

After this encounter, a sense of calm pervaded my entire being. I thought to myself that perhaps what I needed was indeed to lose my sight and physical perception of a world that I was all too familiar with, before I would be able to step into a different dimension and see things as they truly were.

“John, did you know that we were praying for you earlier?” a friend asked matter-of-factly when a group of them visited that night.

"I know," I mumbled weakly under my breath. In my heart, I knew that the chanting that I had heard earlier was their prayers for me. For the first time, I had experienced and acknowledged the power of distance healing via prayers. In my heart, I knew that their prayers had been my saving grace that evening. If anything, I was all the more convinced by the power of prayers.

I am my own healer

I may have surreptitiously escaped a near death, but the thought of dying did not leave me completely. Although death would have been an easy solution, I knew that life was what I was stuck with.

If anything, my near-death experience reinforced my understanding that the kind of life we have led cannot be judged by the material possessions that we accumulate or the power that we command. At the moment of death, we are answerable only to ourselves for our thoughts, words and deeds. This realization gave me the resolve to recover so that I would have a second chance to live life. However, the decision to recover was one that I had to make many times a day. This was especially so when the doctors, who are often looked upon as figures who provide hope for the patients, became the very ones to undermine my resolve.

> "... my near-death experience reinforced my understanding that the kind of life we have led cannot be judged by the material possessions that we accumulate or the power that we command."

When the doctors finally came back to my family and me with a full report on my condition, they disclosed that they had never come across a condition similar to mine. According to their prognosis, they suspected that besides the outer layer of the nerves being damaged, the axons, or the cores of the nerves in my body, had either been severely damaged or had somehow disappeared. The damage to my body was extensive.

Based on my understanding of the anatomy of a human body, I knew that nerves work very much like electrical wires, and are responsible for sending signals from our brain to different parts of our body. As such, they are responsible for the transmission of the basic senses: touch, vision, hearing, taste, smell, and cognition and perception. Consisting of two parts, the outer part of the nerve, known as the myelin sheath, is made of fatty acids and is like the rubber coating of an electrical wire. Its function is to insulate the core. Meanwhile, the axon, or the core of the nerve, which is mainly made of protein, is like the copper conductor of an electrical wire.

So, when the doctors told me that most of my nerves were transmitting little or no signals, it meant that the axons were most likely damaged and I knew that my nerves no longer served a purpose, which explained why my body was so severely impaired. I also knew that, unlike the myelin sheath or other parts of the body that are capable of regenerating themselves, the axon of a nerve can no longer repair itself once it is damaged.

According to the doctors, the results obtained from the nerve conduction tests on both my optical nerves inside my eyes, my spinal cord, as well as the peripheral nerve regions in my body, revealed extremely low and in some cases, almost no nerve electrical signals. That led them to postulate that my body might have lost significant axonal matter and function, and that I would be likely to remain bedridden for the rest of my life, or at best, be severely handicapped.

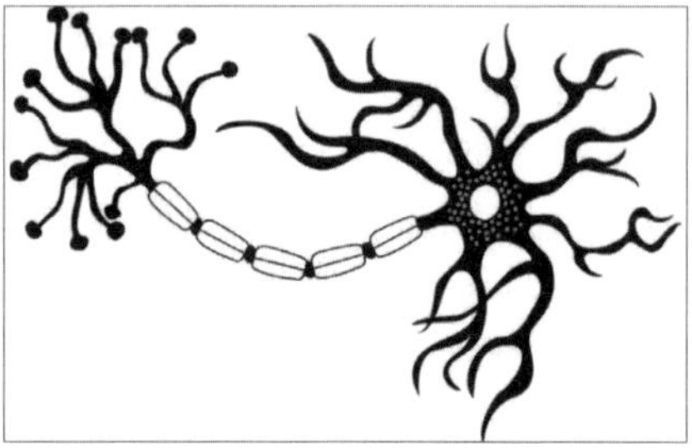

Figure 5-1 Pictorial representation of a nerve fiber

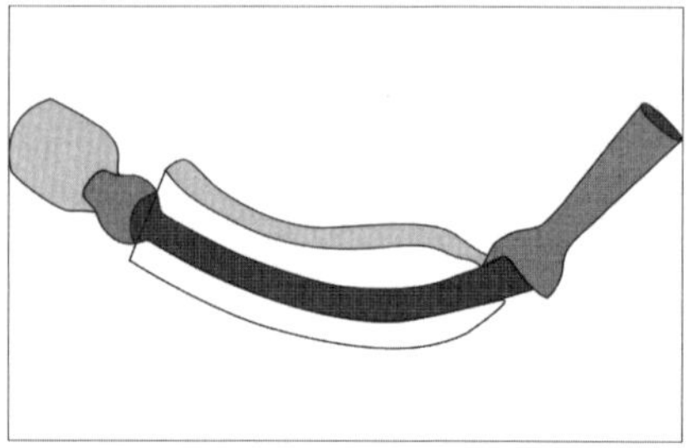

Figure 5-2 Pictorial representation of a nerve and inner axon

More on My Medical Report

SENSORY NERVES:	Lat [ms]	SD	Amp [uV]	SD	CV [m/s]	SD	Amp% [%]	SD
Right Median WRIST - DIG II	10.6		4.5		12.3			
Left Median WRIST - DIG II	7.8		3.0		16.7			
Right Ulnar WRIST - DIG V	2.7		2.8		40.7			
Left Ulnar WRIST - DIG V	—		—		absent			
WRIST - DIG IV	—		—					
Right Peroneal Stim 2 - Rec 2	—		—					
ANKLE - LEG	—		—					
Left Peroneal ANKLE - LEG	3.1		3.6		38.7			
Right Sural ANKLE - LEG	3.1		4.1		38.7			
Left Sural Stim 4 - Rec 4	3.1		4.3		38.7			

Figure 5-3 Extract from John's sensory nerves conduction report

According to my sensory nerves conduction report above, my results revealed a very low and, in some cases, even an absence of sensory transmission signals within most, if not all parts of my body. While the latitude, or speed readings, of such transmissions (as shown in the second column from the left) should reportedly be from many tenths to a hundred for a normal individual, some of my readings ranged from a mere 2.7m/s to 10.6 m/s.

MOTOR NERVES:	Lat [ms]	SD	Amp [mV]	SD	CV [m/s]	SD	Amp% [%]	SD	F [ms]	SD
Right Median									30.5	
WRIST - APB	4.1		1.7							
ELBOW - WRIST	9.2		1.5		47.1		-7			
Left Median									28.9	
WRIST - APB	4.0		2.3							
ELBOW - WRIST	9.3		1.7		47.2		-26			
Right Ulnar									27.1	
WRIST - ADM	2.8		7.9							
ABV ELB WRIST	8.7		6.8		50.0		-13			
Left Ulnar									27.2	
WRIST - ADM	2.7		7.1							
BEL ELB - WRIST	6.0		6.0		51.5		-16			
ABV ELB - BEL ELB	8.9		5.4		48.3		-10			
Right Tibial									58.8	
ANKLE - AH	7.2		7.2							
P FOSSA - ANKLE	18.4		5.3		32.1		-26			
Left Tibial									56.2	
ANKLE - AH	8.3		6.6							
P FOSSA - ANKLE	18.4		3.4		34.7		-48			
Right Peroneal										
ANKLE - EDB										
Left Peroneal					absent					
ANKLE - EDB										
Right Lumbrical inte										
Pos. 1 - Rec pos	4.1		0.2							
Pos. 2 - Pos. 1	4.2		0.9				306			
Left Lumbrical inte										
Pos. 1 - Rec pos	4.1		0.4							
Pos. 2 - Pos. 1	4.0		1.6				308			
Right Peroneal--TA										
Pos. 1 - Rec pos	3.8		2.1							
Pos. 2 - Pos. 1	5.6		2.3		44.4		11			
Left Peroneal--TA										
Pos. 1 - Rec pos	3.9		2.4							
Pos. 2 - Pos. 1	5.8		2.5		44.2		7			

Figure 5-4 Extract from John's motor nerves conduction report

A similar result was also obtained for my motor nerves conduction test, which explained why I was unable to respond to my senses or move about freely.

Comments:
The ERG responses in the right eye were all reduced in amplitude without any delay. The left eye scotopic response was decreased, but other parameters were within normal limits. The PERG showed a mild optic nerve dysfunction. The VEP response was reduced and delayed in both eyes. There was no interocular or inter-hemispheric asymmetry which could be used to localize the disease to specific pre-or post-chiasmal area.

Figure 5-5 Extract from John's Singapore National Eye Centre (SNEC) report

The above report was conducted on my eyes in 2005, revealing that my eyesight was severely compromised for reasons that were unknown even to the doctors.

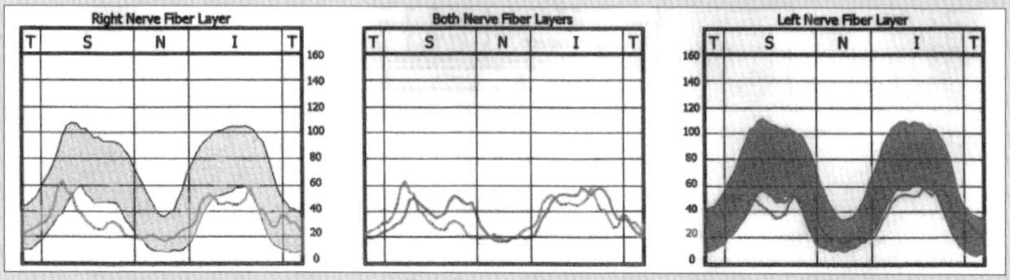

Figure 5-6 Results from John's SNEC report, revealing lower than average nerves density levels in both the right and left eyes

While the average result for a normal person falls within the shaded range, my results were at the extreme lower limit for nerve density in both eyes, as shown in the two graphs on the extreme right and extreme left.

"... I tried to talk myself into unlearning the rationale of medical science and convinced my family and myself that there could still be hope."

As you can imagine, the news was a tremendous blow to my family and I, as it meant that all hope of recovery was lost, whether we liked it or not.

Given my hardwired background in science and human physiology, it was especially hard for me to convince myself that I would be able to defy the laws of medical science and get well, even when all else showed otherwise. Yet, I tried to talk myself into unlearning the rationale of medical science and convinced my family and myself that there could still be hope.

The process was long and it was both mentally and emotionally torturous. Having to let go of my own long-held belief in science and empirical knowledge meant that I had to dissolve my own identity – an identity that had been molded through years of exposure to information and logic. Whether you could call this simply fear of changing the status quo, or a diminishment of my ego, the conflict within me was no less agonizing.

To alter my belief system, which I discovered was pivotal for any kind of transformation to take place, I had to garner much courage and spiritual humility, and had to remove my sense of self, or ego, that was based on what I had learnt and believed of this world. Instead of believing in the limiting convictions held by medical science, I veered towards a greater faith that I would be able to heal myself, as I was as much a part of the forces of nature as they were a part of me. I adopted a new perspective whereby I told myself that all things can be changed under the hands of the Divine in us, if we were to have total faith in it. I convinced myself that nothing was as infinitely powerful as the workings of Mother Nature or the Divine itself, and that we are the image and manifestation of the Divine.

For days, weeks and months, I worked at reinforcing this new found belief. I had to consciously peel away my old beliefs and re-emerge with a different set of beliefs that would be less limiting. Many times, I was reluctant to let go of my old sense of self and its beliefs, as the abandonment of this anchor in my life, which had defined my very being, left me with an acute sense of lost. Despite my insecurities, I persevered, as I knew deep down that our beliefs can hardly be absolute or immutable, given the vast diversity of beliefs in the world.

"Instead of believing in the limiting convictions held by medical science, I veered towards a greater faith that I would be able to heal myself, as I was as much a part of the forces of nature as they were a part of me."

But living that conviction that I would eventually heal was truly hard work, especially when there was no real sign of improvement. At times, all I could do was mutter a few words, which would leave me exhausted for the rest

... my mother was one of the few angels around me who held on to my dream of recovery, despite the odds presented.

of the day, or I was able to just see the faint outlines of shadows. But, at other times, I was completely speechless and back in the world of near complete darkness. Within the span of a day, my mood would fluctuate in relation to my physical condition, from being mildly positive to being inconsolably negative. When my body showed no signs of improvement for days, weeks and even months, I had no choice but to learn to deal with my expectations and cope with my emotions.

"Will I be able to walk?" I would pester the doctors, on days when I found the strength to speak.

"I don't think so," the doctors would reply curtly.

Even though it was probably right of the doctors not to offer any false hope in order to help me manage my own reality and expectations, those words felt harsh and cold and carried such weight that I could not help but feel sentenced to a lifetime of misery and agony.

"Even when everyone else has given up on me, do not give up on me!" I would beg my mother, at times when even I found it brutally hard to go on.

At that point in time, my mother was one of the few angels around me who held on to my dream of recovery, despite the odds presented. Even though she was equally ridden with doubt and fear, on top of her own bout of menopausal problems and a large growing tumor in her uterus, my mother would reassure me, "Don't worry son. I will get you out of here."

Determined to have the best medical treatment available, my family and I sought the opinion of several reputable eye specialists to explore ways to restore my vision. However, many of them did not believe that I could ever recover after reading my medical report. After months of futile observation, one particular senior eye consultant finally told me that I had to accept the fact that I would never be able to recover and regain my eyesight. When I told him that I wanted to see the world again and return to work, he even asked me to see a psychiatrist, to help me cope with accepting my disability both emotionally and mentally. But I refused as I was certain that I would return to a normal life on day.

At the same time, I began to consult some private and even overseas neurologists to gather more opinions on my condition. In the hospital, I was subjected to more painful and terrible tests that were not very different from the ones that I had done previously. During that period of time, my blood was tested so many times a day that they had to draw my blood from other parts of my body, as my fingers and arms had become so badly scarred. What made it worse was when trainee doctors came to take the blood samples and I would be left screaming in pain due to their lack of experience in the procedure.

Not wanting to leave any stone unturned, I attempted every single treatment that the doctors suggested. I went from embarking on a course of chemotherapy and steroids to taking multiple kinds of immunosuppressants, which had the potential of increasing my risk of cancer if took them over the long term. But still, I reaped no sign of improvement. I figured that if my disease did not cause me a slow and torturous death, the terrible side effects from all the drugs I was taking would eventually wear me out. But what was most frustrating was that none of the doctors knew what I was suffering from. The best that they could offer was that my condition could be anything ranging from Miller Fisher Syndrome (MFS), to Chronic Inflammatory Demyelinating Polyneuropathy (CIDP), to Guillain–Barré Syndrome (GBS), to myeloma.

When every other treatment under the sun seemed to fail me and the cause of my condition remained unknown, I knew that I had only myself to depend on. In spite of being bedridden, I attended daily physiotherapy sessions. As in the earlier period, I was not able to stand or even sit up. The sessions were grueling to say the least, but I tried my utmost to stretch my threshold for pain and pushed my physical boundaries for improvement. Each time the therapists moved my body the slightest, a wave of pain, like a nasty electrical shock, pierced though my body. Such was the extent of the pain that I would scream and wail hysterically, but I would ask the therapists to continue. Apart from the tremendous and inexplicable pain that I had to endure, I was not spared from the frustration that welled within me every now and then, which left me in more tears.

But I vowed to preserve and even told the staff at the rehabilitation centre not to give up on me. Fortunately, my physiotherapist and the rest of the staff were very empathetic towards my plight. They were very obliging towards my requests to do more exercises and were very encouraging.

"Your display of fighting spirit is an inspiration to all of us here," a member of the staff once told me during a physiotherapy session.

Even though they never once told me that I could walk again, their gestures and words of encouragement meant a lot to a patient for whom most medical professionals did not have high hopes at all.

That made me even more determined to heal myself. During the early period of my stay, nurses suggested that they insert a tube into my nose to allow liquid food to pass through, but I was quick to object. And when eating was so painstakingly slow that no nurses wanted to feed me, my parents were patient enough to feed me at every meal. As I had little control of my mouth and my tongue, I would often bite my own tongue, which sent blood trickling out of my mouth. As gruesome as it was, I would swallow my food together with all that blood.

But that did not bother me. Instead of mulling over the things that I was unable to do, I started to focus on the little things that I could do then, as well as the things that I might be able to do in the near future.

When I was alone, I would once again journey into my mind. But this time around, I asked myself deeper questions about life as I began to look back at my past with new insight.

> "... the key to unlocking the healing power in my body was through my mind – the gateway to my spiritual beliefs."

What is my true purpose in life? Why am I here? Why do I have such a strange and severe illness? Why is there suffering? Why are there conflicts in this world?

As I spent more quiet time reflecting on all the facets of life, I gradually understood that all conflicts in life stemmed from fear and stupidity, led mostly by wrong beliefs. In my current state, I had become a bystander, seeing all this from the outside for the first time. But I also realized that, as flawed as it is, being a part of this society was most certainly a privilege. Relative to what I was experiencing then, the mundane, everyday problems that arise from our work, finances, relationships and family are actually a blessing to a normal and healthy individual.

Deemed a total invalid in the eyes of others, I realized that I was not even in a position to participate in the dynamics of such problems. To have to tackle such burdens in our lives means that we are at least still in a good shape to face and own them. As I pondered over this, I felt certain that I would treat such problems in life lightly should I ever have the opportunity to return to the world.

When I was not thinking about life, I started to think about my maker or the origin of life itself.I remember considering that if I were created in the likeness of the Source, then I was most certainly bestowed with equal power to perform the unthinkable, like the Source. And if I were indeed created in the likeness of the Source, I could perform seeming miracles, like regeneration, repair, creation and giving energy and meaning to life.

> "Between spirituality and science, I continued to make a conscious and difficult decision to discard what science had taught me about the limitations of my body and chose to embrace my spiritual belief that the Infinite or the Divine is within all of us."

At that moment, I realized that the key to unlocking the healing power in my body was through my mind – the gateway to my spiritual beliefs.

Science often contradicts spirituality. However, supposedly well-grounded scientific and medical facts or dogmas are constantly revised when newer insights are born – some of which derive from our spiritual beliefs. Therefore, I then recognized that mankind's understanding of the workings of Mother Nature have been progressive but not infallible.

The historical pursuit of science to understand the workings of nature can be classified into two general schools of thought. The Plutonian school of thought takes into account the spiritual realm to explain the workings of Mother Nature. The thinking and beliefs adopted tend to be holistic and ecological on all perceived and conceived phenomenon. However, as time passed, the Newtonian school of thought has formed the mainstream pattern of scientific thinking over the last three centuries. It focuses solely on empirical, material and physical proof. Under this school of thought, what cannot be physically proven or empirically formulated cannot be real as yet.

As much truth as it offers, I knew that the Newtonian school of thought is not all-encompassing, as there are still countless phenomena that cannot be explained by its principles. This led me to believe that both schools of thought are equally important and powerful in learning and unearthing the mysteries of this world. Coincidentally, this is also in line with the ancient belief in balance or the Middle Way in Buddhism, or the philosophy of Yin and Yang in Taoism.

Between spirituality and science, I continued to make a conscious and difficult decision to discard what science had taught me about the limitations of my body and chose to embrace my spiritual belief that the Infinite or the Divine is within all of us. As science was not able to offer me a solution to my problem, I decided to seek inner divine intervention to make the seeming impossible, possible.

My first Transcendental Connection

With that insight, I kept telling myself that I had to connect to my Source every day.

Do you hear me? Are you aware of my pain? How do I connect? I would ask, hungrier than ever to communicate with my Source.

After some time, in March 2005, I finally learnt that I did indeed have an audience...

> The source of this wisdom seemed to connect me to the cosmic space that had always existed in and outside of me.

It was an ordinary afternoon. Within the confines of my bed, I could hear the usual flurry of activity outside as nurses went about their routine duties. Through the window of my room, I could hear the vehicles on the road outside. A strong gust of wind blew and I heard the rustling of the leaves. In spite of all that was happening outside, it was still in the ward where I was alone. All by myself, I instinctively asked my Source to eventually heal me as I continued to seek for a miraculous breakthrough. As I kept praying, chanting and speaking to my Source in the silence of my heart, I found myself surrendering to a higher power which was oddly also a part of me.

Suddenly, I felt my spirit filled with a blissful surrender as a surge of cosmic wisdom came upon me. The source of this wisdom seemed to connect me to the cosmic space that had always existed in and outside of me. And I knew intuitively that this was the Source, which had existed inside and outside of me and had been listening to me all this while.

Accustomed to living in a dark, dim and unresolved world, my vision became all of a sudden brighter and clearer. I felt my being soar with an incredible sense of lightness and I felt engulfed by a love that was immeasurably profound and universal. Unknowingly, I had stepped into a realm where the rhythm of life danced around me and I was filled with a child-like excitement. Lying on the same bed where I had been subjected to immense pain, all I felt was love at that moment. I was so filled with love that it felt sufficient to engulf everything and everyone in the entire world. I could feel and sense every being on this planet – their every breath and every heartbeat. It was all so intimate and so clear. Even though my sensory faculties were neurologically damaged and I was desensitized from all feeling in my body, I could somehow sense and connect with the air and space around me.

At that moment, I also became aware that I had entered into an expansive and enormous realm where everything is connected. My world started to expand beyond the ward I was confined to. I was suddenly clear as to who I was. My heartbeat was in perfect synchrony with the heartbeat of everyone on this earth and in this universe. There was no exception; the trees, the ocean, the birds, the air, the soil, the planets, the stars and everything else was in fact one. Essentially, I became aware that we are all linked by a Transcendental Connection to one collective consciousness.

And it dawned upon me that I was now one with the Source or the cosmic truth – a truth or law that has the infinite power to do anything and it is likened to a boundless ocean. And since I was now part of this cosmic ocean of truth, I would possess similar powers to heal myself if I could access this connection with my Source. It occurred to me that I could and should connect with my own emaciated body, organs and nerve cells, and command them to heal themselves.

For the first time in months, I smiled to myself.

Chapter Six
My Road to Recovery

Decoding the blueprint for disease

My Buddhist faith began to take on a renewed meaning and more profound dimensions for me. Whatever I was taught doctrinally, I started to see in a new spiritual light and could relate them to things that were happening around the world. Although there were no significant improvements to my condition, I kept telling my parents and myself that I would not be forsaken by my faith. At some of the most depressing moments, when I really felt like throwing in the towel, I fought even harder to keep the faith alive in my heart.

Hope kept me sane and gave me the will to live on while trapped in a debilitated body. And that hope to recover one day was housed in my faith in the universal law – the Source – that we are all one, linked by a Transcendental Connection.

As a Buddhist, I was taught to chant in prayer. But in the quiet of my ward, I was often in too much pain and was too physically weak to chant out loud, let alone speak clearly.

"Hope kept me sane and gave me the will to live on while trapped in a debilitated body."

How can I pray effectively when I am not able to chant out loud or practice any rituals? How do the mute, mentally challenged and the severely sick chant? I thought to myself when I felt incapable of chanting effectively.

Saddled with so many questions about my faith, I came to realize that I was unsatisfied with my own interpretation of spirituality and prayer. I also realized that I held a rather superficial understanding of faith, prayer and spirituality.

Is there a universal way for all sentient beings to pray, regardless of their condition? Is there a supposedly right way to pray?

I desired so much for an answer, so that I could have the peace and clarity needed to transform my own condition. Relatives, friends and even strangers visited me in the hospital and asked me to chant or pray harder. But they did not understand that I simply was not fit enough to do so. Although they had only good intentions for me, their advice drove me to further frustration as I felt that they were not in my shoes and could not understand my difficulties.

"And the key to a true prayer is to connect from one's heart; it is not based on one's mental fitness or level of concentration or capacity for logical understanding."

But my connection with my Source that fateful afternoon led me to realize that one must hold the intention to connect to one's higher self when praying. And the key to a true prayer is to connect from one's heart; it is not based on one's mental fitness or level of concentration or capacity for logical understanding.

Many of us perform our religious rituals diligently but fail to go deeper to connect to our higher self while praying. I discovered that being aware and holding the intent to make a connection is paramount. With that insight, I discovered a deeper meaning to prayer and I prayed fervently for an improvement in my condition. But that was not all that I prayed for.

Being a Buddhist, I hold the conviction that we abide by an absolute and infinite cosmic law that presides in us and outside of us. I also believe that the universe is governed by the cosmic laws of cause and effect. With this knowledge, I intuitively understood from my higher self or deeper consciousness that when we directly or indirectly hurt other people or the environment around us, we in turn inflict hurt on ourselves. And as a result of this cosmic law of cause and effect, our every thought, word and deed is capable of generating cosmic energies that are stored in our much deeper subconscious minds, which in turn affect us mentally, emotionally, genetically and physiologically (see Chapter Seven).

With this new insight, I reflected upon my life and began to repent all my past shortcomings. I sought forgiveness from the all-encompassing divine for the times when I had been angry and resentful towards my parents. I also expressed my deepest remorse for my spiteful and rebellious ways. And I pledged to help others and share with them the potential power of Transcendental Connection in their lives.

> "... as a result of this cosmic law of cause and effect, our every thought, word and deed is capable of generating cosmic energies that are stored in our much deeper subconscious minds, which in turn affect us mentally, emotionally, genetically and physiologically"

The more soul searching I did, and the more I repented, prayed and stayed connected to my higher self, the deeper I communicated with my inner being and the space around me. It was as though I was harnessing an unknown universal force from within me. I felt an inner sense of liberation that lifted me through my hours of distress.

And, in spite of the difficulties that still stood before me, I was fortunate to have family and friends of different faiths who prayed for me and granted me the strength to persevere. I vowed to have a wide and open heart to receive divine healing from anyone who offered me their well wishes. I knew and felt the power of their prayers fuelling my life force during my weakest moments.

As much as I still felt let down by my body, I marveled at how it could, on the one hand, provide us with the freedom to engage in the many pleasures of life, while, on the other hand, cause pain and suffering when not properly taken care of. I had learnt the hard way that one must strive to be in harmony with oneself and the environment to nurture a wholesome well-being.

Unbeknown to me, I had stumbled upon invaluable life lessons that transcended beyond the body to encompass the mind and the soul, even though my focus had been primarily on the former.

One such lesson that I learnt during this journey of recovery was that every part of my body, from my organs, to my nerves and my tissues, is made of subatomic particles that are in turn just made of common energy wave fields and are essentially one entity.

As a matter of fact, many quantum physicists speculate that nothing is truly solid, regardless of whether it is considered to be matter at the atomic or subatomic level.[4] Instead, everything could be made of a wavelike energy field that vibrates at different frequencies and dimensions. It is then theorized by some authors that the sensory experiences that we perceive from the things around us, be they a soft fabric or a hard table, could actually be holographic. In other words, such sensory experiences are

"... every part of my body, from my organs, to my nerves and my tissues, is made of subatomic particles that are in turn just made of common energy wave fields and are essentially one entity."

merely the result of energy signals being sent to the brain. And the brain, in turn, is actually made of the collective energetic information of matter and energy entities.

The smallest unit in the world is believed by some scientists to have its own behavior and is like a world of its own, in terms of how its energy interacts.[5-6]

Other theories in quantum physics, such as the unified field theory, string theory and quantum field theory, also suggest that matter is merely an inter-connective energy field in time and space. Based on these collective theories, the mind and the body, which are made up of tissues, are essentially nothing but connective energy fields, in the deepest sense, scientifically speaking. And if the mind and body are made of the same energy force, then they are indeed the same entity but manifested differently. Essentially, the mind and body are one. And so, the mind and its thoughts would be able to impact its surroundings.

When my condition remained stagnant, or even worse, deteriorated, I reminded myself of two of Dr Daisuka Ikeda's sayings that echoed this same belief that the mind and body are indeed inseparable.

"When you set your resolve and are determined to do something, every nerve and fibre in your being will set itself to that direction."

"One thing is certain: that the power of belief – the power of thought – will move reality in the direction of what we can believe and conceive. If you believe you can do something, you can. That is a fact."

The long-awaited breakthrough

By March 2005, I was finally clear of my direction and approach towards reinventing my body for the first time. Although I was still fighting my own skepticism about a complete recovery, I took heart in the fact that I was no longer drowning in the dark waters of fear and doubt.

Since I am one with a universe that is omnipotent, please make me whole once more.

Disregarding my doctor's claims that I would no longer be able to get onto my own two feet to work or drive again, I started to use my mind to influence the physical condition of my body, since body and mind are one, as I had come to understand. Every day without fail, I would visualize myself standing up and eventually walking. Not only did I repeat visions of myself standing up and walking in my mind's eye, I most importantly held the vision in my heart. I was so immersed in choreographing these visions that I not only saw it in my mind, but also felt it in my heart. I not only recalled how I walked, but also what it felt like to walk. In my waking hours, I would summon my cells to regenerate my afflicted body. And in my sleep, I also dreamt of walking and seeing again.

Surreptitiously, I managed to sit up in bed and even garnered enough strength to sit up in a wheelchair by mid March 2005. Although that was still a long way from my aim of walking, I acknowledged the fact that every hint of improvement was a milestone that marked a huge stride towards my recovery. Most importantly, it told me that my approach was certainly paying off and that my efforts were not in vain after all.

"Every day without fail, I would visualize myself standing up and eventually walking."

From sitting up, I next endeavored to haul myself up. As effortless as it was for me to simply imagine myself getting up from the wheelchair and walking again, I simply could not get beyond my physical inability to do so. Try as I might, my legs could not feel the ground and would simply crumble under the weight of my body. Yet, I continued to practice during the physiotherapy sessions, as well as within the four walls of my ward. As I slowly regained my health and picked up the pieces of my life, I felt like an infant who was learning everything, all over again.

I recall that I did not succeed in standing up during the initial days. So, I increased the frequency of my practice until I was capable of repeating the very same act of standing up, for up to a hundred times a day. But each time, I was left slumping back into the wheelchair, more exhausted than ever. During those times, I felt that all my efforts were being dwarfed by a body that was out to thwart me.

But I never gave up. Despite the inner conflict that I was subjected to during my stay in the hospital, I resolved to track my progress and detail the beginning of my recovery process. I asked my family to record video clips of me reporting my progress, if any, as well as my thoughts and emotions. Even though my speech was oftentimes unclear, I suspect that it was also my way of releasing the pent up energy inside my body. It was perhaps also a way to put my journey towards a potential recovery in a context that would allow myself and others to better grapple with the reality of my condition.

But what optimism I had towards recovery did not rest well with others, especially with some doctors and friends. Once, a doctor chided me when she found me reporting my progress on video.

"What are you doing? You should accept the reality that you may never recover," she said vehemently.

Undaunted by her harsh words, I replied, "This video will be helpful to others and even yourself, when I do eventually recover."

Later, my family told me that they had spotted the doctor at a corner, with tears welled up in her eyes. Perhaps, she was touched by my sincerity to help others in spite of my sorry condition. Perhaps, she was moved by my determination and courage in adversity. This, I will never know.

But, however strong I appeared to be, my conviction that I would eventually recover was not always unshakable. Every day, I felt like I was fighting a new battle, physically, emotionally and mentally. Every day, I had to brace myself to confront my fears and doubts. Sometimes I won. At other times, I lashed out with screams of desperation and despair. In fact, the thought of giving up was constantly lurking at the back of my mind and I was always fighting to subdue it through prayers.

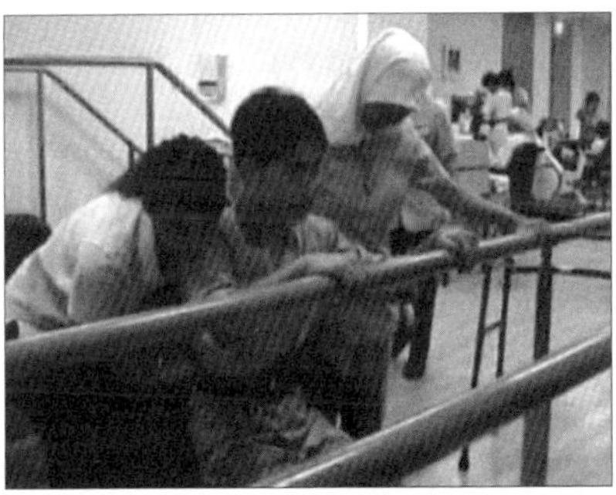

Figure 6-1 John showing signs of recovery at a physiotherapy session at Singapore General Hospital in 2005

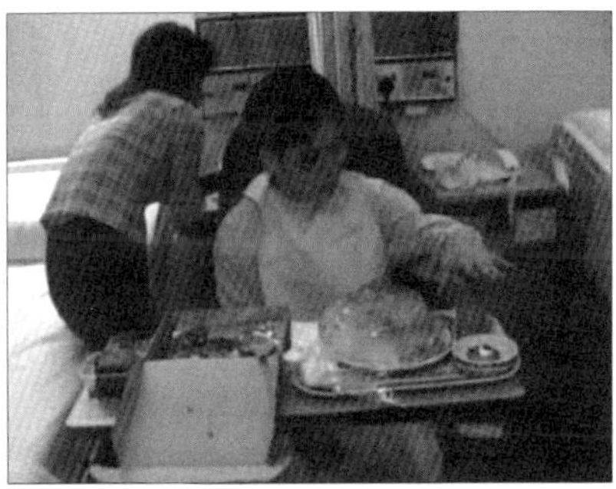

Figure 6-2 John requested to be strapped to a chair when taking his meals because he was unable to sit normally in 2005

After many months of struggle, I finally reached a breakthrough in my condition that took even me by surprise, in April 2005.

Every day, I was at the rehabilitation centre with my physiotherapist, Chloe, where I would practice getting up on my feet. After practicing for a few months, I was beginning to feel that I was getting somewhere with my progress. When I was back at my ward, my family and I would implore my doctors to discharge me. Certain that I would not be able to do it, the doctors told me in jest that they would discharge me if I could briefly stand up by myself from a wheelchair.

After countless mental and physical practices, I was grateful when the time had finally arrived.

On 1 April 2005, something miraculous took place. Under the encouragement of my family members, I braced myself and took a deep breath as I heaved myself up with as much might as I could muster, half expecting nothing out of the ordinary to take place. With my hands vaguely able to feel how they were pressed against the armrest of the wheelchair, I watched in amazement as I slowly lifted my body out of the wheelchair. For a good four seconds, I maintained that position much to the astonishment of my rehabilitation doctor, physiotherapist and myself, before I sank back into the wheelchair. Although I felt spent of whatever energy I had left, I was over the moon with what I had just accomplished.

Everyone in my ward who witnessed my feat got excited for me. My rehabilitation doctor, in particular, was elated. As though I was a proud exhibit on display, he started to wheel me around the hospital to share the good news with all the doctors whom had thought that I would never live to see this day. Not surprisingly, all the doctors and nurses were positively dumbfounded.News of my unbelievable feat spread like wildfire through the hospital and many of the staff rushed by to see me. As I sat on the wheelchair beaming with pride, I felt like I had finally departed hell and had just set foot in heaven. It truly was a triumphant moment and a turning point in my quest for recovery. Till that moment, I had never realized that victory could taste so sweet!

Coincidentally, a three-centimeter tumor that had previously been found in my mother's womb and was due to be removed by her doctors under their orders, suddenly disappeared.

Three steps forward, two steps backward

Upon witnessing an unexpected breakthrough in my condition, my rehabilitation doctor and physiotherapist, together with my family, supported me in an appeal to the hospital for me to be discharged.

When the moment for me to be discharged eventually arrived in the first week of April 2005, it was hard to believe that such a day would have ever come, after months of being enclosed within the walls of the hospital. That day, my family and I were in high spirits. To me, it meant that I was slowly rebuilding the life that had been seized from me.

I can finally see the light at the end of the tunnel! I thought to myself with joy.

Encouraged by my recent leap in progress, I felt motivated to strive harder at recovering and was hopeful that my health would pick up in no time. But what I did not know was that the road to recovery was still an uncertain, long and winding one.

At home, we were without the aid of nurses, so my family hired a maid to attend to my daily needs. To facilitate my movement around the house, my family bought me a walking frame, wheelchair and a gait belt that they had to lift to support the trunk of my body while I practiced standing and at a later stage, walking. But, as day slipped into night, my initial joy slowly dimmed. By that very first night, I realized that even though I was in the familiar quarters of my home, my misery was far from being over.

Although my speech was clearer, it was still sometimes difficult for others to fully comprehend what I was saying. Sometimes, I could not speak due to breathlessness or pain. Sometimes, for unknown reasons, I simply could not express myself verbally for days or even weeks. It was very painful and frustrating when I could not interact with others and enable them to understand what I wanted. My parents and maid struggled to understand my instructions and I became frustrated when our conversations became peppered with many miscommunications. And at some point, my girlfriend could no longer shoulder the emotional and mental burden of my condition and we eventually parted. Although I had mixed feelings then, I knew that it was in our best interests to part and I was thankful for her support and care during the times when she had stood beside me.

Although there had been a breakthrough in my condition, my body was not spared from its usual extreme aches, feelings of discomfort and everyday glitches. Back in the comfort zone of my home, I was not released from the grating discomfort that came with my problem urinating, as well as a bulging and unresponsive bowel. But if anything, I knew that this was better than staying in the hospital.

“... I continued to visualize my nerves regenerating, in spite of the established belief that nerves can never grow back when they are severely damaged.”

Within the confines of my home, I continued to visualize my nerves regenerating, in spite of the established belief that nerves can never grow back when they are severely damaged. Every single day, I would command my nerves to branch out and grow. During that time, I began to wonder if my condition was, in fact, truly an autoimmune disease, created by my own immune system and which, instead of protecting me, was mistakenly attacking my nerves throughout my body. I remember thinking that if this was indeed the case, then the internal balance and harmony of my body and mind must be restored as soon as possible; the memories of one's cells, DNA, blood and physiology must also be corrected.

My body is in perfect harmony and is filled with love. I repeated to myself on a daily basis.

In July 2005, I returned to my doctor so that she could review my progress. As I had failed the knee reflex test on every occasion before, my doctor was so certain that I would once again fail the test that she told her two accompanying junior doctors to forgo it. But while my doctor was busy taking down some notes on my condition, the two junior doctors went ahead to perform the knee reflex test on me anyway. Serendipitously, my knee showed signs of response when they tapped on it gently. Upon seeing this, my doctor exclaimed, "My God! Your nerves are regenerating!"

After this encounter, I was all the more convinced that I was treading the right path towards recovery.

Without fail, I continued to practice trying to stand up with the help of my family and my maid. On some days, I found myself unable to pick myself up from the bed and, on other days, it was hard to get up from the wheelchair. Faced with these seeming setbacks in my recovery, I would spiral into yet another streak of inconsolable despair.

To make matters worse, my condition would seemingly relapse from time to time and I had to be hospitalized on several occasions, much to my disappointment. Such trips back to the hospital marked further episodes of anguish, where I was subjected to further pain from more tests and procedures that were conducted on me.

Once, my stomach, intestines and bowels were in very bad shape. My body was flooded with extreme pain from within, affecting my day-to-day progress. A doctor was checking the inner lining of my stomach when the dose of sedative wore off prematurely while the steel hose was still in my stomach via my mouth. Although I was numb to most sensations on the outside, I was still acutely aware of the pain internally. When the anesthesia wore off too early, I was jolted by a rupturing seizure that sent a splitting pain straight to my head. Such was the extent of the pain then that I swore I could have killed the person who had miscalculated the dosage of anesthetic needed for the procedure.

On another occasion back in the hospital, I was made the subject of a test procedure to be demonstrated to a group of trainee doctors. Unable to protest to the indignation that I was made to suffer, I was laid out stark naked with my legs wide open, while a steel rod was inserted into my genitals to test my bladder pressure. Apart from being excruciatingly painful, the whole experience was regrettably also the most humiliating.

Once, the urologist insisted that I use a catheter again at home to expel my urine, or I would not be discharged. However, my rehabilitation doctor and I managed to convince the urologist that I would not need to depend on a catheter to urinate. As my hands were still void of most sensation and muscular control, I asked my maid to press on my bladder at the hospital and again when I was back home, so as to train my bladder muscles to contract, enabling me to urinate. Something that any ordinary man would take a mere ten seconds to do while standing, took me about half an hour to an hour to do, while in bed or in a wheelchair, and after that, I would be exhausted and perspiring from the effort. To complicate matters, I had this unquenchable thirst that required me to drink up to 10 liters of water per day, which increased the frequency of my urination every day.

Though simply urinating posed such a huge problem to me, moving my bowels was an unimaginably more difficult task. In order to ease my bowels, my maid had to assist me in inserting a liquid or solid laxative directly into my rectum every day. On many occasions, I was totally drained after trying to purge out the feces using my last ounce of strength. But in the end, my effort was often in vain and I was only left with disappointment and exhaustion.

On top of all that, eating continued to be a chore for me. Each time I ingested food, I felt like there were a thousand coarse stones cutting my gut. The discomfort that resulted from a simple meal often left me curled up in tears and the mere thought of consuming food left me feeling revolted.

Until my health had been threatened, it was hard to imagine that such seemingly ordinary tasks, such as urination, moving my bowels and eating, could amount to such distress and difficulty. But, in spite of the daily pain, inconvenience and complications that I faced, I started to visit troubled friends in my spiritual community in the latter half of 2005, or even strangers that I had come to learn about, to offer them encouragement. Even though such trips left me completely exhausted and often plagued by fever the next day, I remained steadfast to my promise to help others, as well as to offer meaning to my own troubled existence.

"Until my health had been threatened, it was hard to imagine that such seemingly ordinary tasks, such as urination, moving my bowels and eating, could amount to such distress and difficulty."

On a daily basis, I continued on my course of steroids and immunosuppressive drugs, as well as a dozen other medicines, which were believed by my doctors to alleviate my symptoms. Eventually, I came to suspect that these drugs were, in fact, causing my body to regress. During the later part of 2005, I could not talk again, breathing was hard, and I could hardly get out of bed. I was constantly curled up in pain, as my organs almost felt like they were on fire and were melting away. My vision was also not improving much. I was so weak that I was not able to conduct physiotherapy at home. As a result, I had to cancel my weekly trips to the Society for the Physically Disabled for subsidized therapy, where I usually met up with other middle-aged professionals and elderly individuals, who had become equally detached from life due to a stroke or a severe accident.

As time passed, my parents and I grew more apprehensive about my stagnation and sometimes even, the aggravation of my condition. In spite of my suspicions that the medications were actually too strong for my body and were causing serious side effects, my neurologist insisted that I had to continue to take all the medications or be bedridden and blind again.

My family and I were at a dilemma as to what to do as I clung onto my every breath with pain in bed and was not even able to get out of my bed and or perform my exercises. My body was wasting away one more time. Deep down, I did not agree with what the neurologist had suggested. Yet, I did not know what to do, or even if she was indeed right.

My family and I prayed fervently for a way out of this deadlock. For many weeks, I had to endure excruciating pain from the very moment I awoke. I could not chant out loud, but I prayed and connected from my heart. Given our dilemma over my condition, my family and I were so emotionally drained that we really felt like giving up sometimes.

Speak to me please! I implored in the silence of my heart as I called upon the universe for an answer to my problem.

One fateful afternoon, a few days later, my mother was walking home from work, when she encountered a lady who was sitting by the side of the road. She stopped my mom gently and told her that our family's act of praying was a deed that was good and benevolent. She told my mother to continue to pray fervently and that I was to remember the heavenly grace bestowed onto me when I recover someday. With those few words, the lady walked away as quietly as she had appeared. Although my mother and I never learned who the lady was, we were nevertheless dumbfounded and amazed by this seemingly chance encounter. But most importantly, we felt encouraged even amid our setbacks.

Shortly after, our prayers for a turnaround in my condition were finally answered when my mother's friend, Chwee Hoon, recommended another neurologist to us. Initially, we had our reservations about seeing another neurologist as we had sought other professionals some time ago and they were all equally clueless. But we learnt that this particular neurologist had a lot more experience and was also a mentor to many other existing neurologists. After observing me and studying my medical records, he told me that I did not have Chronic Inflammatory Demyelinating Polyneuropathy (CIDP) as suspected previously, although he could not confirm it at that point in time. Based on his preliminary deductions, he then instructed me to progressively stop all the medications that I had been taking, as I did not need any medication at all. We were shocked by his curt but confident response.

When my family and I voiced our reservations about his suggestion, the neurologist retorted, "You are recovering and it does not matter what your disease has been labeled by others! You can either choose to believe other people's medical opinion or mine. The choice is yours!"

Even though my family and I were rather hesitant about stopping the various medicines that my doctor had previously prescribed, we finally reached a decision to follow my new neurologist's instructions, as we believed that he was the answer to our prayers.

I decreased the intake of my medications to allow my body time to adjust to the change. And, lo and behold, my condition improved and I was once again able to continue with my daily exercises.

Within months, my body started to respond to some of my mind's desires. Over the course of the next year, my awkward staggers gradually extended to more purposeful strides. From being able to walk only a meter, I was slowly able to walk up to one hundred meters, and then, a thousand meters without resting.

During that period of time, I also had to relearn the basics. Bit by bit, I learnt how to be independent all over again. I learnt to feed myself by first strapping the spoon to my hand with a rubber band, and when given a pen, I scribbled like a toddler, trying to teach my fingers the fine art of wielding a pen once more. On top of that, I trained my tired eyes to make the most of what I could see, as my vision improved very slightly.

During that time, many friends would visit me. Some, at a later stage, even tried to take me to the beach and eat out at restaurants, to reacquaint me with society. A good friend even went so far as to encourage me to learn to ride a bicycle again, even though I could hardly walk or see well!

Returning to a seemingly normal life

By March 2006, my condition had shown steady signs of improvement, even though my vision was still very poor and my steps still weak. Considering how even this level of normalcy in my life had been deemed impossible, my improvement was so heartening to my new neurologist that I was strongly encouraged to return to work.

"Just do it. Take the chance," he said when he saw the hesitance in my eyes.

Although I was initially skeptical, I decided to take the plunge, since my ultimate goal had always been to return to a normal life.

Even though I was far from normal, my boss decided to take me in and allowed me to resume my former position, managing regional business operations in a division within the company. Apart from my boss, none of my colleagues were aware of my condition. Since I appeared to be normal on the outside, their only suspicion that something could be amiss was from my speech, which was still very weak and soft. What they did not know was that my vision was partially impaired in the day and close to useless in the night. And my ability to walk steadily was still weak.

As I was barely able to make out details in front of me, I had to count the number of steps on a flight of stairs, so that I would able to walk with ease up and down those steps throughout the rest of the day. To get around my clients' offices and laboratories, I had to secretly visit their site the day before to familiarize myself with the place and memorize all the corners and turns, as well as the number of steps on each flight of stairs, so that my movements would appear fluid on the following day. On top of coping with these seemingly trivial matters that were essential for me to get by at work on a day to day basis, I still had to cope with my daily bouts of fever, breathlessness and tiredness.

As my feet still lacked much sensation and my vision was cloudy, it was difficult for me to determine the type of surface I was walking on. On top of not being able to see, moving around in new places was a rather daunting task. Many a time, I tripped over curbs, walked into the ladies toilet by mistake, slipped on wet floors, bumped my head against doors, and even drank from the wrong cup at the table!

As I was in charge of regional matters, travelling was frequently on my agenda. Since I was not able to rehearse such trips beforehand, my overseas trips were often peppered with difficulties and mishaps.

At the airport, I was always the last to pick up my luggage from the belt and the last person to leave the immigration counter. It took me a long time to figure out where I was, when in a bustling airport. As I was slow when walking and usually trailed behind others, it took me a long time to find the signs that would lead me to the correct direction or even the exit.

Once, when I was in Vietnam, I even had to pay a beggar off the streets to lead me across a busy road to have my dinner. And when I returned to the hotel that evening, utterly pleased with myself for having ventured out into the dark and hectic streets of Vietnam, I walked right into the glass door of the hotel!

Sometimes, the people around me laughed jokingly at my silly blunders, but at other times, they mistook my actions and were offended. As I seemed perfectly normal to them, my inadequacies often led others to believe that I was either rude or indecent. Some particularly memorable instances of this were when I accidentally walked into a lady in a crowded bus one morning, and when a client placed his hand out to shake mine and I failed to reciprocate the gesture. At other times, I had to squint to see and people would wonder why I was looking at them in a strange manner. In spite of my eye specialist's recommendation that I consider getting a social identity card for the visually handicapped, I resisted.

What would my colleagues think of me? I wondered. *And would people accept me for who I am, even with my physical flaws? Will I lose my job if colleagues find out about my state?*

Even though my family and close friends expressed their worry that I might meet with an accident that would simply make things worse, I persisted in trying to lead as normal a life as possible, as I was anxious to make the most out of the time that this renewed chance had given me. In fact, my parents, therapists, and some social workers were of the view that I should just get a simple job in a factory like other disabled people. But I chose to ignore them. Although driven by a genuine concern for me, the incessant nagging from my loved ones and friends often drove me up the wall.

"Owing to this belief that I could heal, I took on an active role in introducing changes to my life to facilitate my recovery."

Why can't they understand me? I kept thinking.

Sometimes, the pressure from work became too overwhelming for me to cope. And when I did put in more hours to catch up with my work, I would suffer from a high fever the very next day. My inability to measure up to the responsibilities given to me at work sometimes made me angry with myself. Stressed over the limitations that still defined my life, I broke down in the office toilet many times. After which, I would remind myself to be thankful for the progress that I had made thus far.

In spite of all the frustration I faced, as well as the vicious comments that were made as a result of my blunders, I derived strength from my connection to my Source through my prayers, which enabled me to get back on track whenever I was off-course. Although I was embroiled with much struggle at work, I realized how important it was for me to realign myself spiritually. I continually reminded myself not to overreact to situations and to remain clear-headed. Whenever, I came short of these goals, I would repent and continue to work on bettering myself.

Apart from devoting more time to fervent prayers, I believe that having the mindset that I could heal myself was perhaps paramount to my recovery (see section on Void in Chapter Eight). Owing to this belief that I could heal, I took on an active role in introducing changes to my life to facilitate my recovery. Whether on a physical, emotional or mental level, I researched widely on different modalities of science and spiritually to ensure that I had all the ground covered to bring my health to an optimal state. During that period, I experimented with what was working for my body and what was not and I made adjustments to my life accordingly.

For a start, I abstained from eating red meat, especially pork. And when my body grew accustomed to a reduced meat intake, I began to veer my palate towards more green food during more meals (see section on Earth in Chapter Eight).

Through the course of my work at that time, I got acquainted with the subject of water and environmental safety, and was made aware of the connection between our consciousness, water, health and the environment. Based on my knowledge of the importance of water to our body and how water can be improved to promote further well-being, I made a conscious decision to switch towards drinking cleaner, energized water (see section 8.2 on Water in Chapter Eight). I also took great care to make certain that I got sufficient sleep at night to allow nature to work its restorative powers on my body (see section 8.3 on Wood in Chapter Eight). I was also more aware of my body and introduced changes to my breathing pattern to transcend and connect to all parts of my body, as well as to the things around me. I also made a more conscious decision to improve the quality of the air that I breathe.

Slowly but surely, my willingness to take responsibility for my own healing process, alongside the physical improvements that I had made, gave me a greater sense of empowerment over my body and things around me. Even though I had not completely recovered, I felt this overall sense of well-being and slowly returned more and more to the life I had lived before.

Looking back, I sometimes feel that my disease was perhaps the universe's way of slowing me down, as I was by nature an impatient person who wanted things and wanted them now. Or perhaps, it was the universe's way of putting me on a spiritual and emotional path that would teach me the importance of harmony in one's life. Even though my go-getter attitude had brought me some level of success in my life, I eventually learnt that true success lies in striking an overall balance in life.

Being one with the Source

From being completely bedridden to eventually finding my way back into society, the long and arduous process was one that probably would not have materialized if not for my dreadful illness.

Looking back, my connection with the Source certainly marked the turning point of my condition. It was then that I began to perceive myself and my body in a new light. And it was that connection that inspired me to take a second chance at life, even when no one else shared my vision.

In the midst of my struggles, I discovered that when one is attuned to one's higher self or connected to the Source, one is able to subconsciously influence the body, mind and soul according to one's deepest desires. By being transcendentally connected to the Source, the gateway to miracles and dreams are then opened for one to reach. When we are connected to the Source, we place ourselves in a realm where we are able to receive the infinite power of the Divine. And from this place, we can tap into the divine universal force and command our cells to regenerate.

The power that awaits a Transcendental Connection is immense and one does not need to go through what I did to be able to harness its benefits. Similar examples of a Transcendental Connection can be traced throughout the history of mankind. In fact, such a seemingly supernatural connection has been taught by many revered spiritual teachers and notable philosophers, though presented in different ways across different religions, spanning the centuries.

In Buddhism, Siddhartha Gautama, otherwise known as the Buddha, termed this connection the Buddha Nature of man, and anyone can attain this highest state of being. In Taoism, Lao Tzu described this connection with the Source as the Dynamic Balance or enlightenment. This connection is similarly recorded in the Bible in Ephesians 4:24, when Jesus said, "…and put on the new self, which in the likeness of God has been created in righteousness and holiness of the truth." And, in Islamic Sufism, it is taught that "the oneness of God starts from within oneself and one's heart and connects to everything."

Throughout the Eighteenth and Nineteenth centuries, the essence of this message was likewise conveyed by celebrated philosophers, such as Immanuel Kant (22 April 1724 - 12 February 1804), Henry David Thoreau (12 July 1817 - 6 May 1862) and Ralph Waldo Emerson (25 May 1803 - 27 April 1882), who were awakened to the concept of a higher self, as well as their interconnectedness to everything around them.

In more recent times, when Sathya Sai Baba, the Indian guru and spiritual teacher, was asked by a man whether he was God, he answered, "I am God and so are you; except that you are not aware of it."[7]

And, notwithstanding the keen perception offered by religious leaders and ancient philosophers, science – particularly in the field of quantum physics – has similarly shed some powerful insights on this. So, backed by both spiritual and scientific wisdom, the phenomenon known as Transcendental Connection is most certainly real.

To better understand its significance and achieve Transcendental Connection in our lives, I shall introduce two interrelated concepts that can help in our comprehension and application, namely 3,000 Realms in a Single Living Moment and the Five Mutual Elements. These provide us with activities of a Transcendental Connection that can be used to attain harmony and balance in life.

---

[4] *Joseph Polchinski, String Theory (Cambridge: Cambridge UP, 1998) 1-30.*

[5] *Richard Feynman, QED: The Strange Theory of Light and Matter (Princeton: Princeton UP, 1988) 30-50.*

[6] *Hubert F. M. Goenner, "On the History of Unified Field Theories," Living Reviews in Relativity 7 (2004). Web. 1 Oct. 2010. <http://www.livingreviews.org/lrr-2004-2>.*

[7] *Betty Khoo-Kingsley, Conversation with my Spirit Guide (Singapore: Magnum, 1996) 13.*

PART II
Understanding Healing by Transcendental Connection

Atoms or elementary particles themselves are not real: they form a world of potentialities or possibilities rather than one of things or facts
– Werner Heisenberg (1901-1976), Nobel Prize Winner in Physics, 1932

Chapter Seven
3,000 Realms in a Single Living Moment

The principles of 3,000 Realms in a Single Living Moment

The environment influences the lives of people, while people mold and shape their society and their environment at the same time. Derived from ancient oriental thinking and partly influenced by some Buddhist doctrines that originated to explain cosmology and worldly systems, this principle is reflective of the belief that there is a oneness between your life and your environment, and it is this principle that governs the dynamics of *3,000 Realms in a Single Living Moment*.

The concept of *3,000 Realms in a Single Living Moment*[8,9], brings definition to the potentialities and possibilities of the state of our lives at every single moment. It relates to our emotions and thoughts, and describes how our overall well-being results from these. This principle of a single moment in life being manifested in 3,000 distinct possibilities and potentialities shed light on how our lives influence everyone and everything at every moment of life, therein demonstrating the connectivity of all things.

According to this ancient principle, there are 3,000 realms or possible states that we can manifest at any single moment. A dynamic principle, *3,000 Realms in a Single Living Moment*, presents the deep understanding that in every single or present moment, we have the power to choose and alter the state of our lives towards a direction that we desire. This principle also explains that every single moment in our lives is the moment where change can take place and where we should anchor ourselves. It also represents a power that can be found in every present moment. Today, German spiritual teacher Eckhart Tolle shares the same message when he teaches the importance of being in the now, or the single present moment, to be empowered.

So why are there 3,000 realms?

It is believed that each of us, in the course of our lives, experiences one of ten possible states of existence, which shifts from moment to moment depending on the circumstances we are facing. As we experience each of these states, we also experience one of ten associated states (this will be explained in greater detail in a subsequent paragraph), resulting in at least one hundred possible states of existence at any given moment of our lives. Next, these one hundred possible states of existence are affected by ten factors of life that contribute to how our lives interact and change (to also be explained in greater detail in a subsequent paragraph), resulting in at least one thousand possible states of existence at any given moment of our lives. As these one thousand possible states of existence are affected by the three realms of existence – us, our society and our environment – this means that there are, in total, three thousand different possible realms of existence in any single living moment.

The first ten possible states of existence are the most volatile states of our lives. These ten states are: hell or pain; hunger; animality; anger; humility; rapture; learning; realization; compassion or nobleness; and connectedness or enlightenment.

Within these ten states exists another layer of the same ten states that are related but independent. For example, a mother is angry (anger state) when her young son runs across the road without looking out for traffic first, but such a reaction is based on her underlying love for him (compassion state). In another instance, a businessman is delighted (rapture state) after securing a big contract, but, at the same time, schemes as to how to best exploit his staff to gain more profit (hunger state). Finally, a man is suffering from the pain caused by his cancer (hell state) but he is accompanied and cared for by his love ones. Such suffering could evoke his empathy for others who are equally, if not more, dejected (compassion state).

Within these one hundred possible realms of existence, the highest dual state achievable is the state of connection within the state of connection. When one resides in this state, an open and all-directional mind wave from one connects to every cosmic corner of the Source. This is also the state when miracles take place and healing of our body and mind happens in the most profound manner.

The ten factors of life – appearance, nature, entity, power, influence, internal cause, relation, latent effect, effect, and consistency from beginning to end – are the most

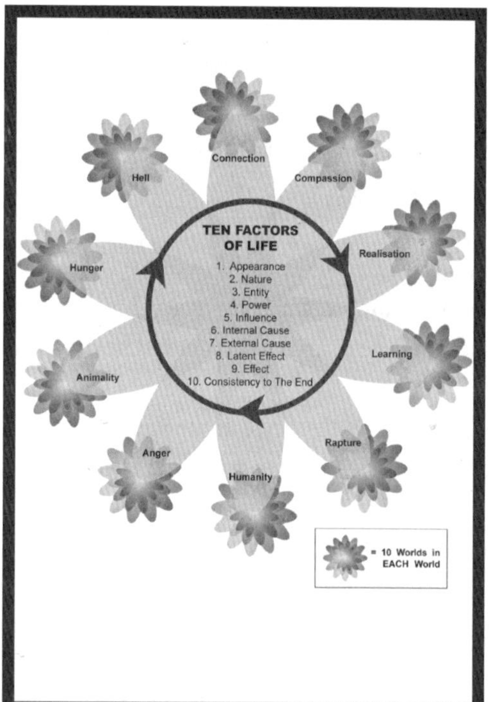

Figure 7-1 Diagram of *3,000 Realms in a Single Living Moment*

basic and natural components of life, within each of the one hundred possible states of life condition. Each state carries the same ten factors or activities of life, whether we are angry or happy or indifferent. These ten factors of life exist like an endlessly activated program that runs constantly in the background of our conscious beings, and are essentially governed by the basic laws of cause and effect.

Out of the ten factors of life, appearance, nature and entity represent life itself, while the remaining factors – power, influence, internal cause, relation, latent effect, effect, and consistency from beginning to end – represent the workings of life and its influences. This, in fact, summarizes how the world we all live in works.

Finally, in the concept of *3,000 Realms in a Single Living Moment*, there are three realms of existence, comprising the Being, collective beings, and the environment. Each of these three realms is mutually interconnected and each will affect another in profound ways.

The Being, also the most important and basic realm of the three, refers to ourselves and our minds. The Being consists of form, perception, conception, volition and consciousness.

Collective beings, on the other hand, refer to the people around us and the society in which we live. Here, the thoughts, words and actions of one Being can affect the collective beings, or our society, in other words. As such, it is futile to look towards a change in our society, if there is no change at the Being level, since the power of one's thoughts and feelings is capable of generating a resonance or energy field, which is interconnected to and can influence the people around us. Examples of this connection include the good or bad vibes that you may receive from another person, or the synchronicity that occurs when someone you suddenly thought of gives you a call. The concept of collective beings can also be used to understand how collective cells, tissues and organs in our body work together harmoniously.

The realm of environment refers to the matter and space that we reside in. It also represents the climate, weather, geography and cosmic system. Just like how the Being affects the society in which we live, our actions similarly affect the environment in which we live, both directly and indirectly. One such example is how the actions of man are capable of causing pollution and harm to the Earth. And, as a result of this change in our environment, problems such as global warming or water pollution result, which in turn, causes men and animals to fall sick.

The concept of environment can also be seen as our body's relationship with our Being. In this context, the environment refers to the vast cosmic space that we are in, which includes the body we inhabit. Since our minds give out resonance and vibration energy to the universal energy field, the cosmic energy field, or environment, is capable of storing unlimited amounts of intelligence and memories derived from our lives.

Our minds and our bodies interact with the universe at every single moment. And that universal consciousness functions like a disc that stores and plays back our lives, deeds and thoughts constantly. Long after we are gone, all that we have done and considered is stored perfectly – both the good and the bad.

In sum then, each possible realm is the result of ten possible states of existence, multiplied by an interrelated ten other possible states of existence, multiplied by ten factors of life, and finally, multiplied by three realms of existence, resulting in 3,000 possible realms existing in any single moment.

How this concept can be used to explain Transcendental Connection

Based on the principle of *3,000 Realms in a Single Living Moment*, the Being connects and influences the collective being, as well as its environment, in a transcendental manner. These three realms are mutually interconnected in very profound and complex ways. When the three realms communicate, they are based on thoughts, words and volitions, or deeds, which manifest as any possible form of energy.

This concept of inter-connectedness was also illustrated in the book *The Hundredth Monkey* by Ken Keyes Jr. Here, the book describes how one macaque monkey discovered how to wash dirty sweet potatoes in a river and soon other monkeys copied him. And by the time the one hundredth monkey had learned this new skill, it was discovered that other monkeys across the sea and at other locations had somehow instantaneously learned the same skill.

From a scientific point of view, this principle can be substantiated by an understanding of quantum physics, which is essentially about the relationship between energy, space and time, which occurs both within us and outside of us.

Albert Einstein spent the later years of his life using the unified field theory in quantum physics to try to explain that we actually belong to one energetic entity in the ocean of the universe's energy field. Based on the unified field theory, it has been revealed that energy, time, space and our consciousnesses are collectively one, and interconnected through space and time. As such, our thoughts can influence matter regardless of time and distance. Many human beings just do not know it or feel it yet.

In more recent times, the concept behind Einstein's favorite unified field theory was further developed when two groups of famous quantum physicists in Europe led by Aspect and Tittel showed that the movement of a particle poses a simultaneous effect on its cousin particle even when they are held at separate locations.[10,11] Not only was the effect simultaneous, it was in fact faster than the speed of light.

In 1997, a simple teleportation experiment was finally successfully carried out on a simple photon and particle which once again reinforced Einstein's unified field theory.[12,13] Thereafter, this simple teleportation experiment paved the way for many more successful and elaborate teleportation experiments.

To further illustrate this unified connection between one's thoughts and its effect on the environment, as proposed by the concept of *3,000 Realms in a Single Living Moment*, the double slit experiment, frequently conducted in physics laboratories, shows that particles can transform into waves and exist in a parallel time and space.[14,15] The test was most famously carried out and explained well by Nobel prize-winning laureate Dr Richard Feynman. Most importantly, the experiment revealed that human thoughts influence the behavior of waves changing back into particles. In doing so, this experiment reiterates the point that our thoughts have a profound effect on the matter that exists around us. And there have been many significantly positive experiments performed repeatedly by physicians, scientists and parapsychologists to prove that telepathic activity exists in humans.[16,17,18]

But how does the principle of *3,000 Realms in a Single Living Moment*, as well as the findings of quantum physics, validate the concept of Transcendental Connection, and how does it bring healing, love or abundance to your life, you might ask.

Well, based on the principle that one's thoughts can affect one's surroundings, the principle of *3,000 Realms in a Single Living Moment* and the associated findings in quantum physics echo related beliefs in mind-body medicine and distance healing, and support the claims that prayers indeed do work.

Whether viewed from a spiritual or scientific angle, a Transcendental Connection is the most powerful thing that we can possibly have and discover. But just like how we do not necessarily need to know the mechanics behind how food nourishes us to benefit from a good diet, we do not have to fully grasp the dynamics of a Transcendental Connection to reap its power. All we have to do is to believe in it, practice it, and use it daily. It is the explanation and the key to the Law of Attraction.

If anything, every change that we yearn to experience in our lives starts with our minds or our consciousness. If science states that human beings use only five to ten percent of their mental and genetic capacity, can you imagine what we would be capable of if we are to use all one hundred percent of our mental and genetic capacity?

But what if I am very troubled and cannot reach this divine connection, you might then ask.

Your faith essentially is the key, regardless of your religion. Only your faith, inner dialogue or prayers are effective vehicles to raise you to a higher state of being. Even when one of your ten states of existence is hell, you have a second set of ten states within your hell state, which can potentially raise your state of being. To raise your state of being, you have to surrender your ego self, practice your faith, and find a true and positive purpose for your life, as you endeavor to push your limitations and sufferings away.

To prepare yourself to enter a state of Transcendental Connection:

- Breathe in and out slowly and deeply for 3 secs each way. Express gratitude that we are still alive.

  Feel the present moment and be only aware of your breathing, the people on this planet and the space which is also your own consciousness. Do this for at least 5 minutes. A connection will take place within you.

- Recognize that our belief system is the root of our thoughts and feelings. Find a noble goal that you feel passionate towards achieving in life.

- Be aware of the present moment and stay in it. Focus on the now and not the past or the future, as they are just mere projections. Continue breathing and be aware of your present heartbeat.

- Understand that your life is made of thoughts and feelings. They are energy. They connect and influence other energy entities (e.g. your environment, other people, etc.) and the cosmic space.

- Be aware that you can connect to three thousand possible realms of existence at any given moment, regardless of your place or location.

- Enter the highest life states by using your inner positive belief or prayer. Remember, it is only in the present moment that you can connect to all the realms or the Source itself.

---

[8] *Jacob Neusner, and Bruce D. Chilton, Altruism in World Religion (USA: George Town UP, 2005) 139.*

[9] *Peter Johnson, The Buddhism of T'ien T'ai (2001). Web. 1 Oct. 2010. <http://www.tientai.net>.*

[10] *Alain Aspect, Philippe Grangier, and Gérard Roger, "Experimental Realization of Einstein-Podolsky-Rosen-Bohm Gedankenexperiment: A New Violation of Bell's Inequalities," Physical Review Letters 49.2 (1982): 91-94.*

[11] *Ryszard Horodecki, Paweł Horodecki, Michal Horodecki, and Karol Horodecki, "Quantum entanglement," Reviews of Modern Physics 81.2 (2009): 865-942.*

[12] *Richard Feynman, QED: The Strange Theory of Light and Matter (Princeton: Princeton UP, 1988) 30-100.*

[13] *Dik Bouwmeester, Jian-Wei Pan, Klaus Mattle, Manfred Eibl, Harald Weinfurter, and Anton Zeilinger, "Experimen tal quantum teleportation," Nature 309.6660 (1997): 575-79.*

[14] *Carlo Rovelli, "Relational quantum mechanics," International Journal of Theoretical Physics 35.8 (1996): 1637-78.*

[15] *Richard Feynman, The Feynman Lectures on Physics, Vol. 3. (USA: Addison-Wesley, 1965) 1-8.*

[16] *Montague Ullman, Stanley Krippner, and Alan Vaughan, Dream Telepathy: Experiments in Nocturnal ESP (Boston: Hampton Roads, 2003) 169.*

[17] *Dean Radin, The Conscious Universe: The Scientific Truth of Psychic Phenomena (New York: Harper Edge, 1997) 59.*

[18] *Rupert Sheldrake, and Pamela Smart, "Experimental tests for telephone telepathy," Journal of the Society for Psychical Research 67.3 (2003): 184-99.*

Chapter Eight
Five Mutual Elements

On a larger scale, the concept of *3,000 Realms in a Single Living Moment* brings out the mutual interconnectivity between man, society and the environment. On a more personal level, the principle of the *Five Mutual Elements* – symbolically represented as Void, Wood, Water, Fire and Earth – demonstrates the mutual relationships between the different aspects of one's life. Essentially, these five elements are the five vital and tangible components that constitute and sustain any human life. When balanced, they bring harmony to one's being.

Of course, the concept of *3,000 Realms in a Single Living Moment* exists for each of the five elements as well. After all, since the five elements are tangible, they are also changeable; this implies, therefore, that we can change our lives when we make changes to these five patterns of living. And in so doing, we can heal any illness and transform the way we live.

But it is important to note that the *Five Mutual Elements* that I am talking about here are different from the systems of Traditional Chinese Medicine and Chinese Feng Shui. Viewed as an ancient universal allocation system, the *Five Mutual Ele-*

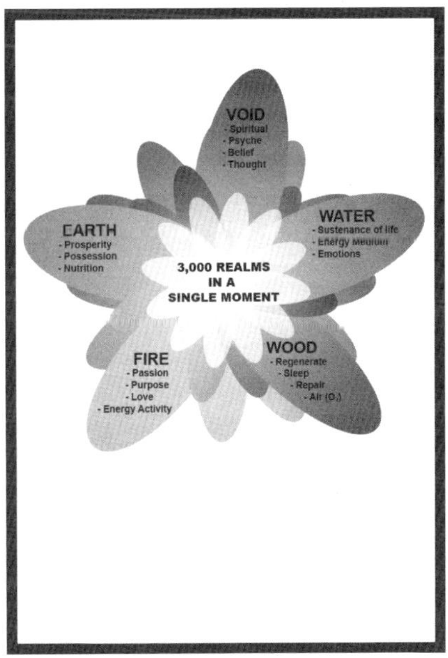

Figure 8-1 Mutual interaction between *3,000 Realms in a Single Living Moment* and the *Five Mutual Elements* in Transcendental Connection activity

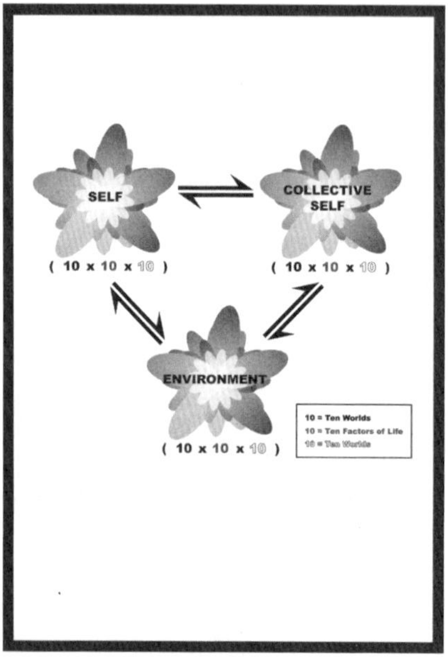

Figure 8-2 Mutual interaction between the Three Realms of Existence – The Being, Collective Beings and The Environment

ments is used to describe the interaction and integration of activities. In this case, each of the five elements represents a specific energy that interacts with each of the others and constitutes a living state. For example, Void represents one's psyche or spiritual state, while Water represents one's emotions. Wood represents one's regenerative potential and Qi, Fire represents energetics, one's goals or passions, and Earth represents the nutrition one receives and one's material wealth.

Void

Like the *3000 realms in a single living moment*, Void is also a spiritual aspect. Any change must start from us altering the very blueprint of our thinking pattern. Here, the Void element refers to one's psyche, spiritual belief, faith, belief system and thoughts. The Void element is also the initial gateway to transcending oneself to the oneness that is in resonance with the Divine rhythm or grace. Here, the Void element is pure and non-physical, and it is best used to describe one's purest state of mind – one that is most aligned to the cosmic rhythm. For any change to take place within oneself, one is required to first and foremost alter one's psyche or thoughts. Since these are also a form of spiritual energy, this energy can travel from one place to another – into your organs and cells, into others around you, and even into the environment – in the manner shown by the principle of *3,000 Realms in a Single Living Moment* (read Chapter Seven for more details on this).

Since words, thoughts and actions permeate the energy field that connects us all in time and space, the sound of words can also change one's state of mind and one's energy flow based on the phenomenon of Transcendental Connection. As such, sincere prayers – whether they are spoken out loud or whispered internally – are vital to bringing about a change to one's psyche, which in turn affects and brings about a balance to the other four mutually interconnected elements.

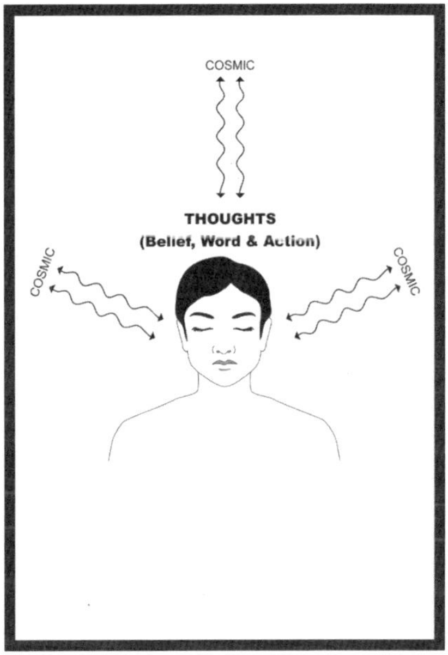

Figure 8-3 Thoughts and beliefs

Similarly, the power of thoughts penetrates time and space, and plays a part in affecting the results we want. Obviously, good thoughts give rise to good outcomes, while bad thoughts give rise to less than desirable outcomes. And, as such, good intentions and a sound moral code do not merely determine how we think, react and take action, they also benefit us directly through the positive results that they bring to our lives.

Among the *Five Mutual Elements*, Void is the most important. Here, Void represents the gateway to enhancing the rest of the four worldly elements which, when brought to a harmonious balance, will lead to the completeness of one's existence in this world. Unless Void is purified and aligned to the cosmic rhythm of the Source's sole intention in creation, one's connection will never be complete.

Water

According to Leonardo Da Vinci, "Water is the driving force of all nature." As we all know, water is necessary to sustain all life on Earth, since all living things are made up of seventy to ninety percent water. Humans, in particular, are made up of about seventy-five to ninety percent water. Physically speaking, we are then mainly water. And, since we are made mostly of water, the quality of the water that we drink affects the quality of our bodies.

This is important because, biologically-speaking, water has the following important functions:
1) Serves as a medium to transport nutrients, oxygen, waste and toxins from the blood, tissues, organs and cells of the body.
2) Serves as a medium for lymphatic system transport and drainage (immunity).
3) Serves as a medium for the excretion of toxins in the form of urine and feces.
4) Provides structural support for the body as a whole, as it comprises more than seventy percent of the body's mass.
5) Serves as a medium for communication in all bodily activities. For example, one's nervous system, circulatory system, cell signaling network and meridian lines.

Considering the role that water plays in sustaining our physical health, it is important that we drink the right water. From a chemical point of view, studies around the world have shown that the municipal water supplied to homes in some countries contains traces of chemicals.[19] Such chemicals range from pharmaceutical drugs (e.g. antibiotics, antiseptics, anti-depressants), to those found in personal care products (e.g. methylparaben, triclosan, polymers), to endocrine disruptors usually found in food waste (e.g. bisphenol A, dioxin), to chlorination agents and other chemical agents. According to these studies, there are close to 90,000 commercial chemical agents used around us daily and these agents frequently find their way into the environment, polluting our drainage systems, soil, underground water and reservoirs.

Due to this concern, in some parts of the world, the authorities have had to step in to use the most sophisticated processes available, such as ultrafiltration, to remove or reduce the concentration of chemicals in the municipal water supply, so that water becomes safe and suitable for daily consumption. However, some of these contaminants may not be present in the water during the process of ultrafiltration or may even disintegrate of their own accord into harmless matter. In any case, it is always highly advisable for us to do a final filtration of our water at home before consuming it. After all, water that is safe to drink may not necessarily be entirely healthy to drink.

Likewise, drinking distilled water is not recommended for health reasons as there are no added benefits to the body. The best water is pure and natural, where the good healing properties of the water – and its optimal mineral composition – have been retained, though the water has been filtered to keep it free of harmful microbes and their metabolites. The water's natural, optimal mineral content always gives the water a specific energy property in addition to its expected nutritional value to the body. The healthy microbes and their wholesome metabolites also contribute to the water's wholesome healing properties, derived from natural springs, underground water or upstream glacier rivers.

Here, the Water element is also representative of one's emotions. Research studies have revealed that water responds more strongly to one's emotions than to other energy sources, like light or sound. And so it can be theorized that one's emotions can control and influence the energy of water and its memory states.

As reflected in the principle of *3,000 Realms in Single Living Moment*, one's emotions and feelings emits bioresonance within one's body and subsequently, the environment. Our emotions are the main indicator whether we are on the right track towards total wellness and whether our thoughts are beneficial to our being. But to be emotionally positive, one needs to strive to lead the best possible life in every moment of every day.

At a quantum level, the world-renowned scientist Professor Masaru Emoto has proved that water has memory. He proved that water receives and gives resonance to its surroundings.[20] According to his studies, water, like man, has memory. When he played a beautiful song or attached any positive words like 'love' or 'gratitude' to some samples of water in his laboratory, the water revealed the presence of beautiful crystals, when studied under a microscope. When he wrote negative words like 'hate' or 'kill', the structure of the water crystals were discovered to be chaotic and ugly, similar to those in waste water. Also, the 'positive' water was observed to allow for the beautiful fermentation of rice compared to the 'negative' water, which caused the rice to become black and pungent after fermentation.

In fact, the structure of the crystals that formed when positive words were used on the water in the laboratory were as beautiful as those found in holy water from Lourdes, spring water from the Himalayan mountains, as well as water blessed by compassionate prayers. Through Prof Emoto's studies, we have learnt that the ability of water to respond to writings, thoughts and music, and its stored 'memory', teaches us that we need to be mindful of our words, thoughts and deeds. If even words and thoughts can produce latent effects in water, imagine how they could affect our bodies.

Such scientific findings perhaps support stories where people have felt better or healthier just from taking holy water or simply, wholesome natural water. From these laboratory studies, one can deduce that the positive energy in water can have a positive effect on one's body. In short, water has a profound link to one's emotions. Emotions affect water molecule clusters and their energetics in the body, which will in turn affect one's oxygen dynamics or *Qi* (a function of the Wood element), as well as one's ability to self-heal or sleep properly (again, of the Wood element). And so, the chemical make-up and physical chemistry quality of the water we drink directly affects the quality of our lives since the biological make up of a human being comprises mainly of water.

Demonstrating the mutual connection between the different elements of the *Five Mutual Elements*, the Metal element (which represents one's mind or psyche) enhances the Water element (which represents one's emotions), which is in turn linked to one's overall well-being.

Wood

The Wood element refers to the regeneration of oneself and the oxygen, air or *Qi* (flow of energy) permeating throughout us. To bring about harmony to one's Being, it is important that we take good care of our body, since it is interconnected to and is also one with our mind and soul. Often an aspect that most of us neglect, until it threatens to affect us significantly, is that of a good night's sleep. Our body requires sufficient sleep and an ample oxygen intake to sustain its overall well-being and support the regenerative process within us.

My unexpected recovery and the regeneration of nerves may be viewed by some scientists as the miraculous reactivation of my adult stem cells, which assisted in the growth of my nerves. Such a deduction is plausible as stem cells in an embryo can change into any cell. The same can be said for adult stem cells, which explains why there has been a heavy interest in stem cell therapy and research, in the hope of curing numerous disorders, including cancer, multiple sclerosis, blindness and diabetes. But the problem is that, as we get older, there are fewer and fewer adult stem cells in our body. So, should there have indeed been a massive reactivation of my adult stem cells, which led to the considerable regeneration of my nerves and bodily functions, the Transcendental Connection that made this miracle possible must have been truly powerful in its potential.

The importance of good sleep

Research has revealed that a lack of sleep has a detrimental effect on one's health. Research on laboratory rats that were deprived of sleep revealed that they lived only a staggering two to three weeks instead of the average lifespan of three years.[21,22] Studies have also repeatedly shown that a lack of sleep indirectly causes weight gain, reduced immunity and a large range of devastating diseases, like diabetes, heart disease, autoimmune diseases, neurological degeneration, depression, weight gain and accelerated aging.[23,24]

In spite of the great amount of research conducted, the complexity and dynamics of sleep are not yet fully understood by scientists. However, scientific findings have gone as far as to reveal that the brain undergoes five repetitive stages in the sleep cycle throughout the night: stage 1 involves a slowing and calming of the brain's activity (creating a transition period between wakefulness and sleep); stage 2 involves rapid, rhythmic brain wave activity and a slowing heart rate; stage 3 is when deep, slow brain waves, known as delta waves, begin to emerge; stage 4 is a period of deep sleep (also known as delta sleep, because of the delta waves that occur during this time); and lastly, stage 5 is the most paradoxical form of sleep because, while the brain and other body systems become more active (usually resulting in dreaming due to the increased brain activity, as well as rapid eye movements and an increased respiration rate), voluntary muscles become more relaxed. Stage 5 of the sleep cycle is frequently referred to as rapid eye movement (REM) sleep, for obvious reasons.

Amongst these five stages, REM sleep seems to be the key in reorganizing and sorting one's memories. One's mental prowess and concentration in the day is best when the REM stage is not disturbed. And, further studies have also linked the REM process to stronger immunity and better physical health.

The importance of getting sufficient sleep is often overlooked in our hectic lives, even though sleeping is, in fact, a very important and vital process in the renewal of our bodies. When we are asleep in the night, regenerative processes – like the repair of wear and tear to our body's tissues and organs, and hormonal adjustments and regulation, as well as the recharging of the immune system – take place. This profound healing process happens mostly in the REM stage of one's sleep, which is the deepest and hardest to reach, if not enough time is given to transcend the stages of sleep.

When we deprive ourselves of sleep during the night, we basically interrupt the body's natural mechanism for repair and regeneration. In fact, studies have shown that nerve damage, premature aging, cancer and blockages of the blood vessels in the heart and brain are strongly linked to a lack of sleep. In the absence of sufficient sleep, the body is also subjected to unnecessary stress and this shows up quickly through common signs, such as sores, ulcers, poorer vision and lower back ache. Those who lack sleep are also prone to having bad breath due to erosion of the lining of one's gastrointestinal track, causing bad microbes to thrive. On top of that, the accumulation of metabolic toxins inside the body makes one's breath even more unbearable.

During my early working years, my lack of sleep became the norm as I worked through the night, finally leaving the office at 3 or 4am, only to return to work later in the morning and press on throughout the day. After learning the correlation of a good sleep to one's health, I strongly believe that my condition was partly – either directly or indirectly – the result of lack of sleep.

Supporting the importance of sleep, some traditional physicians also believe that regular and proper sleep habits are necessary to regulate the body's internal biological rhythm according to the laws of the circadian meridian. The circadian cycle describes the way the body follows a rhythmic pattern to repair different organs at different times of the day. For example, when one is asleep from 1am to 3am, regenerative activities in the body are being channeled towards the liver. And, at other hours in the night, other organs begin their respective regenerative processes according to a schedule set by the body's own internal circadian rhythm.

As such, one needs to receive adequate sleep at night to ensure the restoration of all major organs that are mutually connected to one another; should one organ suffer, the rest will eventually follow suit. As a general rule of thumb, to best harness the benefits of sleep, it is recommended that one sleeps at about 9pm and wakes up before the break of dawn, at about 4am to 5am. If you are able to follow this sleeping pattern, you will feel a big difference in your health after some time. Sleeping well will give your body longevity and improve your quality of life.

Lastly, it is important to note that the magnetic field of the earth as it revolves around the sun has a profound effect on bio-magnetism, and the body's circadian rhythm and meridian flow, and as such, has an influence on our bodies and sleep patterns. Such is the connection between nature and man that it reinforces the principles of *3,000 Realms in a Single Living Moment* at a transcendental level, where man is intimately related to the cosmic rhythm and the activities of the environment.

The importance of proper breathing

The Wood element involves air or *Qi*. As important as sleep is in the regeneration of one's body, it is best accompanied by taking in good quality air and adopting good breathing techniques that will encourage the thorough absorption of good oxygen into every corner of one's tissues and organs, which is the key to keeping diseases at bay and maintaining good overall health.

We all know that one can live without food for weeks or even without water for days, but it is not possible to live without oxygen for minutes, let alone weeks or months. Such is the importance of air and its quality that our body relies on it for its mere survival.

According to noted physiologist Dr Arthur C. Guyton, "All chronic pain, suffering and disease are caused by lack of oxygen at the cell level." In fact, Dr Harry Goldbatt, another celebrated physiologist, went so far as to say that "lack of oxygen clearly plays a major role in causing cells to become cancerous."

Today, research has repeatedly shown that many types of cancer cells cannot survive or flourish in an oxygen-rich environment.[25] Supporting this view, Nobel Prize laureate, Dr Otto Warburg, from the renowned Max Planck Institute, discovered and linked the growth of cancer cells to the lack of an oxygen-rich environment. Thus, it has been postulated that the correct and efficient intake of oxygen can prevent cancer.[26]

Not to be mistaken for the amount of oxygen that is being inhaled, the term "oxygen content" here refers to the concentration of oxygen that is distributed in every part of our tissues, in order for the cells to breathe. Here, the concentration of oxygen that reaches every cell homogeneously, is influenced by factors such as the type of water that we drink, our diet, stress levels, thinking patterns, our subconscious (which influences our breathing patterns), energetic vibration of one's psyche as well as the amount of pollution in our environment.

Furthermore, medically speaking, a high concentration of oxygen in your blood does not necessarily mean that other parts of your body, such as the tissues far from your lungs and blood vessels, will have sufficient oxygen, due to the possible presence of toxins, tissue obstruction and poor blood capillary circulation. As such, factors like sufficient sleep, proper weight management, good drinking water, a good diet, and proper breathing go a long way in enhancing one's physical constitution and physiology.

In the *Huangdi Neijing* (commonly known in English as the "Yellow Emperor's Inner Canon" – a primary source text for Chinese medicine) which originated thousands of years ago in China, it was in fact stated that the highest healing power can be found in correct breathing (*Qi*), followed by acupuncture and then, medicinal products.[27] In fact, proper breathing is the most effective way to good health and also the cheapest mode of healing available. Learning from a reputable *qigong* or meditation teacher can also help to increase the distribution of quality air within the body. There are many breathing techniques – some are simple, while others are more complex – but a Transcendental Connection involves simple breathing techniques that enable one to connect to the mind and body to heal.

Apart from the quality and concentration of air within us, it is equally important to take note of the quality of the air outside too. Here, the chemical and physical content of the air that we take in has an impact on our bodies.

In the city, the air contains more chemical vapors. According to the US Environmental Protection Agency (EPA), the air that we breathe can have more than a hundred possible harmful chemicals.[28] Some chemicals – one of them being carbon monoxide – can have a neurotoxin effect in the long term and can affect one's general physiology and even mental health. Thus, reducing the unnatural intake of air pollutants will assist in one's natural healing processes, as well as prevent acute or chronic health problems in the long run. This is because, when toxins reside in the body, the body has to channel most of its reserves, in terms of its activities and energy, to handle the increased level of toxicity. As a result, the body has little reserves left to heal itself.

In contrast to the high levels of pollution in the city, the air in the countryside and deep in the wilderness is vastly superior. Negative ions – found mostly in the air in forests, and near beaches, waterfalls and mountains – bind with positively charged particles, like viruses and dust, making the air that we breathe when we are in the country cleaner and lighter. Breathing cleaner air is important, as the microbes and chemicals that we breathe in become an extra load for the body to deal with. This is especially so during sleep, when many of the body's repair processes are supposed to take place.

Some scholars also argue that negative ions could make the pH of blood increase, making it less acidic. This is important because, if the level of microbes and pollutants is reduced considerably and one's blood and tissue are less acidic, the healing process will complete more quickly as the body does not need to spend so much energy balancing the blood's pH level or eliminating microbes. Therefore, in the long term, if your health is at an optimal level, you will feel more refreshed when you wake up every morning because the repair process that takes place at night was more effective. This explains why many patients are advised to recuperate in the countryside, far from the airborne pollution of the cities, and they normally recover faster than those who do remain in the cities.

In short, a proper deep breathing technique coupled with good air quality will speed up the natural healing process within one. It also enhances health, fosters longevity, prevents sickness and generates wellness.

Here, the Water element, which represents one's emotions, enhances the Wood element, which relates to the ability to sleep peacefully, breathe properly and regenerate. In the absence of positive emotions or positively energized water in the body, it is impossible to achieve the desired Wood characteristic.

Fire

The Fire element represents one's passions, love and energy. It encompasses one's purpose in life or love of someone or something. Here, Fire represents the passions and dreams that reside in one's heart that keeps one's fixed on achieving a mission or an ideal even when one is up against all odds.

However, when this passion becomes too intense, it can easily become a double-edged sword. Too much passion or Fire is seen as dangerous, as this overzealousness can burn out one's life. Therefore, it is important for one to strive to reach a balance or the Middle Way, in order to be successful in life. With the good regeneration of one's body and mind (Wood element), one has the energy or Fire to be propelled towards success. Hence, Wood enhances Fire.

Fire, moreover, also represents love. Constructive Fire can take the form of love of the spiritual true self (universal), self love (the ego), familial love, love of a spouse, and romantic love. Again, too much love can become destructive, obsessive and stifling. For example, overly concerned parents make a child feel suffocated and put him under unnecessary pressure, and overly passionate lovers ignore the realities of life and put their relationship in danger of falling apart later on under the true financial and social strains that accompany marriage and parenthood.

Yet, love is so important to every living being on this planet. Without it, nothing would move or progress. And most importantly, true love for someone can transform into the energy needed to heal oneself and others. This is the love of the spiritual true self, which is all-encompassing and is a way of living out the love of God or the Source in one's own life. This is also a selfless love that one feels for the world, and is one that enables your true self to open the channel to the divine transformational process. And this is also the most perfect love, as this is essentially a love relationship with one's true self or higher self.

On a personal note, it was my parents' love for me that kept me afloat during my darkest hours. Subsequently, it was my sudden, emerging love for this world that drove me to make a Transcendental Connection that began the healing process within me.

Here, Fire also refers to the energetic exchange of life, which encompasses far more than we realize. For instance, financial exchanges, business transactions and the global economy as a whole are all forms of energy exchange (and so are part of the Earth element as well). Indeed, thoughts, words and actions are all energy too.

Most important, however, is the awareness that every form of energy is connected to every other form in a more profound manner than we realize. For example, Prof Emoto's experiment on the response of water molecules' structure to the resonance of words spoken to or written on the containers holding the water, show us how the water's energies are intimately connected to the energies conveyed by the words. And, the principles behind this are just as obvious in the double slit test, and the quantum entanglements created in the Large Hadron Collider; these are all proof of the interconnectedness around us. So here, we see how prayers – healing by channeling or intent – are really only conduits that reinforce the properties of the Fire element on Transcendental Connection activity.

To illustrate this natural phenomenon further, there is the famous experiment by Russian quantum biologist Vladimir Poponin on a DNA strand. First, a strand of DNA was placed in a vacuum chamber. After it was removed, a laser that was passed through the chamber replicated the exact helical structure of the DNA strand that had been in the chamber previously. It was as if the DNA strand, which had been removed, was surprisingly still there when the laser had shone on the spot where it had been. The energy emitted by the laser left a ghost image of the DNA strand even when the physical form of the DNA strand was no longer around. In other words, the energetic image or memory of the DNA strand still remained.

Similarly, numerous studies done on leaves using a Kirlian camera (used to capture the electromagnetic field or aura of a body), where the top part of the leaf has been cut off, still show the image of the removed portion of the leaf for some time after its removal. Here, there seems to be a link between the concept of spirit and body and Dr Rupert Sheldrake's theory of the morphogenetic field.[29] Such studies are proof that we are interconnected, whether we see it or not with our naked eyes; just like how we do not see radio waves but know that they exist and understand how they can be applied in our daily lives.

The body's ability to heal itself is the result of a mix of tangible and intangible energetic activities. They range from the central and peripheral neurological electrical impulses of nerves, and electron transfer needed for cellular respiration and muscular movement, to the biophotonic fields that exist along meridian lines, as well as the quantum energetic information in time and space that exists in DNA's primary, secondary and tertiary structure.[30]

Also, it is believed that there is an interactive resonance and frequency that can be received and transmitted by our chromosomes and DNA structure to surrounding energies and time-space, which could change our DNA. In fact, an increasing number of scientists believe that healing is possible based on this principle of modulating frequencies into our DNA and reprogramming its very structure and content. It is also believed that *Qi* or the flow of energy and health in the body in an anti-clockwise direction produces mobius coil geometry which produces different levels of electromagnetic energy (Fire) in one's body, which affects one's health and vitality.[31] Other scholars called this scalar energy.

We can understand by now that the human body is energetic and since energy is always in a dynamic state, one can use energy to heal oneself, whether one chooses to engage it through qigong, light therapy, sound therapy, resonance therapy, or other forms of energy therapy. However, to get the therapy to work, we need to do it right and with qualified, honest guidance, because, just like all other forms of therapy, improper application of a therapy can have a negative effect on one's health.

Although such therapies are considered alternative healing, more is being done for us to learn and discover their many benefits. And it is through these efforts that we now know more about ourselves and how the powers of Mother Nature have manifested themselves all around us.

Of course, it will always take some time before there is greater validation and acceptance of such alternative therapies and before they are put into use in partnership with mainstream medical practices. But already, alternative concepts, such as meridian lines and acupoints, which were once frowned upon by mainstream medicine, are now widely accepted and acknowledged. And so is hypnotherapy.

Earth

The Earth element refers to prosperity, wealth, and nutrition or food.

However, it is important to note that, here, prosperity and wealth do not refer to an obsessive attachment to one's possessions. In fact, such an attitude is the opposite of true prosperity, because being a slave to one's possessions generates a fear of lack.

However, that being said, being spiritual does not mean being poor. Contrary to popular belief, true spiritual practice in this day and age should attract prosperity, abundance, love and friendship. This is because a connection to the Source within and without provides one with all the wisdom, creativity and resources needed to bring strength, inner joy and abundance into one's life.

Being poor and spiritual does not mean being noble and non-attached. In Taoism and Buddhism, we are taught about balance, harmony and the Middle Way. What these principles have in common is the belief that striking a balance between spiritual and material wealth creates good values in life.

Some of us mistakenly believe that money is the root of all evil, that money is hard to earn and that it is impossible for an 'ordinary person' to ever be rich, that doing business and being a businessman is 'dirty', that having a lot of money is a sign of greed, and so on. However, true balance and harmony with oneself and the universe means understanding that money itself is not the problem per se, as money is simply a collection of inanimate objects (i.e. checks, dollar bills, assorted coins, credit cards, etc.) that we assign value to; rather, the problem is why we want money or why we want even more money than we have now. The universe, after all, responds to our intentions and if our intentions are good and noble, we can harness the energies needed to achieve our goals. For instance, if we aim to make more money so that we can contribute more generously to worthy causes, we are far more likely to achieve our aims. And indeed, scholars and writers have observed that those who believe that money itself is evil usually live a life of poverty and lack, as they fail to understand what is really holding them back.

To heal one's mind, emotions and body, money plays a vital part too. Many people love to deny this or disassociate themselves from it, as it gives them a false sense of humility. But, money really is a basic requirement of life, whether you use it to consult a doctor, engage a therapist, buy supplements, purchase organic food, or attend self-improvement courses. Even building a church, temple, school or hospital requires a lot of money! And there is really nothing wrong with that. As long as the money is being used to do good – to heal our sick bodies, to provide a place for children to learn, and so on – the energy surrounding the use of this money is positive, and the money is far from being evil in its intent.

The main point, therefore, is to realize that whichever of the five elements we endeavor to excel in, each of them can either be positive or negative, depending on why we have chosen the path that we are on. This is reflected in the principle of *Yin Yang* (usually referred to in English as "yin and yang", which describes how forces that appear to be polar opposites are actually interconnected and interdependent), as well as the concept of good (as represented by a God or gods) versus evil (usually embodied by a demon or other similar malevolent force) found in many religions and cultures. Scientifically, this is also reflected in the presence of positive and negative charges, and the concepts of matter and anti-matter in quantum physics. The key, then, is to actively seek balance.

The importance of eating right

Apart from possessions, food also makes up the Earth element. What we put into our mouth plays a part in affecting our body, which in turn has an effect on our mind and soul.

Conducted by the US National Institutes of Health in 2009, the AARP Diet & Health Study reported that the consumption of red meat and dairy products is associated with the increased risk of pancreatic cancer. It was also discovered that there was no known association between fats from plant foods and pancreatic cancer among the 525,000 participants studied.[32]

Elsewhere, the Nurses' Health Study (also by the US National Institutes of Health) found that when a diet that consisted mainly of saturated and trans fats, of the kind found in meat and processed foods, was replaced by a diet rich in monounsaturated or polyunsaturated fat, of the kind found in vegetables, nuts and fish, in 1,500 people over the age of 70 who had Type 2 Diabetes, the change in diet had led to less cognitive decline amongst the subjects.[33]

The American Institute for Cancer Research (AICR) also reported that the consumption of red meat, like pork and beef, is linked to an increased risk of colorectal cancer. In fact, their report even concluded that consuming more than 18 ounces of meat a week leads to a significant increase in the risk of getting cancer.[34] Based on their studies, the AICR in fact recommends eating more plant-based foods, over red meat and processed food, to decrease your body's susceptibility in developing cancer.

Similarly, an article in the June 2009 issue of the Archives of Internal Medicine reported that protein sources from plants help to lower the risk of developing heart disease.[35]

Elsewhere, investigative findings from scientists have also revealed that animals release stress toxins before they are slaughtered. Professor Wilhelm Schulze and Dr Hazim of Hannover University's School of Veterinary Medicine, Germany, compared the response of an animal's brain and heart activity during and immediately after slaughter.[36] According to the results from their electroencephalograph (EEG) and electrocardiogram (ECG) readings, it was revealed that the common method of slaughtering large animals (i.e. the captive bolt) caused severe pain to the animal before it lost consciousness. And, if Prof Emoto has proven that emotions can affect the memory of water, then you can imagine how consuming meat filled with the memory of pain and angst is harmful for the body, as the meat that we ingest is made up of approximately seventy percent water.

Thus, the Halal way of slaughtering meat (i.e. a quick cut to the neck, slicing both the jugular veins and carotid arteries) has its real wisdom. From both a scientific and holistic point of view, the toxins released during the ritual Halal slaughtering process are much less.

Nevertheless, as Leonardo Da Vinci once said, "Truly man is the king of beasts, for his brutality exceeds theirs. We live by the death of others; we are burial places! I have from an early age abjured the use of meat, and the time will come when men such as I will look on the murder of animals as they now look on the murder of men."

Animals that have suffered pain at death have negative memory resonance locked inside their flesh. When we eat them, it is believed that this negativity threatens our physical and mental health.

Perhaps that is why many spiritual teachers, such as Jesus and Buddha, were believed to have abstained from eating meat as much as they could. Through historical research, Islamic scholars have even discovered that the Prophet Muhammad preferred a mostly vegetarian diet. Furthermore, it is probably no mere coincidence that many great thinkers, inventors and scientists, such as Lao Tzu, Confucius, Albert Einstein, Nicola Tesla, Thomas Edison, Isaac Newton, Leo Tolstoy, Gandhi, Martin Luther King and Leonardo Da Vinci, have also been vegetarians. In fact, some of the strongest and most powerful animals on the planet, such as the rhinoceros, elephant and horse, are also herbivores.

If anything, all the above tells us that the consumption of meat poses many problems to one's health.

Furthermore, it is also an old and outdated belief that protein comes solely from meat, as the opposite has been proven to be true. In fact, in many laboratory studies, it has been shown that vegetables can have a higher protein and micronutrient content than meat.

In fact, essential nutrients for our general well-being, such as phytosterols, alkaloids, flavonoids, anthocyanins and many other phyto-organic metabolites, are found in plant parts but never in any animal or dairy products. Such nutrients have not only proven to possess powerful curative properties against cancer, but can also strengthen one's immunity, slow down aging, reduce cholesterol and protect brain tissues, amongst many other benefits. Perhaps owing to such properties, there are many widespread claims that a vegan diet is beneficial for individuals who are suffering from cancer, lupus or multiple sclerosis.

Renowned physician Dr Max Gerson (18 October 1881 - 8 March 1959), an advocate of a plant-based diet to counter disease and provide general well-being, cured the Nobel Prize winner Albert Schweitzer of his Type II diabetes, as well as Dr Schweitzer's wife of tuberculosis. Although his ideas about a plant-based diet were not supported by the healthcare and pharmaceutical industry during his time, Dr Gerson documented many instances when individuals were cured of heart disease, kidney problems and cancer through his devised dietary therapy. Decades after his death, Dr Gerson was finally recognized for his revolutionary insight over the benefits of a plant-based diet and was inducted into the Orthomolecular Hall of Fame in 2005.

Another contemporary advocate of a plant-based diet, Betty Khoo, the author of *Cancer Cured and Prevent* Naturally, also cited many cases where cancer patients experienced a complete remission after starting on a proper plant-based diet.[37] Norman Walker, known to be one of the pioneers of raw vegetable juicing and the fruit diet, was also healed from cancer after he changed his diet.

In 2006, Dr T. Colin Campbell, recognized as one of the giants in nutrition academia, published an outspoken and landmark book entitled *The China Study*, based on decades of research, statistics and data, which revealed that a plant-based diet does help to prevent and even cure chronic illnesses, like diabetes, cancer and heart disease. In this book, he extensively proved the correlation between a predominantly meat-based diet and most of the common modern ailments.

But notwithstanding the type of food consumed, it is equally important to ensure that they are free from high levels of contaminants. Studies have revealed that a certain level of exposure to pesticides can result in anything from mild skin irritation to birth defects, the growth of tumors, blood and nerve disorders, endocrine disruption, coma and even death. In fact, contaminants, such as pesticides, not only alter the biochemistry of plants and the cycle of its ecology as it interferes with the metabolism of the organism, but also results in bioaccumulation in the people and animals that eat the plants.[38]

Long term exposure to high levels of contaminants found in poultry, agricultural products and processed food items – such as artificial coloring, preservatives, antibiotics, sedatives, hormones, pharmaceutical drugs, fungicides, stabilizers and alfotoxins – can also lead to hormonal imbalances, circulatory problems, diabetes, cancer, neurological degenerative diseases and fertility problems, amongst other things.[39]

For this reason, even though a plant-based diet is recommended, not all food plants grown are entirely suited to generating good health. On some commercial farms, the use of contaminants, such as chemical pesticides, poses problems. As the same piece of land is used to grow the same crops over and over again, the soil becomes depleted of its nutrients and life force, and requires the intervention of even more chemical fertilizers to enhance productivity and sustain the continued and rapid growth of crops. Apart from the use of chemical fertilizers, plant growth hormones are also used in commercial farming. And, as these crops are often harvested before they are fully ripe and then preserved – either whole or in a processed form – so that they can survive storage and transport to their final destination, the nutrients and metabolites in these crops are often not fully mature and not at an optimal level.

In contrast to crops that are grown through commercial farming, crops that are grown organically are more nourishing for the body. According to the International Federation of Organic Agriculture Movements, organic agriculture is defined as "a production system that sustains the health of soils, ecosystems and people." It relies on ecological processes, biodiversity and cycles adapted to local conditions, rather than the use of chemical inputs, which have an adverse effect on the body.

Good organic agriculture combines tradition, innovation and science to benefit the shared environment and promote fair relationships and a good quality of life for all involved. It is based on the cyclic pattern of Mother Nature, to grow, nurture and harvest crops naturally. Such farming methods focus on the regeneration and health of the soil, which in turn generate the good health of the plants and animals that feed on it.

To highlight the benefits of organically-grown produce over commercially-grown produce, certified nutrition specialist Virginia Worthington reviewed 41 published studies to compare the nutritional value of the two. Based on her study, she finally concluded that there was 27% more vitamin C, 21.1% more iron, 29.3% more magnesium, and 13.6% more phosphorus in organically grown produce. In addition, organic products had 15.1% less nitrates than their conventional counterparts.[40] Worthington also noted that five servings of organic vegetables (e.g. lettuce, spinach, carrots, potatoes and cabbage) provided the recommended daily intake of vitamin C for both men and women, while their conventional counterparts did not.

Nutritional value aside, Dr Kikuo Chishima from Nagoya Commercial University, Japan, has discovered that the energy vibration or frequency of a food itself is more important than the nutrition inside it. Science has shown that every nutrient (or in fact any molecule) has a unique resonance frequency and that nutrient molecules store and emit certain frequencies (which are part of the Fire element). According to Dr Kikuo, the right combination of good organic nutrients produces a symphony of positive resonating fields to cells and their surroundings. Therefore, when we consume positive food molecules, they create in us a symphony of resonance to heal. Taking properly farmed fruits and plants is, thus, the ultimate choice for an optimized Earth element.

Based on the above findings, it is safe to say that a plant-based, organic diet promotes well-being and assists in fighting the many diseases that plague man in the 21st century.

Having said that, one still has to practice discretion when selecting organic food. After all, not all organic farmed food are of the same quality and to make matters worse, food is sometimes fraudulently labeled to mislead consumers into thinking that it has indeed been produced organically. On top of that, safe packaging of the produce is also another major concern, though it is beyond the scope of this book.

More about the Five Mutual Elements

Each of the five elements in this system relates to a different function of the body. When we abide by the rhythm of all the mutual elements, our body is able to function more effectively to generate a healing process from within.

The *Five Mutual Elements* classification system is flexible as it lends itself to various situations or contexts. However, do note though, that for our bodily functions, there can be no Void element. Instead, here, we have the more tangible Metal element to replace the position of Void.

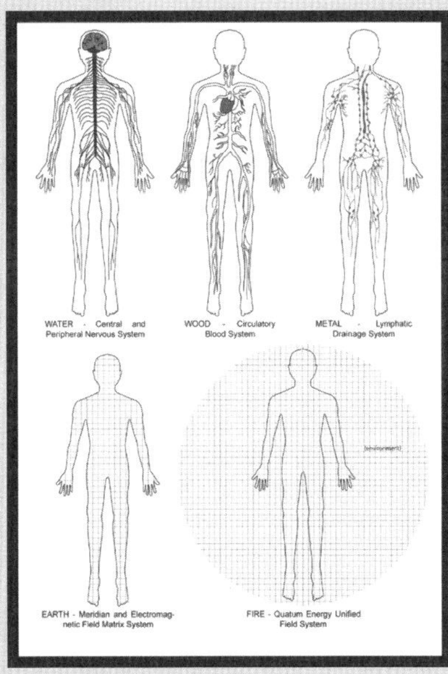

Figure 8-6 Diagram of the human body and the *Five Mutual Elements*

1) Central and Peripheral Nervous System – Water

Represents thoughts, moods and emotions. Contributes to perception, conception of new ideas, and volition or action in life.

2) Circulatory Blood System – Wood

Regenerative channels for repair and the removal of body waste. Brings oxygen into the body system for energy.

3) Lymphatic Drainage System – Metal

Protection of the body from negative physical entities.

4) Meridian and Electromagnetic Field Matrix System – Earth

Controls the communication of electromagnetic waves, polarity and biophotonics, as well as the function of the harmonious field within the body.

5) Quantum Energy Unified Field System – Fire

This is the coherent bio-energy field that connects and communicates to phenomena (which are also energy fields) around us. Our conscious energy and the four above systems are in a unified and mutual relationship with the cosmic energy vibrating around us. This connection explains how personal prayer, qigong masters and metaphysician healers activate the rest of the four elements to produce healing results.

---

[19] *"Sources of common contaminants and their health effects," U.S. Environmental Protection Agency (2007). Web. 10 Oct. 2007. <http://www.epa.gov/superfund/programs/er/hazsubs/sources.htm>.*

[20] *Masaru Emoto, The Healing Power of Water (USA: Hay House, 2007) 31-95.*

[21] *Allan Rechtschaffen, and Bernard M. Bergmann, "Sleep deprivation in the rat by the disk-over-water method," Behavioural Brain Research 69.1 (1995): 55-63.*

[22] *Clete Kushida, Sleep deprivation: Basic Science, Physiology, and Behavior (New York: Informa Healthcare, 2005) 1-2.*

[23] *Shahrad Taheri, Ling Lin, Diane Austin, Terry Young, and Emmanuel Mignot, "Short Sleep Duration Is Associated with Reduced Leptin, Elevated Ghrelin, and Increased Body Mass Index," PLoS Medicine 1.3 (2004): 210-17.*

[24] "No sleep means no new brain cells," BBC News Health (10 Feb. 2007). Web. 1 Oct. 2010. <http://news.bbc.co.uk/2/hi/health/6347043.stm>.

[25] Otto Warburg, "On the origin of cancer cells," Science 123.3191 (1956): 309-14.

[26] Jung-whan Kim, and Chi V. Dang, "Cancer's Molecular Sweet Tooth and the Warburg Effect," Cancer Research 66.18 (2006): 8927-30.

[27] Ilza Veith, trans., The Yellow Emperor's Classic of Internal Medicine (Berkeley: U of California P, 2002): 25-58.

[28] "Technology Transfer Network: Air Toxics Web Site – Pollutants & Sources," U.S. Environmental Protection Agency (24 Mar. 2009). Web. 1 Jun. 2010. <http://www.epa.gov/ttn/atw/pollsour.html>.

[29] Rupert Sheldrake, "Morphic Resonance and Morphic Fields: An Introduction," Presenting the work of Dr. Rupert Sheldrake, Biologist & Author (February 2005). Web. 28 May 2008. <http://www.sheldrake.org/Articles&Papers/papers/morphic/morphic_intro.html>.

[30] Peter P. Gariaev, Boris I. Birshtein, Alexander M. Iarochenko, Peter J. Marcer, George G. Tertishny, Katherine A. Leonova, and Uwe Kaempf, The DNA-wave Biocomputer. Paper. Russian Academy of Sciences, and Wave Genetics Inc, 2002.

[31] Stephen Linsteadt, and Maria Elena Boekemeyer, The Heart of Health: The Principles of Physical Health and Vitality (USA: Natural Healing House Press, 2003) 132.

[32] Anne C. M. Thiébaut, Li Jiao, Debra T. Silverman, Amanda J. Cross, Frances E. Thompson, Amy F. Subar, Albert R. Hollenbeck, Arthur Schatzkin, and Rachael Z. Stolzenberg-Solomon, "Dietary Fatty Acids and Pancreatic Cancer in the NIH-AARP Diet and Health Study," Journal of the National Cancer Institute 101.14 (2009): 1001-11.

[33] Elizabeth E. Devore, Meir J. Stampfer, Monique M.B. Breteler, Bernard Rosner, Jae Hee Kang, Olivia Okereke, Frank B. Hu, and Francine Grodstein, "Dietary Fat Intake and Cognitive Decline in Women With Type 2 Diabetes," Diabetes Care 32.4 (2009): 635-40.

[34] "For Red Meat, Another Red Light," American Institute for Cancer Research (May 2007). Web. 1 Oct. 2010. <http://www.aicr.org/site/News2?page=NewsArticle&id=11809>.

[35] David J. A. Jenkins, Julia M. W. Wong, Cyril W. C. Kendall, Amin Esfahani, Vivian W. Y. Ng, Tracy C. K. Leong, Dorothea A. Faulkner, Ed Vidgen, Kathryn A. Greaves, Gregory Paul, and William Singer, "The Effect of a Plant-Based Low-Carbohydrate ("Eco-Atkins") Diet on Body Weight and Blood Lipid Concentrations in Hyperlipidemic Subjects," Archives of Internal Medicine 169.11 (2009): 1046-54.

[36] Sahib M. Bleher, trans., Experiments for the objectification of pain and consciousness during conventional (cap tive bolt stunning) and religiously mandated ("ritual cutting") slaughter procedures for sheep and calves, by W. Schulze, H. Schultze-Petzold, A.S. Hazem, and R. Gross, Deutsche Tierärztliche Wochenschrift 85 (1978): 62-66. Web. 1 Jun. 2010. <http://www.mustaqim.co.uk/halalstudy.htm>.

[37] Betty Khoo-Kingsley, Cancer Cured and Prevented Naturally (Singapore: AKLTG, 2009) 201-57.

[38] "What Are the Potential Health Effects of Pesticides?" Community Guide to Recognizing and Reporting Pesticide Problems. California Department of Pesticide Regulation (2008). Web. 1 Jun. 2010. <http://www.cdpr.ca.gov/docs/dept/comguide/effects_excerpt.pdf>.

[39] "Sources of common contaminants and their health effects," U.S. Environmental Protection Agency (2007). Web. 10

Oct. 2007. <http://www.epa.gov/superfund/programs/er/hazsubs/sources.htm>.

[40] *Virginia Worthington, "Nutrition and Biodynamics: Evidence for the Nutritional Superiority of Organic Crops," Biodynamics 224 (1999): 58-69.*

Part III
How Others Have Healed Themselves

Through their healing, we have learnt that people of any faith or belief system – even atheists – are capable of recovering miraculously.

Chapter Nine
Passing the Light On

Looking back, I see how this healing system has been revealed to me through moments of understanding here and there in my life, like a jigsaw puzzle that has slowly taken shape over a span of more than a decade. Looking back, I recognize that it was not my condition that had given me a deeper insight into life. Rather, it was my journey of internal resolve, from fear to hope, with its many questions and answers, as I progressed from failure to triumph, that has enabled me to emerge with a greater sense of clarity. Looking back, I cannot help but be amazed at how my life was interrupted by innumerable episodes of trial and tribulation, until I had grasped the significance of achieving harmony in life and a connection from within and around me.

The lessons learnt during this process of recovery became the source of my service towards others who were similarly plagued with seemingly incurable illnesses. Driven by this spur to reach out to others, I simply made myself available to those in need, even though I was clueless as to how to help them initially. But I soon learnt that just by telling my story, I served as a source of inspiration for them. By placing myself in their shoes and approaching them with heartfelt compassion and love, I was able to connect with them at a deeper, and oftentimes, transcendental level.

By word of mouth, more people from my circle of friends, hospital acquaintances and fellow members of spiritual communities approached me to visit someone whom they knew was in need of help. Just like that, I became more involved in reaching out to others through one-to-one sessions. Gradually, my days were filled with more visits and follow-up sessions with individuals, both young and old, who were either terminally ill or had been pronounced incurable by doctors.

Despite my own set of physical limitations then, as I had only just recovered, I continued to share with others how I had shed my own paralysis and blindness to become a healthy, functioning member of society once more. I helped them to understand how I had changed my own life, and how they could change theirs. And, while some of them made steady improvements over a long period of time, others experienced almost miraculous recoveries from their illnesses rather quickly.

Through their healing, we have learnt that people of any faith or belief system – even atheists – are capable of recovering miraculously. With this understanding, I know that a Transcendental Connection can be achieved by anybody. And, when I realized that this connection could bring about an improvement in the condition of those who had been deemed incurable, I was all the more convinced that I had stumbled upon a natural healing system, whose powers had been revealed both in ancient philosophies and recent scientific discoveries about how the body truly works.

Below are some selected stories about how I tried to pass this light on.

Fighting genetic defects

I met Luke (not his real name) in 2005, while I was still attending physiotherapy sessions at the Society for the Physically Disabled (SPD). At that point, Luke had already been suffering from an incurable genetic disorder called neurofibromatosis (NF) for the past twelve years.

He had once been a normal and healthy boy, until he discovered tumors growing in his body when he was in his early teens. Luke's condition was one where tumors would grow not only inside but also outside of the body. In fact, such was the severity of his condition that, when I met him, his body was riddled with hundreds of tumors. Some were as big as golf balls. Due to the uncontrolled and widespread growth of these tumors, doctors had decided not to remove the tumors surgically anymore. As the tumors were even growing inside his central nervous system, his hearing and speech were badly impaired. And if his condition were to worsen, he would even lose his eyesight.

When I first met Luke at the SPD, he was completely paralyzed from the neck down. Due to the overproduction of melanin in his body, as a result of his disease, his skin was dark and looked somewhat like the wrinkled skin of an old elephant. In addition, Luke often experienced sudden muscle spasms, due to his nerves being compressed by the numerous tumors all over his body. Such was his discomfort that his mother had to quit her day job and adjust his ailing body in bed and in his wheelchair every half an hour.

During that time, I also learnt that we shared the same Buddhist faith. During our sessions at the SPD, our mothers would talk to each other and that was how I got acquainted with him and I even gave him my wheelchair when I was somewhat able to walk.

Even after I stopped going to the SPD for treatment, I did not forget about Luke. Instead, I took the initiative to approach his family and joined them in their prayer sessions for Luke every Saturday morning, together with a group of my Buddhist friends. During those prayer sessions, I kept reminding his family to continue to have faith that they could change Luke's genetic makeup and make him better, even though, compared to other ailments, hereditary genetic disorders are the hardest to reverse and heal. I helped them to understand that they needed to connect their intent to their higher self while praying and even after prayer.

Just two months later, Luke started to experience a strange bout of fever, excessive perspiration and severe diarrhea. According to his mother, Luke's stools were also unusually smelly and of an odd color. It was as if his body was dispelling the toxins within, and Luke's skin began to heal shortly after. In just two months, the tumors on his face and scalp had shrunk. Soon, Luke was even able to move his neck and his fingers. Today, he is working with a network marketing company, and earns a decent income. And today, he has reached the stage where he is even able to move his torso slightly.

The will of a young man

I first met Jonathan (not his real name) when he was just 21 years of age. At that time, in 2006, I had just returned to work and I was rather weak. But through the request of a friend, I made a trip to the National University Hospital to visit this young man.

He had already been in the hospital for a week by then. The cervical region of Jonathan's neck had been severely crushed during a regular rugby game, and even after undergoing surgery by a top local surgeon, Jonathan was left completely paralyzed from the neck down.

During my first visit to see Jonathan, it was clear that he was unable to move, was down and very despondent. Seeing his dejected look as he lay motionless in bed, I could only imagine what a tremendous blow it must have been for an active man like him to lose his mobility at such a young age.

During that visit, Jonathan's parents, obviously devastated by what had happened, told me that according to his doctor, Jonathan would most likely never be able to lift his hand, let alone get up and walk. When I heard their comments, I instinctively rebuked them. "No, he can move his hands," I pointed out. Lying there quietly in bed, Jonathan heard what I had said and somehow believed that he could in fact move his hands.

During each of my visits that week, I told Jonathan and his family to pray for his recovery. I told them that it did not matter if Jonathan was a Christian and that his parents were Buddhists, so long as they had faith in their prayers. I told Jonathan the importance of facing his difficulties with the right mindset (i.e. a desire to heal himself), and that when he was in the right rhythm of things, he would then attract people or things that would assist him in his recovery. I also taught him the power of belief and visualization, and how the mind and body are inseparable.

Fortunately, Jonathan was an extremely intelligent and strong-willed young man to begin with, and was determined to recover. In fact, such was his conviction in his ability to heal himself that whenever I asked him if he believed he would be able to walk again, he would reply without hesitation, "Yes, I will walk again one day."

Coupled with the strong support that he received from his family, especially his mother, who went to great lengths to ensure that Jonathan was eating right, he started to show strong signs of improvement very quickly.

In less than a fortnight, the unthinkable happened when Jonathan was able to move his hands, albeit slightly. Today, Jonathan is able to sit up in a wheelchair and push himself up to a standing position with assistance. He is able to move about in bed, make phone calls and send text messages by himself. Instead of shutting himself out from the rest of the world due to his physical disabilities, Jonathan even provides tuition to younger students, and manages an investment and trading portfolio online. Even though he is still some distance from his goal of being able to stand up and walk, the improvement in Jonathan's health has already far exceeded the expectations of most of his doctors and is a fine example of how miracles are real and achievable. To date, I am assured to know that he is making obvious progress whenever I visit him every few months.

Taking the first step towards recovery

Through a distant referral, I was introduced to Stacey (not her real name), a lady in her fifties, in April 2009. At that point, Stacey had already been diagnosed with severe transverse myelitis – a condition where the spinal cord has multiple lesions and the myelin sheath of the nerves has been damaged. Due to her condition, Stacey was paralyzed from the neck down and had to be hospitalized.

During Stacey's stay at the hospital, the doctors placed her under observation and administered the usual anti-inflammatory drugs and immune suppressants to keep her condition from worsening. By her seventh month in the hospital, Stacey was asked to stop her physiotherapy sessions and was about to be discharged by the hospital. According to her doctors, Stacey had passed the timeline for recovery with no sign of improvement, which led her doctors to believe that she was unlikely to get back onto her own two feet.

When I first met Stacey, she was still in hospital, in her seventh month of stay. During my first two sessions with Stacey, I failed to make a connection with her, try as I might. None of what I said resonated with her. So, during my third visit, I was all the more determined to strike a connection with her, so that she could, in turn, establish a connection with herself.

I told her more about my story, and told her about the improvements that I and others had made simply by changing our belief system, diets and sleeping habits. I shared with her the miraculous stories of recovery of people I had met or had heard of. I told her about the need to be aware of her emotions as they could affect her health. Most importantly, I endeavored to alter her self-limiting belief that she would not be able to recover by telling her about my acquired insights into science and spirituality and how we can all create miracles in our lives.

This time around, Stacey finally displayed a genuine interest in what I was saying.

"How do I connect to heal?" she asked.

"Begin by asking yourself what is your true purpose in this world."

"How do I know what is my true purpose?"

"Do you have message for this world?" I probed.

"I do not know."

"Find the answer within," I suggested gently.

By intuitively asking Stacey for her purpose in life, I was trying to get her to look inwards to find a meaning to her existence. By asking her if she had a message to share with this world, I was trying to help her find direction in life. At the end of the day, I was trying to direct her to the door to a deeper connection, but she had to walk through it by herself.

After a moment of silence, tears started to well up in her eyes. "Yes, John. I understand what you are saying. I believe that I can do it now."

"So, what is it that you want to do?"

"I want to stand up in a month's time!" Stacey announced with new-found purpose and resolve.

Heartened by her response, I promised to pray for her during the one month when

I would be away in Boston. Recognizing the power of prayers, I prayed fervently for Stacey and her husband, Mark. I knew that Mark was also praying hard for Stacey as he wanted, more than anything, for them to live a fulfilling life together. And so, as a Buddhist, Mark kept chanting *Nam Myo Ho Renge Kyo* as he prayed fervently and determinedly for Stacey to recover.

Lo and behold, Mark called me a month later, after I had returned to Singapore. "Stacey managed to stand up! The staff at the hospital were amazed. They were so surprised and excited, John!"

Shortly after making that first step towards recovery, Stacey progressed so quickly that, by the following month, she could walk up to a hundred meters around the hospital's grounds. Today, she no longer has problems with walking, even though her hands are still slightly weak but recovering well. In any case, she has shown unbelievable improvement and remains optimistic about her recovery. The Stacey that I now know sees this world in a different light and lives to serve a purpose.

If you do not mind, it does not matter

Darryl (not his real name), aged 44, was an experienced optometrist, having practiced for many years. As his parents had passed on when he was young, he lived the life of a bachelor, comfortable but alone.

In 2003, Darryl was diagnosed with Parkinson's disease, followed by nose cancer in 2009. In order to keep his Parkinson's disease under control, the drugs he took resulted in him having severe cramps many times a day.

Doctors could not explain why his cramps were so severe and frequent that they affected his daily life. But deep down, I intuitively knew that his psychological state and bad diet might have also contributed to his unusually severe cramps. Such was the severity of his condition that he was attacked by painful cramps more than ten times a day and for more than half an hour each time, till he screamed and cried for mercy. As a result of his physical condition, Darryl was told to take leave from work until he had recovered.

When I first met Darryl at his house in late 2008, he was so badly plagued by his cramps that he could barely bring himself to open the door. He was so consumed by pain that he could not even attend to himself or his home. His room had a foul stench and his entire home was a complete mess. He was so depressed, out of synch with life and riddled with pain that he was not even able to carry out everyday activities, like eating, bathing or sitting down properly.

Despite being diagnosed with stage four nose cancer, Darryl was so psychologically consumed by his cramps that he barely gave his cancer a second thought. Perhaps as a result of his not paying any attention to it, his cancer did not manifest itself in any way that caused him discomfort or inconvenience. In fact, considering how advanced his cancer was, it was astonishing how little it seemed to have affected him – much to the surprise of his doctors even.

This is a perfect example of the power of the Void element, showing how one's psyche can determine the manifestation of one's physical reality. In fact, such was his absolute disregard for his cancer that Darryl told me, "Cancer is no big deal. It is nothing! I can live with cancer but I cannot live with these stupid cramps!"

Instead of being concerned about his cancer – a condition which was life threatening – Darryl placed all his focus on his cramps, to the point that he was almost obsessed with them.

When will my next cramp strike? How bad will it be? How would it affect me? Darryl would replay these worries in his head repeatedly.

So, when I learnt about his obsession with his cramps, I began to suspect that on a psychological level, his cramps were partly caused by his constant fear in anticipation of the next one to strike.

Seeing how his mind was so preoccupied with his cramps, I decided to break Darryl's obsessive focus on his cramps by getting him to take part in some activities. During my sessions, I worked on how he perceived himself, to get him to stop his constant obsession with his cramps and to initiate a shift in his belief system.

I once even asked Darryl, "If I can recover, then what about you?" And, from time to time, I would also ask him, "Do you want to recover? How do you want to recover? Who is responsible for your recovery?"

By doing so, I was trying to help him focus on healing from within. I hoped to challenge his old ways of thinking, which were mired in constant fear and agony. I figured that as long as he focused his mind so strongly on his cramps, there was no way that they would ever go away. I also tried to remove his self-limiting belief that he could no longer go out and socialize in case he suffered a cramp while he was outdoors.

Although the change was not easy, he did become more open to the idea of short trips to the library or around the neighborhood. But it was not until he implemented a change in his diet, to remove meat and include more wholesome greens and fruits into his daily meals, that he witnessed a reduced frequency in his cramps within just a month.

Over many sessions, I continued to share with him the ways that he could change his diet, belief system and his psyche in accordance with the principles of Transcendental Connection. Over time, the frequency of his cramps reduced drastically to just once or twice a day. In fact, on some days, he did not suffer any cramps at all.

And, even though his cancer has now spread to other parts of his body, Darryl does not display the physical symptoms of a typical cancer patient. He looks normal, leads an almost normal life and plans to return to work, while he continues to devote time to praying and working on his recovery.

Personally, Darryl's story serves as a testimonial that the power of one's mind or psyche, as well as one's faith, which belongs to the Void element, can truly move mountains and create drastically different outcomes, even when one is seriously sick. Here, the power of the Earth element has also come into play, through a change in his diet, lending to a positive transformation in an extremely short time.

A transformative connection

I was introduced to Kevin (not his real name) earlier this year. A man in his fifties, Kevin was struck by a stroke that had left half his body paralyzed. When I first met Kevin, he appeared lost and jaded.

As a result of his paralysis, Kevin was also frustrated, as he was unable to meet the needs of his family. Not only was Kevin understandably out of a job, his wife had made the decision to quit her job to take care of him, even though it meant that the family ran into such great financial difficulty that they were even unable to foot their monthly utilities bill. With little income to contend with, Kevin and his wife depended on what little their daughter earned for their livelihood.

As if his paralysis was not disconcerting enough, Kevin was piqued that he was unable to swallow any food. And as a result, a feeding tube had to be inserted into his nostril in order to prevent him from choking.

So, when I first visited him and asked Kevin what he wanted to improve on, he promptly replied, "I want to be able to eat again." And, sensing the strength of this desire, I told him to work on achieving just that.

In my first session with Kevin, I shared with him how I had defied medical science and overcome my paralysis and blindness. As I was truly speaking from personal experience, Kevin felt that he could relate to and connect with me. By altering his perception towards his paralysis, I convinced him that he could help himself to heal. When I told him about the concept of Transcendental Connection, he was receptive and willing to introduce changes to his life to bring about much needed harmony and balance.

Perhaps also owing to Kevin's strong desire to recover and provide for his family again, Kevin grew increasingly determined to turn his situation around. For him, his first step towards recovery was to be able to eat with his own mouth, instead of depending on a feeding tube. And, true enough, Kevin actually managed to eat food on his own just three days later!

Deeply moved by the sudden leap in progress, Kevin confided in a friend of mine between chokes, "John told me that I could eat again and I did. I believe I will eventually recover."

With that, Kevin continued to press on by exercising more at home. Under the loving care and encouragement of his wife, Kevin showed such improvement merely a month later that he was able to haul himself up from his wheelchair!

Heartened by his improvement, Kevin's wife continued to offer prayers for his recovery. Moreover, I encouraged him and his family to help enhance his Earth element by replacing his predominantly meat-based diet with one that was plant-based. Coupled with all these changes, I also introduced ways for him to improve on his Wood element, such as changing his sleeping and breathing patterns. In a mere 45 days, Kevin appeared stronger and more alert. In fact, such is the improvement in his condition today that he is now able to walk with the aid of no more than a simple walking stick.

First Step to spiritual transformation

Michael, aged 64, had been diagnosed with terminal bladder cancer. A capable and independent man who had held an esteemed position before he retired, Michael was used to being in command of things. Usually the one who was in a sufficiently privileged position to extend help to the less fortunate, Michael never imagined that the tables would turn on him someday. Faced with difficulties in breathing, the discomfort of using a surgical drainage tube to pass urine, and being immobile, Michael could not face the reality that his body had failed him.

Before I met Michael, many concerned relatives and friends had already offered him advice, including turning to a plant-based diet and practicing qigong or meditation, amongst other alternative healing remedies to complement his mainstream medical treatments. But being the stubborn person that he was, Michael argued against the effectiveness of these unorthodox approaches. While Michael's pragmatic, Western-educated ways had served him well throughout his professional life, they had so colored his general perception on matters that it was impossible for him to come to terms with new ideas on medicine and health.

At her wits end, Michael's sister decided to approach me for help.

When I first met Michael, he appeared angry and defeated by his helplessness towards his condition, but did not know how to express his woes or receive help from others. Knowing that any persuasion on my part for him to change his lifestyle would be futile, I decided to engage him spiritually instead of intellectually. Instead of telling him about the benefits of naturopathic treatments, I stressed the importance of having spiritual humility. Instead of convincing him to give alternative treatments a go, I shared how the power of love became the source of inspiration for me when I was at the lowest point of my life. Based on my personal experiences, I explained to him how love had nurtured my soul and how it, in turn, had nourished my body.

The conversation Michael and I had was surprisingly long for someone who was unreceptive, or rather, not used to receiving help from others. Although there was seemingly no significant breakthrough during our conversation, something Michael said assured me that he must have found some solace in what I had shared.

"John, I need to reflect on my life and repent," Michael murmured with pensive eyes.

And before I left, Michael's sister claimed it was already a miracle that I had managed to engage him in a sharing for so long.

True enough, a miracle had indeed taken place. Just days after my meeting with Michael, his sister rang me to say that Michael was a changed man. According to his sister, Michael appeared to be in better spirits after we spoke. And while his relationship with his family had always been close, he now seemed more open about his feelings.

In fact, he had even sent one of his sisters an affectionate message that said, "When are you going to visit me? I miss you."

On top of being more expressive about his feelings, Michael even started to return to his Christian faith through fervent prayers.

Even though his condition has not shown any signs of improvement, it is just as heartening to both his family and himself that his outlook on life has changed for the better. To Michael and his family, this beginning of spiritual awakening is perhaps the crucial step of healing first from the within. Right from the beginning, I had explained to his family that healing one's soul is far more critical than healing one's body, especially in Michael's case.

His physical condition deteriorated months later when I met him again. However, this time, he was more at peace with himself, turned more spiritual and contained lesser anger. He told me he is seeking God every moment. I was deeply gratified when I heard that. We had a soulful connection that evening and one that I will remember forever. Ultimately, the most important thing in our life is how we die and exit this world. Michael had a spiritual transformation and passed away peacefully and was surrounded by many loved ones showering him with prayers and love vibrations. Michael is indeed a marvelous soul I encountered.

Flying free of a mental cage

In 1997, I met Sylvia (not her real name), who was just 16 years of age then. At that time, she was suffering from a mental illness and had already dropped out of school about two to three years previously. On top of the distress that her condition caused her, Sylvia was further overwhelmed by anxiety and frustration as she felt uncertain of her future, or rather the lack of one. Unable to take charge of her mental state and emotions, Sylvia resorted to hiding in her closet. As an outlet for her pent up emotions, Sylvia even turned physically abusive towards herself and her parents.

When I first met Sylvia, she appeared deep in a daze and afraid for no apparent reason. From what I had learnt from her parents, medication did nothing to improve her situation. Over time, Sylvia had simply grown more and more disappointed in herself. And so deep-seated was her frustration that it had led to occasional outbursts of hysteria.

Determined to help her, I would visit Sylvia two to three times a week. During my sessions with her, I would encourage her to pray.

However, at that time, Sylvia was someone of very few words. When I asked her to pray, she would tell me that she was unable to concentrate on praying as her mind was filled with so many negative thoughts.

"It is too late. Praying will not work for me," Sylvia would state dejectedly.

But, I persisted in encouraging her to pray with her heart and connect from within. "I know you are unable to concentrate. So, let your thoughts and questions come and go. Do not fight them."

Even though Sylvia wanted very much to recover from her condition, it was a struggle nonetheless. Only after a very long time, and under the constant encouragement of her family and myself, did she gradually stop obsessing over her thoughts and become more at peace with her condition, and most importantly herself. Slowly, she began to open up and started to communicate more freely with the people around her.

From praying just five minutes a day, she eventually progressed to praying for half an hour every day. Together with her family, Sylvia also made the conscious decision to heal from within, and so, stopped taking any medication, as they found them to be of little or no use to her to begin with.

A year later, Sylvia fully recovered from her condition. Eventually, she went back to her studies and completed her tertiary education. Today, she is no different from any other ordinary working adult.

EPILOGUE

Since time immemorial, instances of Transcendental Connection have dotted the history of mankind. A connection that is non-religious, unbiased and universal, a Transcendental Connection is a natural approach towards harnessing harmony and balance in our lives, and it has been a phenomenon that is inherent in all healing regardless of the modalities or methods pursued.

Owing to its very nature, activities of a Transcendental Connection have always been active within and around every single one of us – in every mountain, every tree, every water droplet, every living thing, every cell, every atom, every electron, every photon, and every quantum mechanical resonance. Found in the silence of every present moment, a Transcendental Connection involves the dynamic relationship between the conscious being (man), collective beings, the environment and their activities, latent or manifested. When we are able to transcendentally connect to everything within and outside of us, we put ourselves in a sacred position, where powerful healing can be channeled for our physical, mental and emotional well-being.

We have all heard of cases where HIV patients, still clinically infected with the deadly virus, have a viral count that is unbelievably low or almost undetectable. Not only are they not plagued by their illness, but are reportedly living long and fulfilling lives. And, let us not forget the many instances when we have heard of the terminally ill suddenly receiving a remission from cancer or other terminal diseases.

Regardless of what these patients' religious beliefs are, miraculous recoveries have been widely reported in the medical world. And the reason for their miraculous healing is because they have been transcendentally connected to the Source.

Much like the many cyclical phenomenon in nature (e.g. cell cycles, water cycles, geological periods, and astrological movements), Transcendental Connection does not merely relate to miraculous healing, as shown extensively in this book, but also contributes to the natural and inevitable cycle of birth, sickness, aging and decline that governs the lives of all of us. Since death is part of our life cycle, entering into death also brings new life. Once we accept and understand that death is part of the cycle of life, the death of someone need not be viewed as a traumatic event, but as the natural ebb and flow of life.

The previous chapter, featuring the stories of individuals who had conquered their ailments, highlighted only some of many who have been touched by a Transcendental Connection in their lives. Among those to whom I have extended my help, some did not choose to recover. However, at the very least, I am glad to know that instead of departing from this world grudgingly and unwillingly, they left this world peacefully and with greater awareness of their own body, mind, spirituality and the Source. As it goes to show, being transcendentally connected does not provide physical immortality or physical perfection but it does create a pure state of mental, spiritual and physical well-being.

Just as there are those who chose to depart from this world peacefully, many also recovered. But did I heal them with some mystical power? No.

As reflected in the principle of *3,000 Realms in a Single Living Moment*, one's state of mind is constantly fluctuating between the ten possible states of existence (see Chapter Seven for details), as it is impossible to maintain the status quo in life and our state is dependent on what is happening both within and around us.

Just like everyone else, my life is flawed and I have had my own set of problems to face. But I have grown to be more conscious of my life choices after my brush with paralysis and blindness, as well as two short-lived marriages. Although my second marriage was regrettably short and hence not brought up in the earlier chapters, it has nevertheless bestowed upon me a precious daughter.

I am not perfect but I am conscious of my flaws. I am not saintly but I am aware. But in spite of my own problems, I never ceased to try to help others in need. In doing so, I have managed to build a deep connection with others that onlookers would not be able to understand the true dynamics of; only the patient and I share this mutual understanding.

Having said this, I must also add that there are often many people who are also involved in the healing process, and they play a dutiful role as friends, parents or spouse. I view myself as only one part of the whole recovery process. Without the help of others around the patient, doing what they are good at, be it caring, cooking or praying for the patient, my role alone is sometimes not enough for the patient to make a breakthrough in their recovery. I only play the role of a healing catalyst and the patient's navigator towards a Transcendental Connection.

There is a saying that when we light a lantern for others, we light our own path too. When we light one more candle with our own candle, the room only turns brighter when both our flames remain lit. Because of what I had experienced in my life, I was filled with empathy for the sick and understood their struggles. As such, I was better able to relate to them and reach out to them in ways that they needed to be touched. And in so doing, I learnt so much from them about the strength of the human spirit – knowledge that cannot be acquired from medical or philosophical literature alone.

While I am an advocate of Transcendental Connection in all healings, I am not saying that a medical approach towards healing is ineffectual. In fact, I fully recognize that mainstream Western medical practices are best in saving lives, in the case of acute medical conditions where immediate medical intervention or even surgery is required. However, despite being a credible source of treatment, Western medical practices still have their shortcomings, as most of their resources are focused on the pathological pathway of diseases (i.e. mechanisms to stop the symptoms of a disease, through the use of synthetic drugs and invasive surgeries), while little is placed in research into the body's natural healing processes, or even the science of biological regeneration and its dynamics. Even though many have reaped the benefits of mainstream medical practices, many are still unable to recover from extreme or unknown medical conditions using these methods. Amongst them, some resort to looking for a solution from within or from alternative treatments in tandem with current medical practices. I am one such living example.

As what Charles Haanel (1866 to 1949), author of the revolutionary *The Master Key System* and the earliest advocate of The Law of Attraction said, "The source of all Power is world within, the Universal Fountain of Supply. The Infinite Energy of which each individual is an outlet."

All of us possess immense power to heal ourselves physically, mentally, spiritually, emotionally and financially. Yet, the majority of us are not aware of it yet. By harnessing the right belief system, developing a positive mental attitude and an unwavering faith (in religion, thinking, prayer and meditation), everything can evolve and gradually be shaped to suit our every intention – an intention that should always carry an altruistic value and love. Only this way, can our thought energy engage the cosmic consciousness around us to allow things to respond and move towards our goals, be they in the areas of health, love or wealth. During my stay in the hospital, I transcended and arrived at a realization that the Cosmic Divine creates out of love. Thus, if we desire to change or create things out of pure love, our intended creations can happen.

Through the stories of medical marvel in my book, as well as the stories of other courageous individuals whom I have met on this journey of discovery, I hope to demonstrate that our acts of miraculous healing are not merely pure coincidences. While there is no denying that our learning journeys are imbued with much pain and agony, overcoming these challenges and our shortcomings can bring us immeasurable blessings and a renewed perception on life. Most importantly, I hope that these stories of faith and hope have reaffirmed the message that new transformations are always on the horizon when a transcendental change takes seed within us.

Just as we are one and connected, it is my sincere desire for you to reap the life-changing blessings of a Transcendental Connection just as I so blessedly have.

ANNEX: TIPS FOR RECOVERY

Healing one's life and lifestyle is far more vital than healing one's physical body. When we take steps to promote a general well-being in our lives, our body is likely to take its cue from these changes and respond accordingly. Besides seeking proper medical treatment, it is essential for us to acknowledge that we are responsible for our own health and recovery. As we embark on our road towards recovery, we need to work on developing our Void element first and foremost, before we proceed to work on the remaining four elements of Water, Wood, Fire and Earth. The reason for this is that our attitude and psyche, as represented by the Void element, are the gateway from which we initiate changes to our body, life and the environment. Without the right psyche or belief system, we do not have the mental capacity to spark off a transformation from within.

1. Void element – Belief and Psyche

- Have you already told yourself that you can completely heal your body or life?
- Are you already convinced that your mind is connected to your body and your surroundings?
- Have you started to believe that there is a Higher Self, Divinity, or a Source residing in you and listening to you?
- Our subconscious runs our bodies and controls the way we react to external factors ninety percent of the time. Are you aware of this and willing to consciously change the way you react to things?
- Do you believe in the power of prayers? Even a sincere internal dialogue is a form of prayer.
- Are you convinced that you are what you believe you are?

2. Water element – Feeling and Emotion

- Your feelings and emotions are actually determined by how you see the world.
- Negative emotions can result in the poor physical health of the body (e.g. illnesses).
- Can you maintain a sense of peacefulness, regardless of the events that take place around you?
- Water can affect your health and emotions. Do you drink healthy water? And do you ensure that you drink enough healthy water?
- Do you bless the water and food that you consume and are you thankful for them?

3. Wood element – Regeneration and Breathing

- With positive emotions, one can sleep well. Deep sleep enables the body to regenerate and heal itself.
- Do you go to sleep early (between 9pm to 10pm), and wake up early (between 5am to 6am)? Internal healing can only take place when we get enough good sleep.
- Do you make it a habit to breathe slowly and deeply? Refer to Chapter 7 on Transcendental Connection Breathing Techniqiues
- Are you convinced that you can send positive thoughts to your body to generate internal healing while you breathe, as suggested above?

4. Fire element – Energetics, Goals and Passion

- With the right breathing techniques, the air (Qi; or breathing) that we take in facilitates the flow of energy inside our body.
- Do you feel that your mental state (Void, controlled by Fire) is clearer and stronger now?
- Set a goal in your heart and mind for the good and benefit of mankind to justify your recovery to the universe. This will help give you purpose and aid in your

recovery, even if no one believes that you can heal. This is vital.

- Are you starting to love everyone you meet and every little that thing you do?
- Do you feel that you are now alive and filled with gratitude?
- All positive lights, sounds, emotions, thoughts and deeds are energy that can heal us. Be a generous giver and receiver of these five energies.

5. Earth element – Nutrition, Abundance and Wealth

- Have you switched to a well-balanced, plant-based diet yet?
- Are you consuming food that contains less pollutants and contaminants?
- Do you have sufficient abundance in wealth, nutrition and love to initiate your own healing journey and sustain your recovery? And, if you do not, do you know that you can attract abundance in wealth, nutrition and love, even if you are sick, so long as the other four elements – Void, Water, Wood and Fire – are realized in your life?
- Do you still suffer from the misconception that money is root of all evil, and therefore stands in the way of your own healing? Or, do you believe that you can attract wealth and abundance from the Source?
- Money itself is neutral. But the value of money is dependent on our belief in how money can control us and how we can use it. The flow of money can also be a positive exchange of energy, when used appropriately and for well-meaning purposes.

ACKNOWLEDGEMENTS

My beloved parents – they live a life of which I am most proud. They teach me what it means to be simple in both one's needs and wants. I love both of you and I am proud to be your child.

My dearest friends, together with my comrades in faith, who have been there to offer my family their prayers, time and hearty cheers during our darkest period in life. They are Weng Leong, Fong Jie, Dianna, Seet Teck Kiang, Mun Chu, Matthew Johnson, Pearl Lee, Liu San, Robin, Dr Ng Yee Sien, Dr Christopher Yang, Chwee Hoon, Tan Mei Mei, Sussana Toi, Slyvia Tan, Dr Chong Peng Neo, David Lim (the Mount Everest Mountaineer), and Jerry Tay.

Dr Daisaku Ikeda– your words have put me on the correct path whenever I was off course. Your words inspired me to hang on and never let go of the coming light, even when the world had struck me off and had given up on me. I have since started to understand what it means to discard the transient self: be true to yourself, love life, and give to the world.

My precious daughter, Vera Wong – daddy loves you so much. I guess I can never express this well enough in words or actions. I wrote this book because you came into my life and have given me a reason to complete my journey. I love you.

Vera's mummy – thank you from the bottom of my heart for your love. The trials and tribulations that we have faced remind me to keep moving forward no matter what and to shed myself of the petty concerns that would hold me back. I have always loved you.

My partner, Josephine Lin – the completion of this book has been possible only with your support, grace, patience and incredible quirky charm, that has brightened my life.

Phoon Kok Hwa and his team at Candid Creation Publishing, especially Corrine Teng and Louise Lim, this book would not have been a success without your help and advice. Thank you!

BIBLIOGRAPHY

"Agricultural pesticides and the atmosphere." Environment Canada, September 2001. Web. 12 Oct. 2007. <http://www.ec.gc.ca/science/sandesept01/article3_e.html>.

Aspect, Alain, Philippe Grangier, and Gérard Roger. "Experimental Realization of Einstein-Podolsky-Rosen-Bohm *Gedankenexperiment:* A New Violation of Bell's Inequalities." *Physical Review Letters* 49.2 (1982): 91-94. Print.

Baxter, Gwen J., Allan B. Graham, James R. Lawrence, David Wiles, and John R. Paterson. "Salicylic acid in soups prepared from organically and non-organically grown vegetables." *The European Journal of Nutrition* 40.6 (2001): 289-92. Print.

Bengtsson, Ingemar, and Karol Życzkowski. *Geometry of Quantum States: An Introduction to Quantum Entanglement.* Cambridge: Cambridge UP, 2006. Print.

Bingham, S. "Pesticides exceeding environmental quality standards (EQS)." Environment Agency (UK), 2007. Web. 12 Oct. 2007. <http://www.environment-agency.gov.uk/yourenv/eff/1190084/business_industry/agri/pests/917555/?version=1&lang=_e>

---. "Pesticides in rivers and groundwater." Environment Agency (UK), 2007. Web. 12 Oct. 2007.<http://www.environment-agency.gov.uk/yourenv/eff/1190084/business_industry/agri/pests/915588/?version=1&lang=_e>.

Bleher, Sahib, trans. *Experiments for the objectification of pain and consciousness during conventional (captive bolt stunning) and religiously mandated ("ritual cutting") slaughter procedures for sheep and calves,* by W. Schulze, H. Schultze-Petzold, A.S. Hazem, and R. Gross, Deutsche Tierärztliche Wochenschrift 85 (1978): 62-66. Web. 1 Jun. 2010. <http://www.mustaqim.co.uk/halalstudy.htm>.

Bousso, Raphael. "The holographic principle." *Reviews of Modern Physics* 74.3 (2002): 825-74. Print.

Bouwmeester, Dik, Jian-Wei Pan, Klaus Mattle, Manfred Eibl, Harald Weinfurter, and Anton Zeilinger. "Experimental quantum teleportation." *Nature* 309.6660 (1997): 575-79. Print.

Campbell, T. Colin. *The China Study: Startling Implications for Diet, Weight Loss and Long-term Health.* Dallas, TX: BenBella Books, 2005. Print.

Chang, Jii-Ju, Joachim Fisch, and Fritz-Albert Popp, eds. *Biophotons.* Dordrecht: Kluwer Academic Publishers, 1998. Print.

Chishima, Kikuo. *Revolution of Biology and Medicine.* Japan: Neo-Haematological Society Press, 1972. Print.

Cloud, John. "Why Your DNA Isn't Your Destiny." *TIME* 18 Jan. 2010: 49-53. Print.

Devore, Elizabeth E., Meir J. Stampfer, Monique M.B. Breteler, Bernard Rosner, Jae Hee Kang, Olivia Okereke, Frank B. Hu, and Francine Grodstein. "Dietary Fat Intake and Cognitive Decline in Women With Type 2 Diabetes." *Diabetes Care* 32.4 (2009): 635-40. Print.

Emoto, Masaru. *The Healing Power of Water.* USA: Hay House, 2007. Print.

Esselstyn Jr., Caldwell B. "Resolving the Coronary Artery Disease Epidemic through Plant-Based Nutrition." *Preventive Cardiology* 4.4 (2001): 171-77. Print.

Felitti, Vincent, Robert F. Anda, Dale Nordenberg, David F. Williamson, Alison M. Spitz, Valerie Edwards, Mary P. Koss, and James S. Marks. "Relationship of childhood abuse and household dysfunction to many of the leading causes of death in adults. The Adverse Childhood Experiences (ACE) Study." *American Journal of Preventive Medicine* 14.4 (1998): 245-58. Print.

Feynman, Richard. *QED: The Strange Theory of Light and Matter.* Princeton: Princeton UP, 1988. Print.

---. *The Feynman Lectures on Physics,* Vol. 3. USA: Addison-Wesley, 1965. Print.

"For Red Meat, Another Red Light." American Institute for Cancer Research, May 2007. Web. 1 Oct. 2010. <http://www.aicr.org/site/News2?page=NewsArticle&id=11809>.

Frampton, Paul H. *Gauge Field Theories.* 2nd ed. New York: Wiley, 2000. Print.

Frank, Philipp. *Philosophy of Science.* New York: Prentice-Hall, 1957. Print.

Frank-Kamenetskii, Maxim D. *Unraveling DNA: The Most Important Molecule of Life.* New York: Perseus Books, 1997. Print.

French, Anthony P., and Edwin F. Taylor. *An Introduction to Quantum Physics.* New York: Norton, 1978. Print.

Gariaev, Peter P., Boris I. Birshtein, Alexander M. Iarochenko, Peter J. Marcer, George G. Tertishny, Katherine A. Leonova, and Uwe Kaempf. *The DNA-wave Biocomputer.* Paper. Russian Academy of Sciences, and Wave Genetics Inc, 2002.

Gariaev, Peter P., K.V. Grigorev, A.A. Vasilev, V.P. Poponin, and V.A. Shcheglov. "Investigation of the Fluctuation Dynamics of DNA Solutions by Laser Correlation Spectroscopy." *Bulletin of the Lebedev Physics Institute* 11-12 (1992): 23-30. Print.

Garjajev, Peter. *Der wellengenetische Code.* Moscow: BackBone Publishing, 1997. Print

Gibson, T.J., C.B. Johnson, J.C. Murrell, J.P. Chambers, K.J. Stafford, and D.J. Mellor. "Components of electroencephalographic responses to slaughter in halothane-anaesthetised calves: effects of cutting neck tissues compared with major blood vessels." *New Zealand Veterinary Journal* 57.2 (2009): 84-89. Print.

Goenner, Hubert F.M. "On the History of Unified Field Theories." *Living Reviews in Relativity* 7 (2004): n. pag. Web. 1 Oct. 2010 <http://www.livingreviews.org/lrr-2004-2>.

Goncharova, Z.A., and V.A. Baliazin. "Risk factors of multiple sclerosis development in the population of the Rostov region." *Zh Nevrol Psikhiatr Im S S Korsakova* 109 (2009): 10-15. Print.

Green, Michael B., John H. Schwarz, and Edward Witten. *Superstring Theory.* Cambridge: Cambridge UP, 1987. Print.

Greiner, Walter, and Berndt Müller. *Gauge Theory of Weak Interactions.* Berlin: Springer, 2000. Print.

Horodecki, Ryszard, Paweł Horodecki, Michał Horodecki, and Karol Horodecki. "Quantum entanglement." *Reviews of Modern Physics* 81.2 (2009): 865-942. Print.

Horowitz, Leonard G., and Joseph Puleo. *Healing Codes for the Biological Apocalypse.* Idaho: Tetrahedron Publishing Group, 2001. Print.

Hunt, Valerie V. *Infinite Mind: Science of the Human Vibrations of Consciousness.* Los Angeles: Malibu Publishing, 1996. Print.

Ikeda, Daisaku. *Buddhism and the Cosmos: Daisaku Ikeda in conversation with Katsugi Masayoshi and Eeichi Shimura.* London: Macdonald, 1985. Print.

Itzykson, Claude, and Jean-Bernard Zuber. *Quantum Field Theory.* USA: Dover Publications, 2006. Print.

Jaeger, Gregg. *Entanglement, Information, and the Interpretation of Quantum Mechanics.* Berlin: Springer, 2009. Print.

Jenkins, David J.A., Julia M.W. Wong, Cyril W.C. Kendall, Amin Esfahani, Vivian W.Y. Ng, Tracy C.K. Leong, Dorothea A. Faulkner, Ed Vidgen, Kathryn A. Greaves, Gregory Paul, and William Singer. "The Effect of a Plant-Based Low-Carbohydrate ("Eco-Atkins") Diet on Body Weight and Blood Lipid Concentrations in Hyperlipidemic Subjects." *Archives of Internal Medicine* 169.11 (2009): 1046-54. Print.

Johnson, Peter. *The Buddhism of T'ien T'ai.* 2001. Web. 1 Oct. 2010. <http://www.tientai.net>.

Johnston, A.E. "Soil organic matter, effects on soils and crops." *Soil Use Management* 2.3 (1986): 97-105. Print.

Kane, Gordon L. *Modern Elementary Particle Physics.* New York: Perseus Books, 1987. Print.

Kannan, G., and J.A. Mench. "Prior handling does not significantly reduce the stress response to pre-slaughter handling in broiler chickens." *Applied Animal Behaviour Science* 51.1 (1997): 87-99. Print.

Kellogg, Robert L., Richard Nehring, Arthur Grube, Don W. Goss, and Steve Plotkin. "Environmental Indicators of Pesticide Leaching and Runoff from Farm Fields." United States Department of Agriculture Natural Resources Conservation Service, February 2000. Web. 3 Oct. 2007. <http://www.nrcs.usda.gov/technical/NRI/pubs/

eip_pap.html>.

Khoo-Kingsley, Betty. *Cancer Cured and Prevented Naturally.* Singapore: AKLTG, 2009. Print.

---. *Conversation with my Spirit Guide.* Singapore: Magnum, 1996. Print.

Kim, Jung-whan, and Chi V. Dang. "Cancer's Molecular Sweet Tooth and the Warburg Effect." *Cancer Research* 66.18 (2006): 8927-30. Print.

Kushida, Clete. *Sleep deprivation: Basic Science, Physiology, and Behavior.* New York: Informa Healthcare, 2005. Print.

Lairon, Denis. "Nutritional quality and safety of organic food. A review." *Agronomy for Sustainable Development* 30.1 (2010): 33-41. Print.

Leviton, Richard. "The Holographic Body." *East West Journal* 18.8 (1988): 42. Print.

"Life Potential." *Words of Wisdom by Buddhist Philosopher Daisaku Ikeda.* Soka Gakkai. Web. 1 Dec 2010. <http://www.ikedaquotes.org/life-potential.html>.

Linsteadt, Stephen, and Maria Elena Boekemeyer. *The Heart of Health: The Principles of Physical Health and Vitality.* USA: Natural Healing House Press, 2003. Print.

Lipton, Bruce. "Insight Into Cellular Consciousness." *Bridges* 12.1 (2001): 5. Print.

---. *The Biology of Belief: Unleashing the Power of Consciousness,* Matter and Miracles. USA: Sounds True, 2008. Audio book.

Lorenz, Eric S. "Pesticide Safety Fact Sheet: Potential Health Effects of Pesticides." *The Pennsylvania State University, College of Agricultural Sciences Publications.* The Pennsylvania State University, College of Agricultural Sciences, Agricultural Research and Cooperative Extension, Pesticide Education Program, 2009. Web. 1 June 2010. <http://pubs.cas.psu.edu/freepubs/pdfs/uo198.pdf>.

Lotter, Don W., Rita Seidel, and W. Liebhardt. "The performance of organic and conventional cropping systems in an extreme climate year." *American Journal of Alternative Agriculture* 18.3 (2003): 146-54. Print.

Mizrahi, Anna, Paul Knekt, Jukka Montonen, Maarit A. Laaksonen, Markku Heliövaara, and Ritva Järvinen. "Plant foods and the risk of cerebrovascular diseases: a potential protection of fruit consumption." *British Journal of Nutrition* 102.7

(2009): 1075-83. Print.

"Module 6: Ecology and Environmental Considerations." *Pesticide Safety Education Program.* Cornell University Cooperative Extension, Pesticide Management Education Program, 2008. Web. 11 Oct. 2007. <http://psep.cce.cornell.edu/Tutorials/core-tutorial/module06/index.aspx>.

Montagnier, L, Aäissa, J et al, "Electromagnetic detection of HIV DNA in the blood of AIDS patients treated by antiretroviral therapy". *Interdisciplinary Sciences: Computational Life Sciences*, 03 July 2009, Volume 1, Number 4, 245-253, DOI: 10.1007/s12539-009-0059-0 Accessed 27 January 2011

Montagnier, L, Aäissa, J et al, "Electromagnetic Signals Are Produced by Aqueous Nanostructures Derived from Bacterial DNA Sequences". *Interdisciplinary Sciences: Computational Life Sciences*, 06 January 2009, Volume 1, Number 2, 81-90, DOI: 10.1007/s12539-009-0036-7 Accessed 27 Jan 2011.

Moss, B.W., and C.H. McMurray. "The effect of the duration and type of stress on some serum enzyme levels in pigs." *Research in Veterinary Science* 26.1 (1979): 1-6. Print.

Neusner, Jacob, and Bruce D. Chilton. *Altruism in World Religion.* USA: George Town UP, 2005. Print.

"No sleep means no new brain cells." *BBC News Health.* BBC News, 10 February 2007. Web. 1 Oct. 2010. <http://news.bbc.co.uk/2/hi/health/6347043.stm>.

"Nutritional Considerations." Organic Trade Association, 7 September 2010. Web. 1 Nov. 2010. <http://www.ota.com/organic/benefits/nutrition.html>.

Oschman, James L. *Energy Medicine: The Scientific Basis.* London: Churchill Livingstone, 2000. Print.

Pace, James C., and Deborah Drumm. "The Phantom Leaf Effect and its Implications for Near-Death and Out-of-Body Experiences." *Journal of Near-Death Studies* 10.4 (1992): 233-40. Print.

Pedersen, T.L. "Pesticide residues in drinking water." *Extonet.* University of California-Davis, Oregon State University, Michigan State University, Cornell University, and the University of Idaho, June 1997. Web. 15 Sep. 2007. <http://extoxnet.orst.edu/faqs/safedrink/pest.htm>.

"Pesticide Registration (PR) Notice 2001-X Draft: Spray and Dust Drift Label Statements for Pesticide Products." U.S. Environmental Protection Agency, 11 September 2007. Web. 19 Sep. 2007. <http://www.epa.gov/PR_Notices/prdraft-spraydrift801.htm>.

Petersen, Maria Skaalum, Jónrit Halling, Sára Bech, Lene Wermuth, Pál Weihe, Flemming Nielsen, Poul J. Jørgensen, Esben Budtz-Jørgensen, and Philippe Grandjean. "Impact of dietary exposure to food contaminants on the risk of Parkinson's disease." *NeuroToxicology* 29.4 (2008): 584-90. Print.

"Pharmaceuticals and Personal Care Products (PPCPs): Frequent Questions." U.S. Environmental Protection Agency, 28 October 2010. Web. 12 Nov. 2010. <http://www.epa.gov/ppcp/faq.html>.

Plenio, Martin B., and Shashank Virmani. "An introduction to entanglement measures." *Quantum Information & Computation* 7.1 (2007): 1-51. Print.

Polchinski, Joseph. *String Theory.* Cambridge: Cambridge UP, 1998. Print.

Popp, Fritz-Albert, J.J. Chang, A. Herzog, Z. Yan, and Y. Yan. "Evidence of non-classical (squeezed) light in biological systems." *Physics Letters A* 293.1 (2002): 98-102. Print.

Popp, Fritz-Albert, and Ke-hsueh Li. "Hyberbolic Relaxation as a Sufficient Condition of a Fully Coherent Ergodic Field." *International Journal of Theoretical Physics* 32.9 (1993): 1573-83. Print.

Popp, Fritz-Albert, and Y. Yan. "Delayed luminescence of biological systems in terms of coherent states." *Physics Letters A* 293.1 (2002): 93-97. Print.

Radin, Dean. *The Conscious Universe: The Scientific Truth of Psychic Phenomena.* New York: Harper Edge, 1997. Print.

Rechtschaffen, Allan, and Bernard M. Bergmann. "Sleep deprivation in the rat by the disk-over-water method." *Behavioural Brain Research* 69.1 (1995): 55-63. Print.

Republic of Uzbekistan, National Biodiversity Strategy Project Steering Committee with the Financial Assistance of The Global Environmental Facility (GEF) and Technical Assistance of United Nations Development Programme (UNDP). "Biodiversity Conservation: National Strategy and Action Plan." *Biodiversity Planning Support Programme (UNDP – UNEP): NBSAP Websites for North East & East Central Asia.* 1998. Web. 17 Sep. 2007. <http://bpsp-neca.brim.ac.cn/books/actpln_uzbek/index.html>.

Reynolds, Jefferson D. "International pesticide trade: Is there any hope for the effective regulation of controlled substances? *Journal of Land Use & Environmental Law* 13.1 (1997): n. pag. Web. 1 Jun. 2010. <http://www.law.fsu.edu/journals/landuse/Vol131/REYN.HTMl>.

Rovelli, Carlo. "Relational quantum mechanics." *International Journal of Theoretical Physics* 35.8 (1996): 1637-78. Print.

Schlebusch, Klaus-Peter, Walburg Maric-Oehler, and Fritz-Albert Popp. "Biophotonics in the infrared spectral range reveal acupuncture meridian structure of the body." *The Journal of Alternative and Complementary Medicine* 11.1 (2005): 171-73. Print.

"Sequoia and Kings Canyon National Parks: Air Quality – Airborne Synthetic Chemicals." National Park Service, U.S. Department of the Interior, 1 August 2006. Web. 19 Sep. 2007. <http://www.nps.gov/seki/naturescience/air_synthchem.htm>.

Sheldrake, Rupert. "Morphic Resonance and Morphic Fields: An Introduction." *Presenting the work of Dr. Rupert Sheldrake, Biologist & Author.* February 2005. Web. 28 May 2008. <http://www.sheldrake.org/Articles&Papers/papers/morphic/morphic_intro.html>.

Sheldrake, Rupert, and Pamela Smart. "Experimental tests for telephone telepathy." *Journal of the Society for Psychical Research* 67.3 (2003): 184-99. Print.

Som, Prantika, H.L. Atkins, D. Bandoypadhyay, J.S. Fowler, A.R. MacGregor, K. Matsui, Z.H. Oster, D.F. Sacker, C.Y. Shlue, H. Turner, C-N. Wan, A.P. Wolf, and S. V. Zabinski. "A Fluorinated Glucose Analog, 2-fluoro-2-deoxy-D-glucose (F-18):

Nontoxic Tracer for Rapid Tumor Detection." *The Journal of Nuclear Medicine* 21.7 (1980): 670-75. Print.

"Sources of common contaminants and their health effects." U.S. Environmental Protection Agency, 2007. Web. 10 Oct. 2007. <http://www.epa.gov/superfund/programs/er/hazsubs/sources.htm>.

Steward, Edward G. *Quantum Mechanics: Its Early Development and the Road to Entanglement.* London: Imperial College P, 2008. Print.

Strachey, James, gen. ed. *The Standard Edition of the Complete Psychological Works of Sigmund Freud.* 24 vols. London: Vintage, 1999. Print.

Susskind, Leonard. "The world as a hologram." *Journal of Mathematical Physics* 36.11 (1995): 6377-96. Print.

Taheri, Shahrad, Ling Lin, Diane Austin, Terry Young, and Emmanuel Mignot. "Short Sleep Duration Is Associated with Reduced Leptin, Elevated Ghrelin, and Increased Body Mass Index." *PLoS Medicine* 1.3 (2004): 210-17. Print.

Talbot, Michael. *The Holographic Universe.* New York: HarperPerennial, 1992. Print.

Tatur, V. *The Secrets of New Thinking.* Moscow: Progress Publisher, 1990. Print.

"Technology Transfer Network: Air Toxics Web Site – Pollutants & Sources." U.S. Environmental Protection Agency, 24 March 2009. Web. 1 Jun. 2010. <http://www.epa.gov/ttn/atw/pollsour.html>.

Terry, Mary Beth, Geoffrey Howe, Janice M. Pogoda, Fang Fang Zhang, Anders Ahlbom, Won Choi, Graham G. Giles, Julian Little, Flora Lubin, Francoise Menegoz, Philip Ryan, Brigitte Schlehofer, and Susan Preston-Martin. "An International Case-Control Study of Adult Diet and Brain Tumor Risk: A Histology-Specific Analysis by Food Group." *Annals of Epidemiology* 19.3 (2009): 161-71. Print.

"The Soka Gakkai Dictionary of Buddhism." Soka Gakkai International. Web. 1 Oct. 2010. <http://www.sgilibrary.org/search_dict.php?id=2376>.

Thiébaut, Anne C.M., Li Jiao, Debra T. Silverman, Amanda J. Cross, Frances E. Thompson, Amy F. Subar, Albert R. Hollenbeck, Arthur Schatzkin, and Rachael Z. Stolzenberg-Solomon. "Dietary Fatty Acids and Pancreatic Cancer in the NIH-AARP

Diet and Health Study." *Journal of the National Cancer Institute* 101.14 (2009): 1001-11. Print.

Ullman, Montague, Stanley Krippner, and Alan Vaughan. *Dream Telepathy: Experiments in Nocturnal ESP.* Boston: Hampton Roads, 2003. Print.

"Vegetarian diets may prevent & treat some chronic diseases. Plant-based diets can meet all current nutrient needs and may lessen disease risk." *Duke Medicine Health News* 16.1 (2010): 1-2. Print.

Veith, Ilza, trans. *The Yellow Emperor's Classic of Internal Medicine.* Berkeley: U of California P, 2002. Print.

Wang, Shiow Y., Chi-Tsun Chen, William Sciarappa, Chien Y. Wang, and Mary J. Camp. "Fruit Quality, Antioxidant Capacity, and Flavonoid Content of Organically and Conventionally Grown Blueberries." *Journal of Agricultural and Food Chemistry* 56.14 (2008): 5788-94. Print.

Warburg, Otto H. "On the origin of cancer cells." *Science* 123.3191 (1956): 309-14. Print.

---. "The Prime Cause and Prevention of Cancer – Part 1." Total Health Associates, 1969. Web. 30 Oct. 2007. <http://healingtools.tripod.com/primecause1.html>.

Watson, Burton, trans. *The Lotus Sutra.* New York: Columbia UP, 1993. Print.

Wegman, Holly, and Cinnamon Stetler. "A meta-analytic review of the effects of childhood abuse on medical outcomes in adulthood." *Psychosomatic Medicine* 71.8 (2009): 805-12. Print.

"What Are the Potential Health Effects of Pesticides?" *Community Guide to Recognizing and Reporting Pesticide Problems.* California Department of Pesticide Regulation, 2008. Web. 1 Jun. 2010. <http://www.cdpr.ca.gov/docs/dept/comguide/effects_excerpt.pdf>.

Wolff, Milo. "Matter Waves and Buddhist Thought – Explaining Tetrode and the EPR Effect." *The Wolff Papers.* 26 July 1998. Web. 1 Jun. 2010. <http://mwolff.tripod.com/tetrode.html>.

Wordsworth, Chloe F. *Holographic Repatterning: Modalities for Transforming*

Resonance Patterns. Arizona: Wordsworth Productions, 1994. Print.

Worthington, Virginia. "Nutrition and Biodynamics: Evidence for the Nutritional Superiority of Organic Crops." *Biodynamics* 224 (1999): 58-69. Print.

---. "Nutritional Quality of Organic Versus Conventional Fruits, Vegetables, and Grains." *The Journal of Alternative and Complementary Medicine* 7.2 (2001): 161-73. Print.

Yanick Jr., Paul. *Professional's Guidebook of Quantum Medicine.* Las Vegas, NV: American Academy of Quantum Medicine, 2000. Print.

The National Neurological Foundation (NNF) would like to acknowledge the following co-sponsors in the fundraising drive during the first print run of this book.

info121

Gaia One

SCIENTIFIC RESOURCES

TRANSCENDENTAL® CONNECTION

Mr and Mrs Chuai Aun, Ooi

Dr Christopher Yang Mao Lin

Mr Tan Meng Gui and Mdm Baby Sim Sharon

Anonymous Supporters of Go Veg, Be Green 2 Save The Planet

Sandra Liew

To connect with the author and to find out more about upcoming talks, seminars, retreats and workshops, check out:

1. On the Web: www.transcendentalconnection.com
   www.gaialifeinternational.com
2. On Facebook: transcendentalconnection
3. On Twitter: JOHNWONGCW

For queries, please email:
ask@transcendentalconnection.com

Джон Берг

ИСКУССТВО В

John Berger
WAYS OF SEEING

В СОЗДАНИИ ЭТОЙ КНИГИ ПРИНИМАЛИ УЧАСТИЕ:

Джон Бергер

Свен Бломберг

Крис Фокс

Майкл Дибб

Ричард Холлис

Джон Бергер

ИСКУССТВО ВИДЕТЬ

Издательство «КЛАУДБЕРРИ»
Санкт-Петербург

УДК 7.01
ББК 85.0
Б48

Перевод с английского Евгении Шраги

Бергер, Дж.
Б48 Искусство видеть / Пер. с англ. Е. Шраги. – СПб.: Клаудберри, 2012. – 184 с.

«Искусство видеть» Джона Бергера (1926-2017) – это одна из самых обсуждаемых и влиятельных книг об искусстве, когда-либо изданных в мире. Она написана по мотивам знаменитого фильма BBC и впервые была опубликована вслед за его премьерным показом в 1972 году. В том же году критик Sunday Times писал: «Бергер не просто открывает нам глаза на то, как мы видим произведения изобразительного искусства, он почти наверняка изменит само восприятие искусства зрителем». Спустя сорок с лишним лет можно с уверенностью утверждать: пророчество сбылось.

ISBN 978-5-903974-02-3

ЭТУ КНИГУ МЫ СДЕЛАЛИ ВПЯТЕРОМ. Точкой отсчета для нее послужили некоторые идеи, сформулированные в телевизионном сериале «Искусство видеть» (в оригинале – Ways of Seeing). Мы попытались расширить и развить их. Идеи эти повлияли не только на то, что именно мы здесь говорим, но и на то, как мы пытаемся сказать это. Форма изложения отражает наш замысел в не меньшей степени, чем приводимые нами аргументы.

Книга состоит из семи пронумерованных эссе. Их можно читать в любом порядке. Четыре из них используют и слова, и изображения, три – только изображения. Эти чисто визуальные эссе (о способах видеть женщину и о некоторых противоречивых аспектах традиции масляной живописи) призваны поднять не меньше вопросов, чем эссе словесные. Иногда в визуальных эссе не дается никакой информации о приведенных в них картинах, поскольку мы решили, что такая информация будет отвлекать от поставленных вопросов. Эти сведения можно найти в списке репродукций, который находится в конце книги.

В собранных здесь эссе рассматриваются лишь отдельные аспекты избранных тем, причем в первую очередь те, что стали особенно актуальными для современного исторического сознания. Главной нашей задачей было начать задавать вопросы.

1

Зрение первично по отношению к речи. Ребенок уже видит и понимает, хотя еще не умеет говорить.

Но зрение первично и в ином смысле. Понимание нашего места в окружающем мире формируется именно благодаря зрению; мы объясняем мир словами, но слова ничего не могут поделать с тем фактом, что мы этим миром окружены. Отношения между тем, что мы видим, и тем, что мы знаем, остаются зыбкими. Каждый вечер мы видим, как садится Солнце. Мы знаем, что это вертится Земля. Однако знание, объяснение все-таки не вполне вяжутся с увиденным. Художник-сюрреалист Магритт сыграл на этом несоответствии между словом и образом в своей картине «Ключ к грезам».

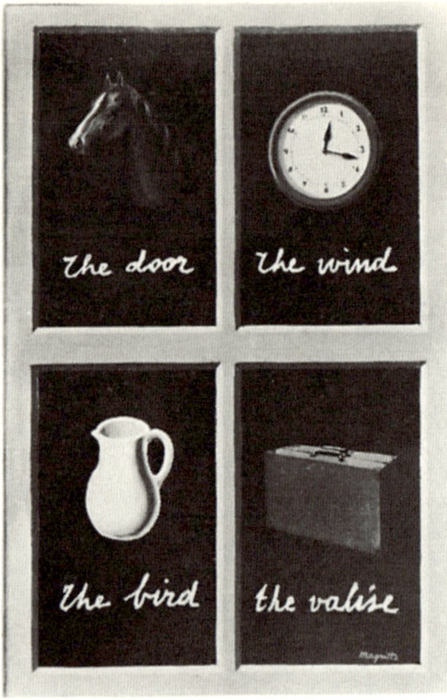

КЛЮЧ К ГРЕЗАМ.
РЕНЕ МАГРИТТ.
1898–1967

То, что мы знаем или во что верим, влияет на то, как мы видим окружающие нас вещи. К примеру, в Средние века, когда люди верили в реальное существование Ада, горящий огонь значил для них нечто отличное от того, что он значит для нас. И с другой стороны, их представление об Аде многим обязано зрелищу всепоглощающего огня и виду остающегося после него пепла, а также боли от полученных ожогов.

Когда человек влюблен, образ любимого обладает тем совершенством, полноту которого не измеришь ни словами, ни объятиями, – его на какое-то время может вместить только любовное соитие.

Однако это видение, приходящее раньше слов и не поддающееся вполне словесному определению, не есть лишь автоматическое реагирование на раздражители. (Так можно поставить вопрос, только если рассматривать совсем крохотную часть процесса, имеющую отношение к сетчатке глаза.) Мы видим только то, на что мы смотрим. А смотреть – это совершать выбор. В результате сделанного выбора то, что мы видим, становится доступным нам (однако вовсе не обязательно физически доступным). Дотронуться до чего бы то ни было означает вступить с этим предметом в некоторые отношения. (Закрыв глаза, пройдитесь по комнате и обратите внимание, насколько осязание похоже на зрение, но только статичное, ограниченное.) Мы никогда не смотрим просто на одну вещь, мы смотрим на отношения между вещами и нами. Наше зрение все время активно, оно подвижно, оно удерживает вещи в пространстве вокруг себя, оно утверждает все то, что существует для нас таких, какие мы есть.

Вскоре после того как мы начинаем видеть, мы понимаем, что и нас можно увидеть. Этот чужой взгляд соединяется с нашим собственным взглядом, чтобы наша принадлежность к видимому миру стала вполне бесспорной.

Если мы осознаем, что можем видеть тот холм вдалеке, то неизбежно предполагаем, что и нас можно увидеть с того холма. Взаимность зрения более глубинна, чем взаимность словесного диалога. И нередко диалог – это попытка вербализовать наше видение, попытка объяснить, как (метафорически и буквально) «ты видишь вещи», попытка выяснить, как «он видит вещи».

Все изображения (в том смысле, в котором мы используем это слово в нашей книге) созданы человеком.

Изображение – это воссозданное видение. Это явление (или множество явлений), изъятое из пространства и времени, где оно впервые явилось, и сохраненное – на несколько мгновений или на несколько веков. Всякое изображение воплощает в себе некоторый способ видеть. Даже фотография. Поскольку фотография, вопреки распространенному мнению, не есть автоматическая фик-

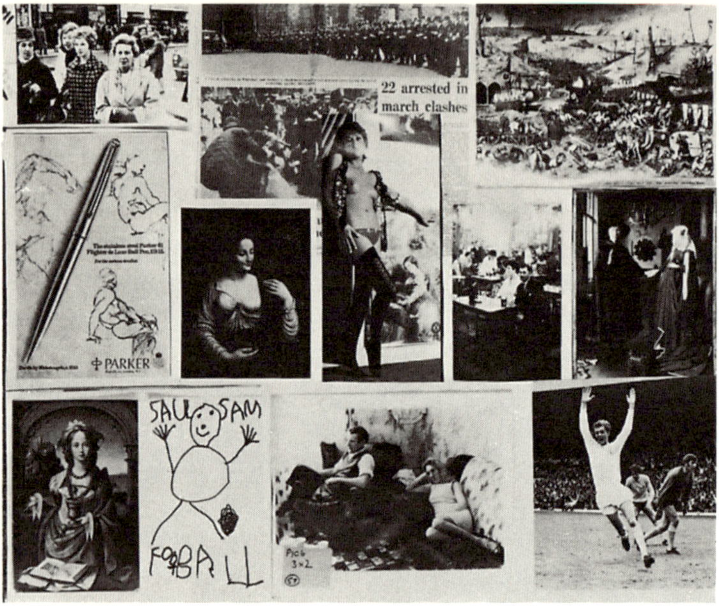

сация. Всякий раз, смотря на фотографию, мы помним (пусть хотя бы краем сознания) о фотографе, выбравшем именно эти предмет и перспективу из бесконечности других возможных предметов и перспектив. Это применимо даже к самому случайному семейному снимку. То, как фотограф видит мир, отражается в выборе объектов съемки. То, как художник видит мир, можно понять по тем следам, которые он оставляет на холсте или на бумаге. И хотя всякое изображение воплощает в себе определенный способ видения, наше восприятие и оценка в свою очередь зависят от нашего собственного способа видеть. (Так, например, некая барышня может находиться в компании двадцати человек, но мы, по собственным субъективным причинам, не сводим глаз именно с нее.)

Первоначально изображения создавались для того, чтобы явить зрителю образ чего-то отсутствующего. Постепенно стало очевидно, что изображение может пережить то, что оно изображает, и продемонстрировать, как что-то выглядело (или кто-то выглядел) когда-то прежде, а следовательно, как изображенное виделось тогда другими людьми. Позднее было осознано, что картина фиксирует в том числе и специфическую точку зрения ее создателя. Картина стала свидетельством того, как А видел Б. Это было результатом возраставшего осознания ценности личности, которое сопровождало возраставший интерес к истории. Будет легкомысленно пытаться точно датировать это последнее изменение. Но, вне всякого сомнения, такого рода осознание в Европе происходило с начала эпохи Возрождения.

Никакие другие реликвии и тексты не способны предоставить нам столь непосредственное свидетельство о мире, окружавшем людей в иные времена. В этом аспекте картины точнее и богаче литературы. Это не значит, что мы отрицаем экспрессивность и художественную силу искусства, толкуя его как исключительно документальное свидетельство; чем более образным и художественным является произведение, тем глубже оно позволяет нам разделить опыт, полученный автором от увиденного.

Однако, когда изображение подается как произведение искусства, на его восприятие влияют наши благоприобретенные представления об искусстве – представления, касающиеся:

КРАСОТЫ
ПРАВДЫ
ГЕНИАЛЬНОСТИ
ЦИВИЛИЗОВАННОСТИ
ФОРМЫ
ОБЩЕСТВЕННОГО ПОЛОЖЕНИЯ
ВКУСА и т. д.

Многие из этих представлений уже не имеют никакого отношения к миру, каков он есть. (Мир, каков он есть, – это не просто факт реальности, он включает еще и сознание.) Не соответствуя правде настоящего, эти предубеждения влияют на представления о прошлом. Искажают его, вместо того чтобы прояснять. Прошлое отнюдь не ждет пассивно, пока его исследуют и признают таким, какое оно есть. История – это всегда отношения между настоящим и его прошлым. Следовательно, страхи настоящего ведут к искажению прошлого. Прошлое нужно не для того, чтобы в нем жить, прошлое — это колодец, из которого мы черпаем воду, чтобы действовать в настоящем. Искажение прошлого культуры влечет за собой двойную потерю. Произведения искусства становятся слишком далекими от нас. И прошлое предоставляет нам все меньше выводов, которые мы могли бы реализовать в действии.

Когда мы «видим» пейзаж, мы помещаем себя в него. Если бы мы «увидели» произведение искусства прошлого, мы бы поместили себя в историю. Если нам не дают его увидеть, у нас отнимают ту историю, которая нам принадлежит. Кому это выгодно? В конечном счете смысл искусства искажается, потому что привилегированное меньшинство стремится создать историю, которая бы оправдывала существование правящих классов (а в современных понятиях такое оправдание уже совершенно невозможно). Именно поэтому искажение неизбежно.

Давайте рассмотрим типичный пример такого рода искажения. Недавно была опубликована двухтомная монография о Франсе Хальсе.[1] На текущий момент это самая авторитетная работа о данном художнике. Как узкоспециальная книга по искусствоведению она не лучше и не хуже любой другой.

---

[1] Seymour Slive. Frans Hals. — London: Phaidon Press Ltd., 1970–1974.

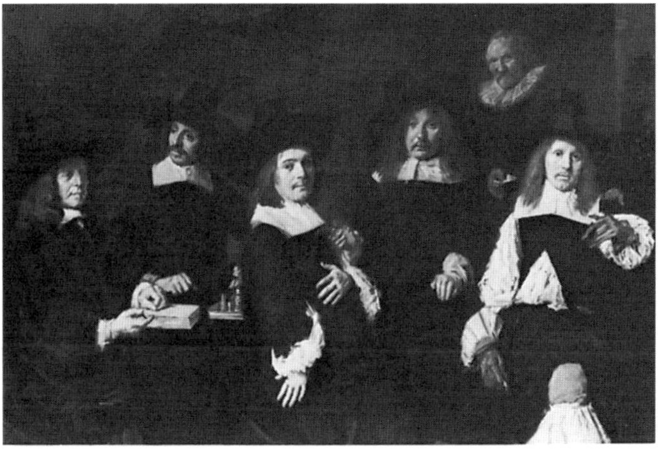

РЕГЕНТЫ ПРИЮТА ДЛЯ ПРЕСТАРЕЛЫХ.
ХАЛЬС. 1580–1666

РЕГЕНТШИ ПРИЮТА ДЛЯ ПРЕСТАРЕЛЫХ.
ХАЛЬС. 1580–1666

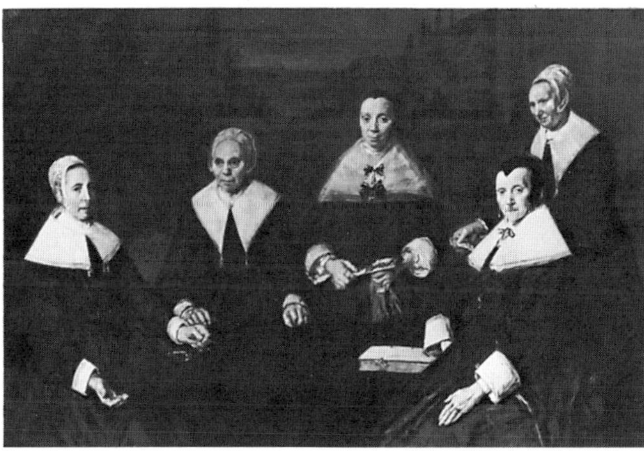

Две последние крупные картины Хальса изображают попечителей и попечительниц богадельни для престарелых бедняков в средневековом голландском городе Харлем. Это были заказные портреты. Хальсу было уже за восемьдесят, и он вел нищенское существование. Большую часть своей жизни он прожил в долгах. Зимой 1664-го, в тот год, когда Хальс начал писать эти картины, он получил в качестве благотворительной помощи три телеги торфа, иначе он умер бы от холода. А те, кто теперь позировал ему, как раз и распределяли такую благотворительную помощь.

Автор отмечает данные факты, а потом говорит, что было бы некорректно усматривать в этих картинах какую бы то ни было критику в адрес изображенных на них людей. Нет никаких свидетельств, пишет он, тому, что Хальс был обозлен и обижен, когда писал их. Между тем автор считает эти картины выдающимися произведениями искусства и объясняет почему. Вот что он пишет о «Регентшах»:

> «Портреты всех этих женщин говорят нам о человеческой природе с равной внятностью. Все они одинаково четко выступают на *крайне* темном фоне, в то же время они связаны между собой очень жесткой ритмической организацией картины и дополнительной диагональю, созданной их головами и руками. Тонкие модуляции *глубокого,* насыщенного черного вносят свой вклад в *гармоничное единство* целого и создают *незабываемый* контраст с *сильными* белыми и живыми телесными тонами, отдельные мазки которых достигают *предельной выразительности и силы*» [Курсив наш].

Разумеется, композиционное единство картины во многом обеспечивает силу того впечатления, которое она производит. Вполне уместно анализировать композицию живописного полотна. Но тут о композиции пишется так, словно она сама по себе несет эмоциональный заряд. Такие понятия, как *гармоничное единство, незабываемый контраст,* достижение *предельной выразительности и силы,* переводят эмоцию, которую вызывает картина, из плоскости переживаемого опыта в плоскость безучаст-

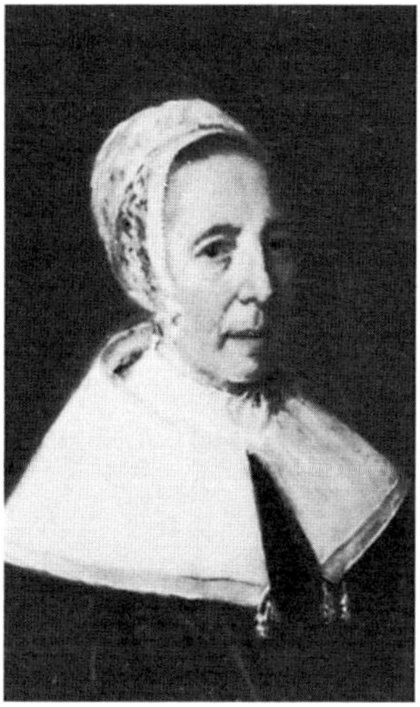 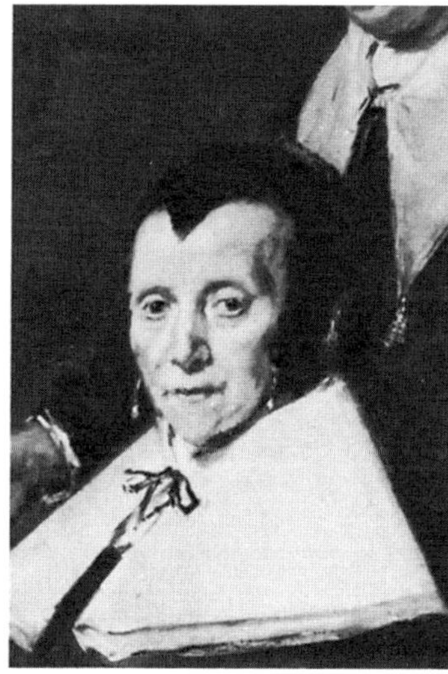

ной «оценки произведения искусства». Все конфликты исчезают. Мы остаемся с неизменной «человеческой природой» и картиной, рассматриваемой как совершенный рукотворный объект.

Очень мало что известно о Хальсе и о регентах, сделавших ему этот заказ. Невозможно предоставить и косвенные свидетельства о том, каковы были их отношения. Но эти картины – тоже свидетельство: группа мужчин и группа женщин, как их видел другой человек, художник. Рассмотрите это свидетельство – и судите сами.

Историк искусства боится таких прямых суждений:

> «Как и во многих других картинах Хальса, детальность и тонкость образов вводит нас в искушение и заставляет поверить, будто мы знаем индивидуальные особенности и даже привычки изображенных мужчин и женщин».

О каком, собственно, «искушении» он пишет? Это не что иное, как воздействие картин на нас, зрителей. Они воздействуют на нас, потому что мы принимаем то, как

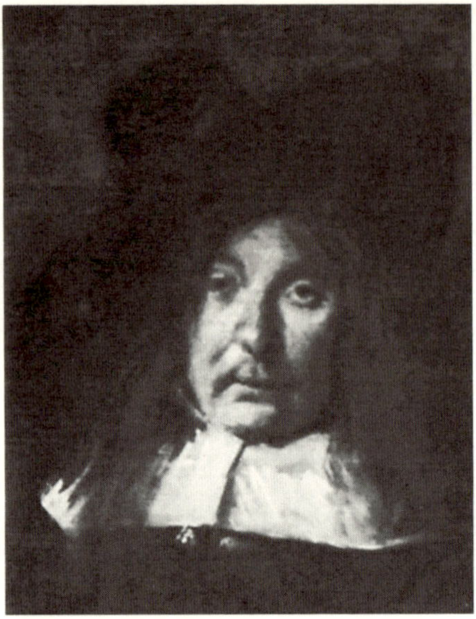

Хальс видит своих моделей. Мы принимаем его взгляд не просто так. Мы принимаем его в той мере, в которой он соответствует нашим наблюдениям над людьми (с их жестами и лицами) и общественными институтами. Это оказывается возможным, потому что мы по-прежнему живем в обществе со сходными социальными отношениями и моральными ценностями. И именно это придает картинам психологическую и социальную актуальность. Именно это (а не мастерство художника как «искусителя») убеждает нас в том, что мы действительно можем знать изображенных там людей.

Автор продолжает:

> «Над некоторыми критиками это искушение возымело полную власть. Так, например, утверждалось, будто регент со странным расфокусированным взглядом, в сдвинутой набок шляпе, едва прикрывающей его длинные, прилизанные волосы, изображен пьяным».

Автор полагает, что это клевета. Он уверяет, что в то время было модно носить шляпу набок. Он цитирует медицинское заключение, дабы доказать, что выражение лица регента могло быть результатом паралича лицевого нерва. Он настаивает, что регенты не приняли бы картину, если бы один из них был изображен на ней пьяным. На обсуждение любого из этих соображений можно потратить много страниц. (В XVII веке мужчины носили шляпы набекрень, чтобы выглядеть авантюристами и бонвиванами. А пьянство было вполне общепринятой практикой. И так дале.) Но эта дискуссия только дальше уведет нас от того единственного конфликта, который имеет значение и который автор стремится обойти.

Это конфликт между регентами и живописцем: первые смотрят на Хальса – одинокого, старого художника, растерявшего славу и живущего за счет общественной благотворительности; а он рассматривает их глазами нищего, который, тем не менее, должен пытаться быть объективным, то есть должен преодолеть свое видение мира, присущее ему как нищему. Вот в чем драма этих картин. Драма «незабываемого контраста».

Искажение вовсе не сводится к используемой терминологии. Искажение – это забалтывание того, что в противном случае было бы очевидным. Хальс был первым художником, изобразившим новые характеры и новые лица, созданные капитализмом. Он сделал в живописи то, что два столетия спустя Бальзак сделает в литературе. Однако автор нашей авторитетной работы, посвященной этим картинам, резюмирует достижения художника, отсылая к:

«решительной преданности Хальса его собственному видению мира, которое обогащает наше понимание людей и увеличивает наше благоговение перед все возрастающей мощью могущественных импульсов, давших ему возможность так близко показать нам жизненные силы бытия».

Это и есть искажение прошлого (которое, кстати, может иметь и псевдомарксисткий характер).

Чтобы его избежать, давайте рассмотрим те отношения, которые существуют сейчас между настоящим и прошлым (разумеется, в интересующем нас аспекте визуальных образов). Если мы сможем видеть настоящее достаточно ясно, то будем задавать правильные вопросы прошлому.

Сегодня мы видим искусство прошлого так, как никто никогда его не видел. Мы даже воспринимаем его иначе.

Эта разница может быть проиллюстрирована на примере того, как в разные времена понималась перспектива. Перспектива – условность, присущая только европейскому искусству и впервые возникшая в эпоху Раннего Возрождения, – центрирует все во взгляде зрителя. Это как луч маяка, только место света, идущего наружу, занимают образы, идущие внутрь. Образы эти принято было называть реальностью. Перспектива делает глаз центром видимого мира. Все сходится в глазу, как в исчезающей точке бесконечности. Видимый мир оказывается устроенным для зрителя, как когда-то Вселенная мыслилась устроенной для Бога.

Согласно условности перспективы визуальность не взаимна. Богу не нужно ставить себя ни в какие отношения с другими: Он везде. Перспектива обладает внутренним противоречием: она структурирует все образы реальности так, чтобы они были адресованы только одному зрителю, но этот зритель, в отличие от Бога, может находиться только в одном месте в данный момент времени.

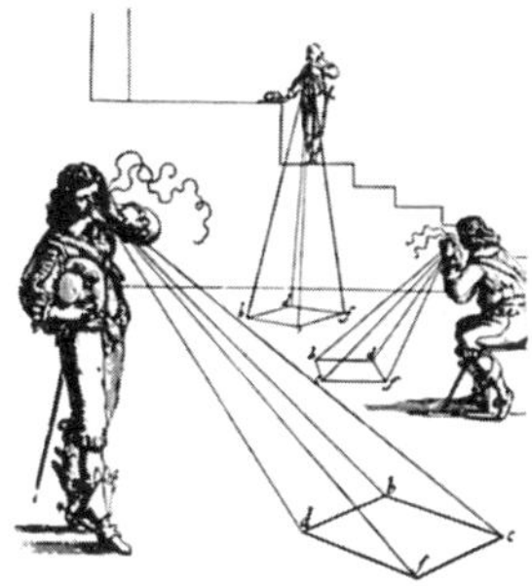

После изобретения камеры это противоречие постепенно стало очевидным.

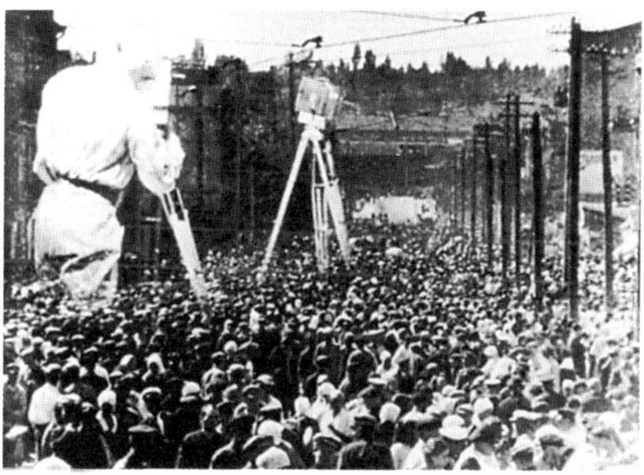

КАДР ИЗ ФИЛЬМА «ЧЕЛОВЕК С КИНОАППАРАТОМ». Д. ВЕРТОВ

«Я — киноглаз. Я — глаз механический. Я — машина, показывающая вам мир таким, каким только я его смогу увидеть. Я освобождаю себя с сегодня навсегда от неподвижности человеческой. Я в непрерывном движении. Я приближаюсь и удаляюсь от предметов, я подлезаю под них, я влезаю на них, я двигаюсь рядом с мордой бегущей лошади, я врезаюсь на полном ходу в толпу, я бегу перед бегущими солдатами, я опрокидываюсь на спину, я поднимаюсь вместе с аэропланами, я падаю и взлетаю вместе с падающими и взлетающими телами. Вот я, аппарат, бросился по равнодействующей, лавируя среди хаоса движений, фиксируя движение с движения от самых сложных комбинаций.

<...> освобожденный от временных и пространственных рамок, я сопоставляю любые точки вселенной, где бы я их ни зафиксировал. Мой путь — к созданию свежего восприятия мира. Вот я и расшифровываю по-новому неизвестный вам мир».[2]

Камера изолировала мгновенные образы и таким образом разрушила представление об их вневременной природе. Или, иными словами, камера показала, что идея проходящего времени неотделима от визуального опыта (это справедливо по отношению ко всему, кроме живописи). То, что ты видел, зависит от того, где ты был и когда. То, что ты видел, стало производной от твоего положения во времени и пространстве. Стало невозможным дальше считать, что все сходится в глазу, как в исчезающей точке бесконечности.

Я не хочу сказать, что до изобретения камеры люди верили, что каждый видит все. Но перспектива организовывала зримое пространство так, словно это на самом деле был идеал. Всякий рисунок или живописное полотно, использующее перспективу, говорит своему зрителю, что он – центр мира. Камера же – а особенно кинокамера – демонстрирует, что центра нет.

Изобретение камеры изменило способ видения мира. Видимое стало значить для нас нечто иное. Это мгновенно сказалось и на живописи.

Для импрессионистов видимый мир уже иной, он не ждет, когда же человек его рассмотрит. Напротив, видимое становится текучим и мимолетным. Для кубистов видимое – это уже не то, что может поймать один взгляд, но все множество возможных взглядов на изображаемый предмет или изображаемого человека.

---

[2] Это цитата из статьи, написанной в 1923 г. Дзигой Вертовым, революционным советским кинорежиссером.

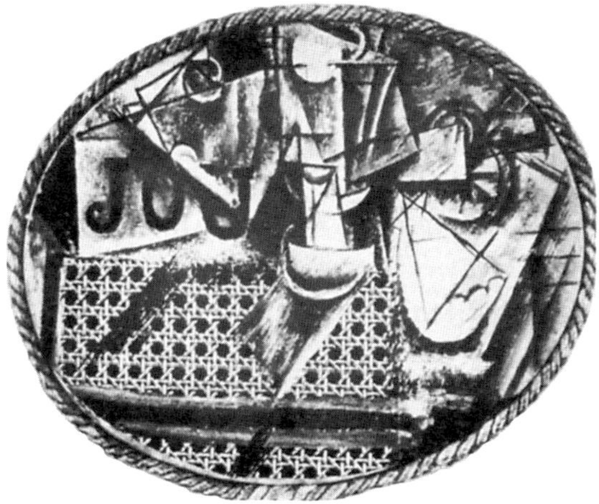

НАТЮРМОРТ С ПЛЕТЕНЫМ СТУЛОМ. ПИКАССО. 1881–1973

Изобретение камеры изменило и способ видения картин, написанных задолго до того, как камера была изобретена. Первоначально картины были неотъемлемой частью здания, для которого они создавались. Зайдя в раннеренессансную церковь или часовню, можно почувствовать, что росписи на стенах изображают внутреннюю жизнь этого здания, что в совокупности они формируют его память – в такой степени они были частью этого здания, и только его.

Уникальность всякой картины была частью уникальности того места, где она висела. Иногда картина перевозилась с места на место. Но никогда ее нельзя было

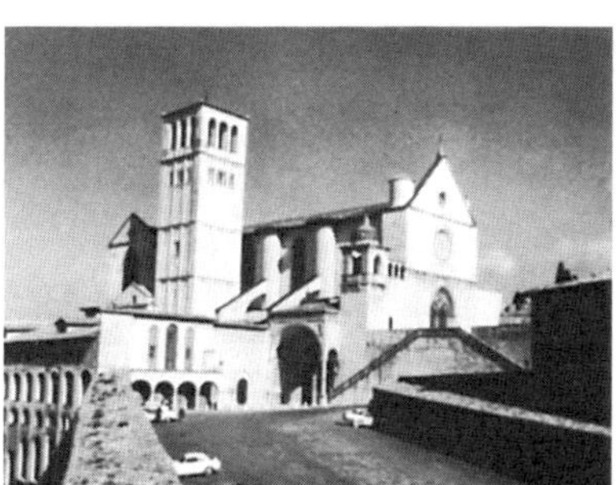

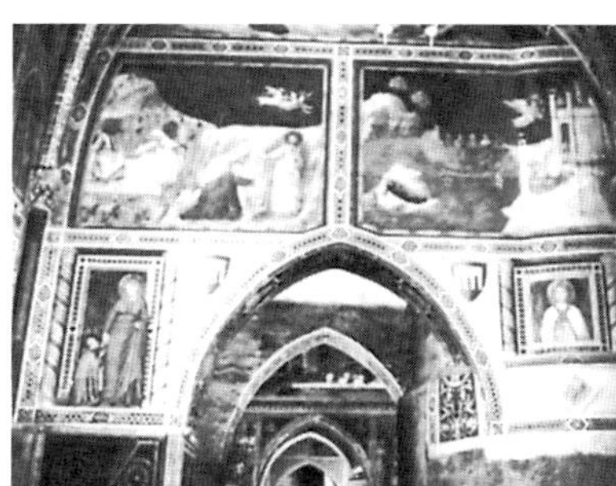

ЦЕРКОВЬ СВЯТОГО ФРАНЦИСКА В АССИЗИ

увидеть в двух местах одновременно. Когда камера воспроизводит изображение, она разрушает его уникальность. В результате меняется его значение. Или, вернее, значение умножается и разбивается на массу значений.

Яркая иллюстрация этому – то, что происходит, когда картину показывают по телевизору. Картина входит в дом каждого телезрителя. И вот она там, у него, в окружении его обоев, его мебели, его воспоминаний. Она входит в атмосферу его семьи. Она становится предметом для их разговора. Она приспосабливает свое значение к их значениям. В то же время она входит и в миллионы других домов и в каждом из них оказывается увиденной в разном контексте. Благодаря камере не зритель приходит к картине, а картина приходит к зрителю. В этом путешествии значение картины меняется.

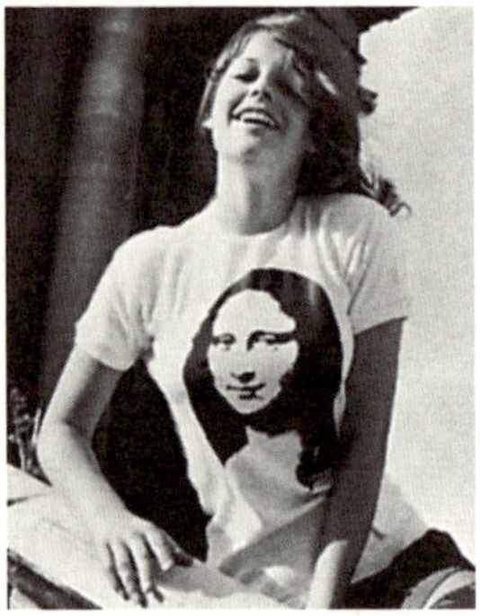

Можно, конечно, доказывать, что все репродукции так или иначе искажают оригинал, а следовательно, исходное произведение в каком-то смысле остается уникальным. Возьмем репродукцию картины Леонардо да Винчи «Мадонна в скалах» [«Мадонна в гроте»].

Увидев эту репродукцию, можно пойти в Национальную галерею, посмотреть на оригинал и выяснить, что же в репродукции оказалось утрачено. Или можно забыть о качестве репродукции и просто вспомнить, уви-

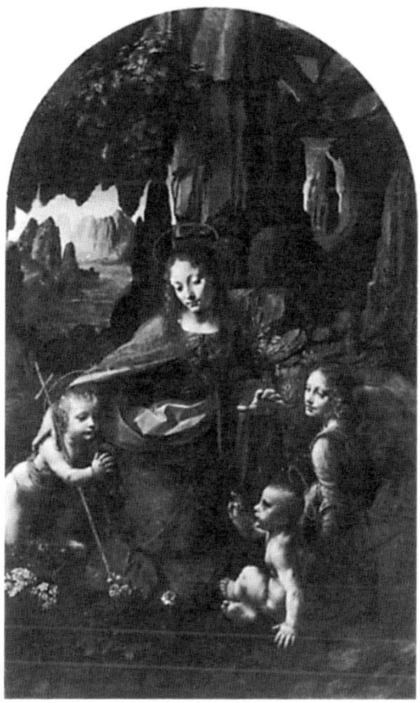

МАДОННА В СКАЛАХ. ЛЕОНАРДО ДА ВИНЧИ. 1452–1519. ЛОНДОНСКАЯ НАЦИОНАЛЬНАЯ ГАЛЕРЕЯ

дев оригинал, что это знаменитая картина, которую ты уже видел когда-то на репродукции. Но в любом случае уникальность оригинала теперь заключается в том, что это *оригинал репродукции*. Воспринимается как уникальное уже не то, что на картине изображено; ее основное значение обнаруживают теперь не в том, что она говорит, а в том, чем она является.

Этот новый статус оригинала – вполне естественное следствие новых способов воспроизводства изображений. Но именно на этой стадии в дело вновь вступает процесс искажения. Значение оригинала теперь заключается не в том, что он, один-единственный, говорит, а в том, чем он, один-единственный, является. Как современная культура оценивает и трактует его уникальное существование? Оригинал воспринимается как объект, ценность которого определяется его редкостью. Эта ценность утверждается и измеряется теми ценами, которые предлагают за него на рынке. Но поскольку это все-таки «произведение искусства» (а принято считать, что искусство выше торговли), то утверждают, что его рыночная цена является отражением его духовной ценности. Однако духовная ценность объекта (отдельно от его смыслового посыла или назидания, в нем заключенного) может быть объяснена лишь в понятиях магии или религии. А поскольку ни то ни другое в современном обществе не является живой силой, то «произведение искусства» оказывается окружено атмосферой почитания, сравнимого с религиозным по силе, но не по содержанию. Произведения искусства обсуждаются и преподносятся так, словно это священные реликвии – первые и важнейшие свидетельства их собственной долговечности. Прошлое, в котором были созданы эти произведения, изучается для того, чтобы проследить их историю и доказать их подлинность. Они объявляются искусством в том случае, если их происхождение оказывается подтвержденным.

Глядя на «Мадонну в скалах», посетитель Национальной галереи (благодаря всему тому, что он слышал и читал об этой картине) будет чувствовать примерно следующее: «Я стою перед ней. Я вижу ее. Эта картина Леонардо не похожа ни на одну другую картину в мире. В Национальной галерее хранится ее подлинник. Если я буду достаточно старательно смотреть на нее, то смогу почувствовать ее подлинность. “Мадонна в скалах” Леонардо да Винчи: она подлинна, а потому прекрасна!»

Отвергнуть такого рода чувства как наивные будет неверно. Они вполне соответствуют многосложному взгляду специалистов по искусству, для которых написан каталог Национальной галереи. Статья о «Мадонне в скалах» одна из самых длинных в нем. Это четырнадцать страниц мелким шрифтом. И ни слова о смысле этой картины. Там рассказывается о том, кто ее заказал, о юридических спорах, о том, кому она принадлежала, о вероятных датах ее создания, о семьях ее владельцев. За этой информацией стоят годы разысканий, цель которых – рассеять малейшие сомнения относительно авторства этой картины. Вторая же цель – доказать, что практически идентичная работа Леонардо, хранящаяся в Лувре, – это копия той, что висит в Национальной галерее.

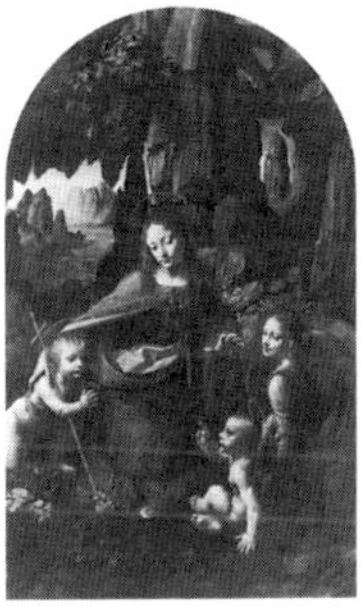

ЛОНДОНСКАЯ НАЦИОНАЛЬНАЯ ГАЛЕРЕЯ

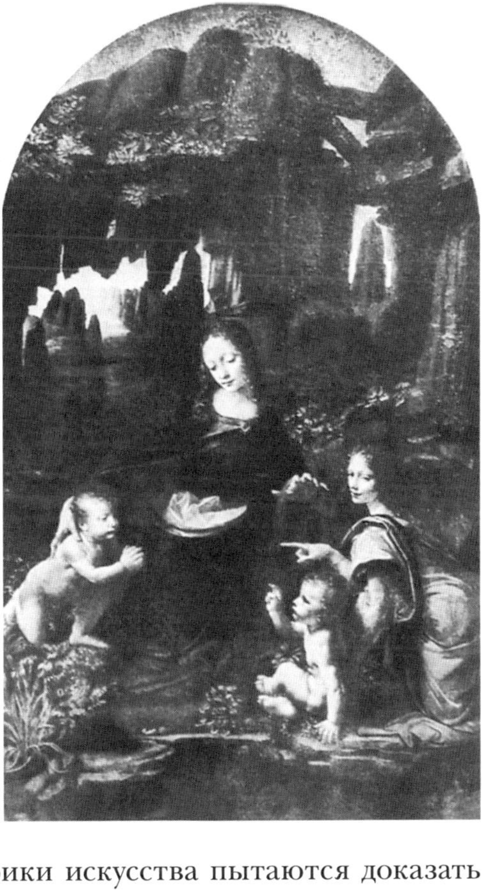

МАДОННА В СКАЛАХ. ЛЕОНАРДО ДА ВИНЧИ. 1452–1519. ЛУВР

Французские историки искусства пытаются доказать противоположное.

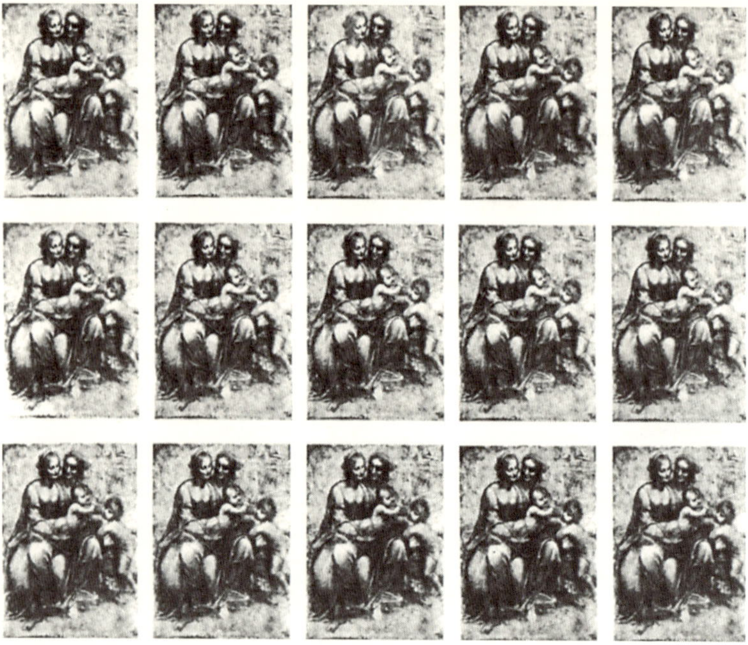

МАДОННА С МЛАДЕНЦЕМ, СВЯТОЙ АННОЙ И СВЯТЫМ ИОАННОМ КРЕСТИТЕЛЕМ.
ЛЕОНАРДО ДА ВИНЧИ.
1452–1519

Репродукции этюда Леонардо «Мадонна с младенцем, святой Анной и святым Иоанном Крестителем» продаются лучше, чем репродукции любой другой картины из коллекции Национальной галереи. А всего несколько лет назад эта работа была известна только специалистам. Она стала популярной благодаря тому, что некий американец хотел купить ее за два с половиной миллиона фунтов стерлингов.

Теперь она висит в отдельном зале. Этот зал напоминает часовню. Рисунок находится за пуленепробиваемым стеклом и стал производить совершенно новое впечатление. Не тем, что он изображает, не своим значением. Он стал таким эффектным и таинственным благодаря своей рыночной цене.

Фальшивая религиозность, окружающая сегодня произведения искусства и в конечном счете зависящая от их рыночной ценности, стала субститутом того, что живопись утратила в тот момент, когда камера сделала ее воспроизводимой. Функция этой религиозности чисто ностальгическая. Это последняя, слабая попытка утвердить ценности олигархической, недемократической культуры. Если изображение перестало быть уникальным и недоступным, то неким таинственным образом таковым должен стать предмет искусства, вещь.

Большая часть населения не ходит в художественные музеи. Следующая таблица демонстрирует, насколько тесно интерес к искусству связан с привилегированным образованием.

Процент от каждой образовательной категории, посещающей художественные музеи

	Греция	Польша	Франция	Голландия		Греция	Польша	Франция	Голландия
Без образования	0,02	0,12	0,15	–	Только среднее образование	10,5	10,4	10	20
Только начальное образование	0,30	1,50	0,45	0,50	Послешкольное, в том числе высшее образование	11,5	11,7	12,5	17,3

Источник: Pierre Bourdieu, Alain Darbel. L'Amour de l'Art. — Paris: Editions de Minuit, 1969. Appendix 5, table 4.

Для большинства является аксиомой та мысль, что музеи наполнены священными реликвиями, и это убеждение опирается на тайну, к которой большинство непричастно, – тайну огромного богатства. Или, иными словами, считается, что подлинное искусство – это прерогатива (в материальном и духовном смысле) исключительно богатых. Следующая таблица продемонстрирует, какие ассоциации вызывает у каждого социального класса художественная галерея.

На какое из перечисленных ниже мест, по-вашему, больше всего похож музей?

	Разнорабочие	Квалифицированные рабочие и «белые воротнички»	Руководство и высшее руководство
	%	%	%
Церковь	66	45	30,5
Библиотека	9	34	28
Лекционный зал	–	4	4,5
Универмаг или вестибюль общественного здания	–	7	2
Церковь и библиотека	9	2	4,5
Церковь и лекционный зал	4	2	–
Библиотека и лекционный зал	–	–	2
Ни один из этих вариантов	4	2	19,5
Воздержался	8	4	9
	100 % – 53 человека	100 % – 98 человек	100 % – 99 человек

Источник: Ibid., Appendix 4, table 8.

В эпоху репродуцируемости образов значение живописного произведения уже не закреплено за ним самим; его значение становится передаваемым: то есть оно становится своего рода информацией, и, как любая информация, оно либо используется, либо игнорируется; информация не обладает никакой особенной властью сама по себе. Когда картина используется, ее значение либо модифицируется, либо полностью изменяется. Нужно отчетливо осознавать, к чему именно это приводит. Речь не о том, что репродукция неспособна верно воспроизвести определенные аспекты оригинала; репродукция делает возможным (и даже неизбежным) то, что образ будет использоваться для самых разных целей, и копия, в отличие от оригинала, сможет приспособиться к ним всем. Давайте рассмотрим несколько вариантов того, как копия приспосабливается к такого рода использованию.

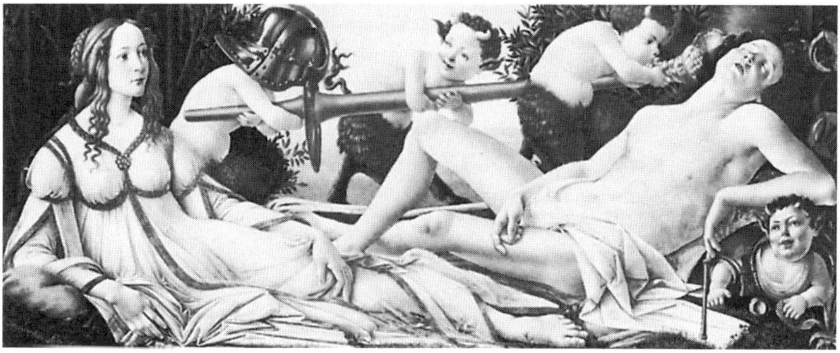

Репродукция изолирует фрагмент картины. И деталь видоизменяется. Аллегорическая фигура превращается в портрет девушки.

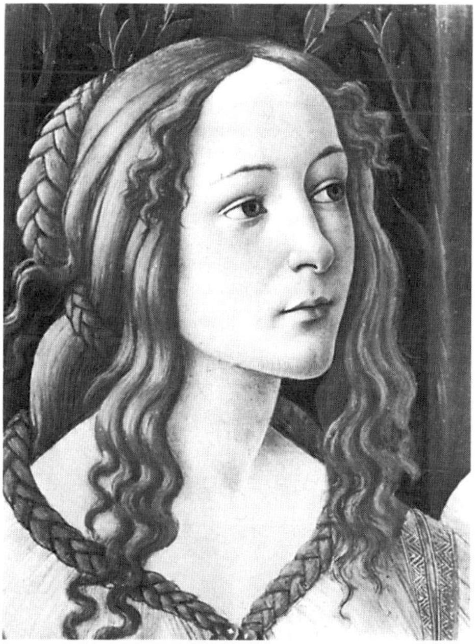

Когда картина воспроизводится при помощи кинокамеры, она неизбежно становится материалом для того, что хочет сказать режиссер.

Фильм, демонстрирующий произведения живописи, ведет зрителя сквозь картину к собственным выводам режиссера. Картина уступает власть режиссеру.

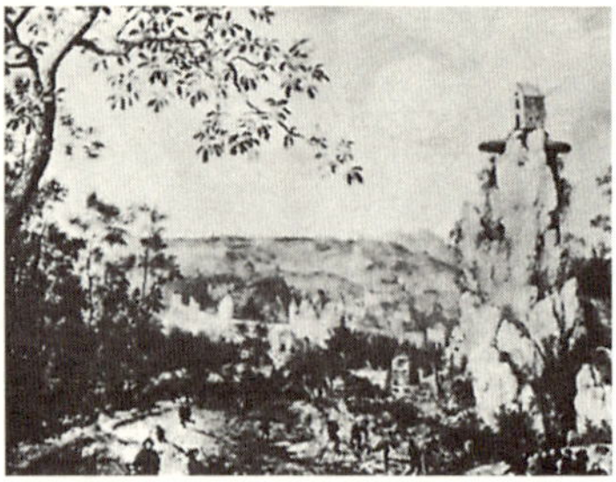
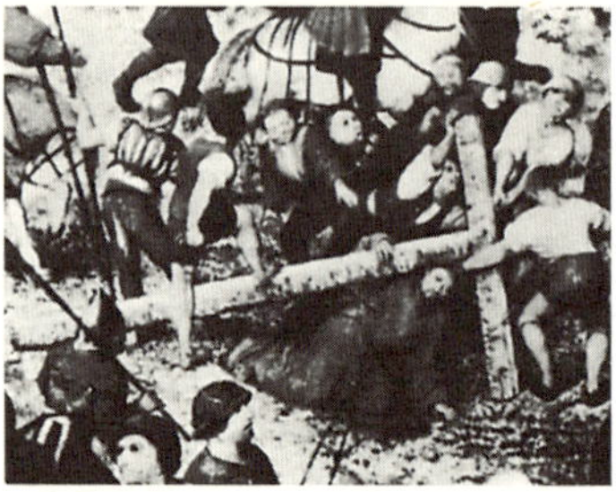

Это происходит потому, что фильм разворачивается во времени, а картина статична.

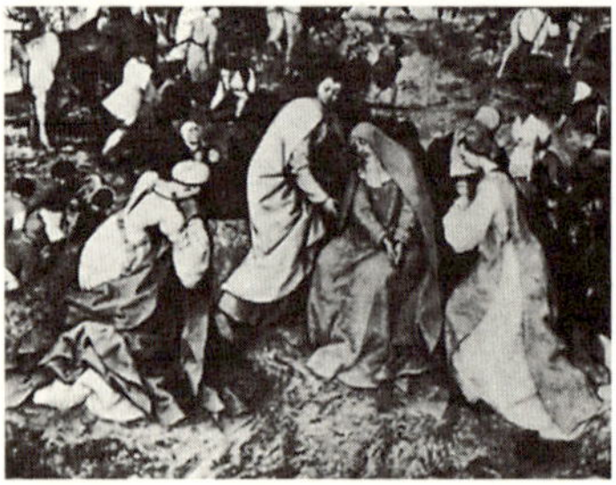
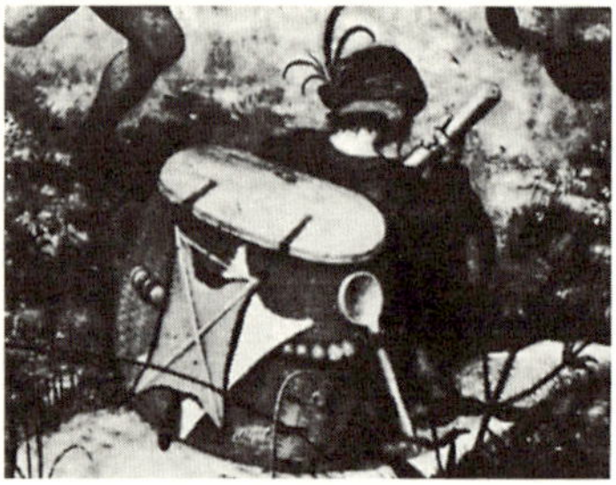

Образы в фильме, которые следуют один за другим, складываются в доказательство, становящееся непреложным.

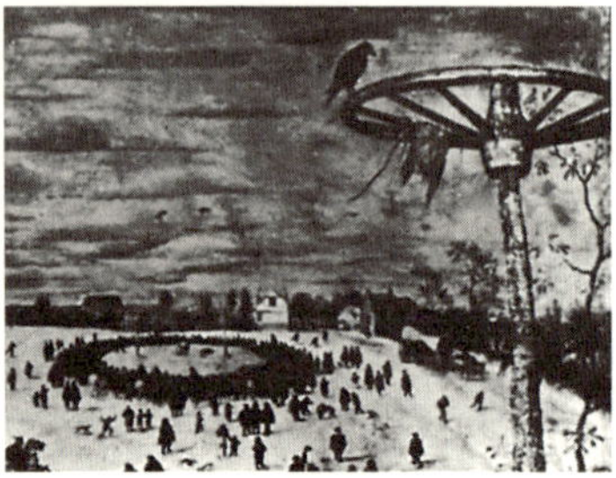
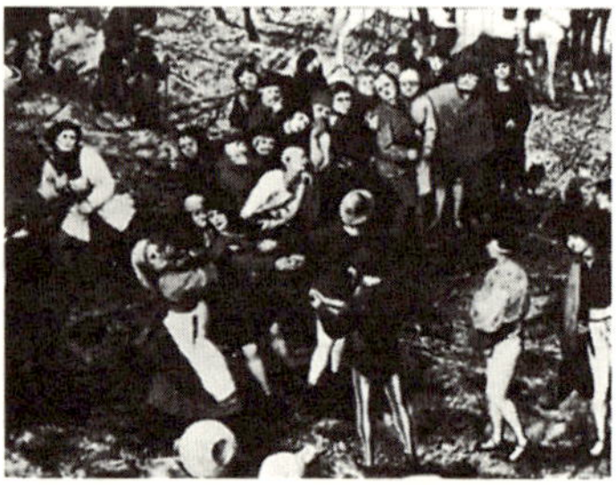

На картине все ее элементы могут быть увидены одновременно. Зрителю может понадобиться время для того, чтобы рассмотреть каждую деталь картины, но когда бы он ни пришел к выводу, единство и одновременность картины всегда может изменить или уточнить этот вывод. Картина сохраняет свою власть.

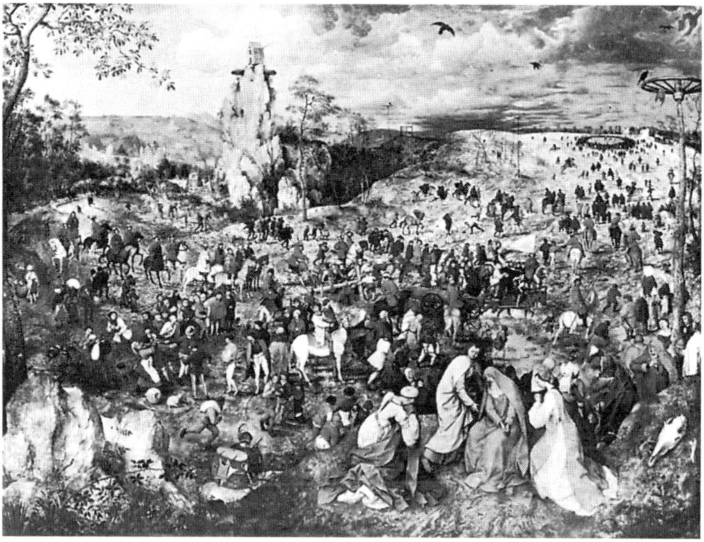

ШЕСТВИЕ НА ГОЛГОФУ. БРЕЙГЕЛЬ. 1525–1569

Репродукции картин нередко сопровождаются словами.

Вот перед вами пейзаж с полсм и взлетающими с земли птицами. Посмотрите на него. А потом переверните страницу.

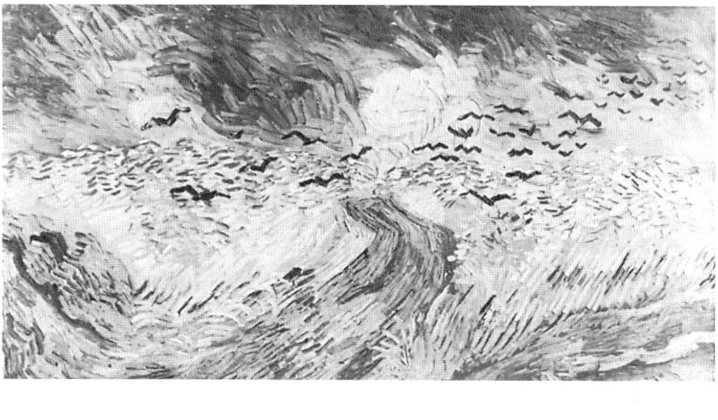

ПШЕНИЧНОЕ ПОЛЕ С ВОРОНАМИ. ВАН ГОГ. 1853–1890

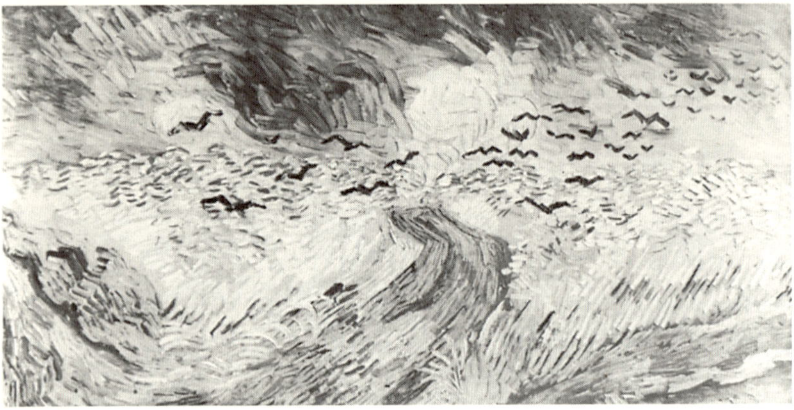

ПШЕНИЧНОЕ ПОЛЕ С ВОРОНАМИ.
ВАН ГОГ. 1853–1890
ЭТО ПОСЛЕДНЯЯ КАРТИНА ВАН ГОГА.
ОН НАПИСАЛ ЕЕ НЕЗАДОЛГО ДО САМОУБИЙСТВА.

Сложно в точности описать, как именно слова изменили картину, но они определенно ее изменили. Теперь картина иллюстрирует некое утверждение.

Все воспроизведенные в этом эссе картины стали частью аргументации, имеющей мало или практически никакого отношения к их первоначальному, независимому смыслу. Слова цитируют живопись, чтобы укрепить свою собственную, словесную власть. (Эссе без слов, включенные в нашу книгу, сделают это разграничение, вероятно, еще яснее.)

Репродукции картин, как и любая другая информация, вынуждены бороться за свое место под солнцем со всей другой непрерывно передаваемой информацией.

Как следствие, репродукция, отсылая к оригинальной картине, сама становится предметом отсылок для других изображений. Смысл изображения меняется в зависимости от того, что можно увидеть непосредственно рядом с ним или что показывается непосредственно

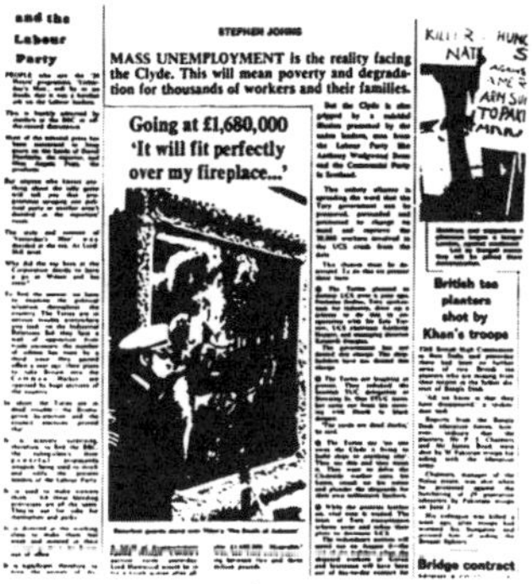

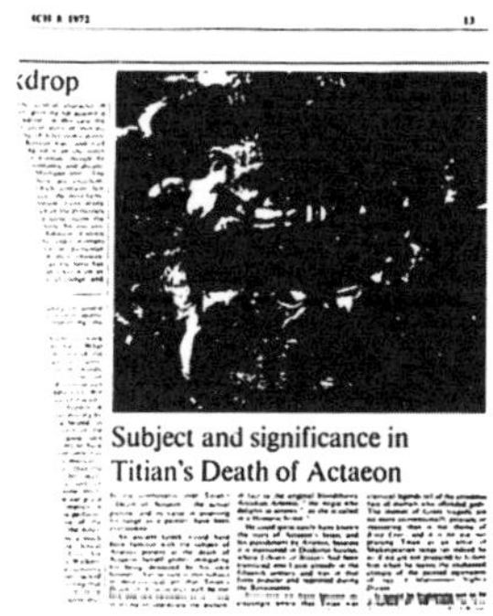

после него. И власть, которой обладает изображение, распространяется на весь контекст, в котором оно обнаруживается.

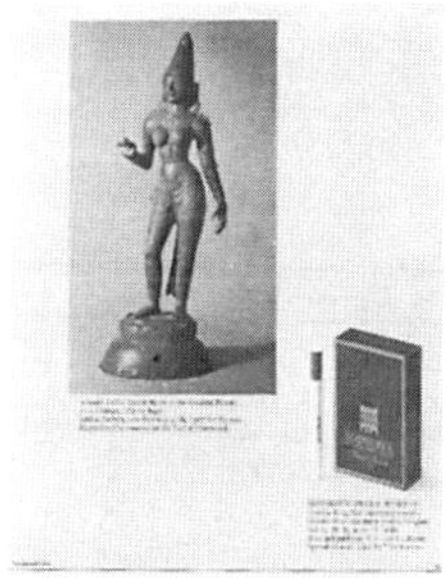

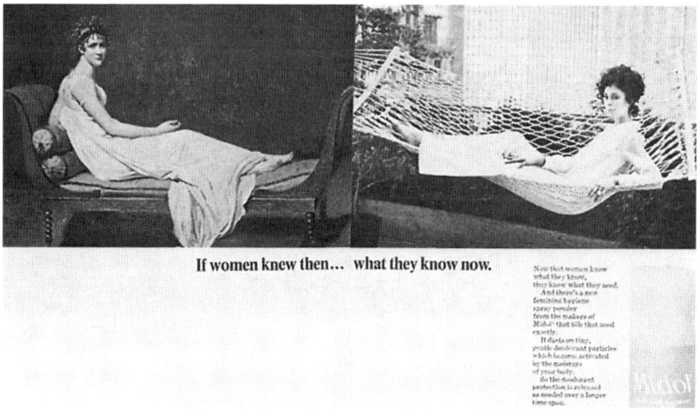

Поскольку произведения искусства воспроизводимы, то теоретически они могут быть использованы кем угодно. Однако чаще всего – в книгах об искусстве, в журналах, в фильмах и в золоченых рамах на стенах гостиных – репродукции по-прежнему используются для поддержания иллюзии, что ничего не изменилось, что искусство, с его уникальной, не ослабшей властью, оправдывает все остальные формы власти, что благодаря искусству неравенство выглядит благородно, а иерархия – волнующе. Например, вся концепция Национального культурного наследия эксплуатирует авторитет искусства для того, чтобы прославлять существующую социальную систему и ее ценности.

Средства воспроизводства изображений используются политически и коммерчески для того, чтобы представлять в ложном свете или вообще отрицать то, что благодаря их существованию делается возможным. Но

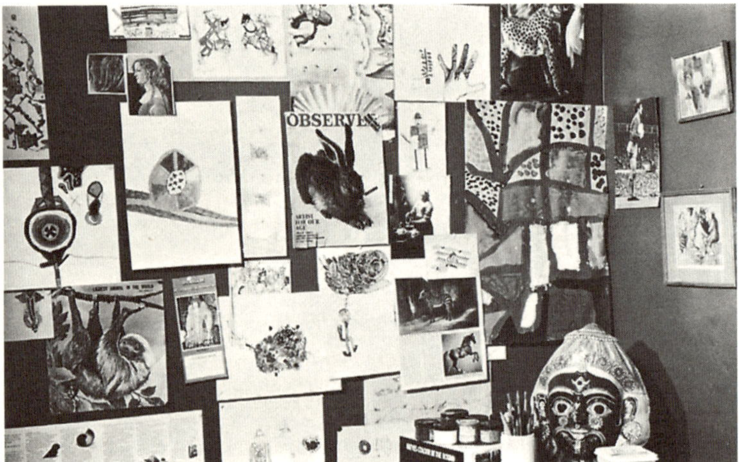

порой отдельные люди используют репродукции иным образом.

И взрослые, и дети иногда устраивают где-нибудь у себя в спальне подобную стенку, на которую они прикрепляют всевозможные бумажки: письма, фотографии, репродукции, вырезки из газет, рисунки и открытки. Все картинки на такой стене принадлежат одному языку – и более или менее равноправны в его рамках, поскольку это очень личная выборка, соответствующая опыту жильца этой комнаты и отражающая его опыт. По логике вещей, такого рода стенды должны заменить музеи.

Что мы хотим этим сказать? Давайте сперва определимся с тем, чего мы сказать не хотим.

Мы не хотим сказать, что единственное чувство, которое можно испытать, стоя перед подлинными живописными полотнами, — это благоговейный трепет перед их долговечностью. Традиционный подход к подлинникам (который мы встречаем в музейных каталогах, путеводителях и аудиогидах) – это далеко не единственный

СЛУЖАНКА С КУВШИНОМ МОЛОКА. ВЕРМЕЕР. 1632–1675

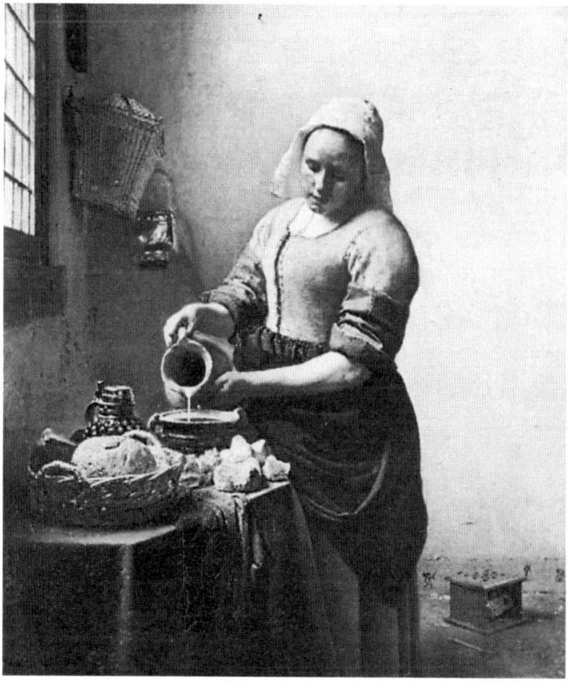

возможный подход. Когда на искусство прошлого перестанут смотреть ностальгически, его произведения перестанут быть священными реликвиями (хотя они и не станут вновь тем, чем они были до эпохи репродукций). Мы не говорим, что подлинники сегодня совершенно бесполезны.

Оригинальные полотна молчаливы и неподвижны. Этим не может похвастаться информация. Даже репродукция, висящая на стене, несравнима в этом отношении с оригиналом, в котором тишина и покой пронизывают сам материал, краску, позволяющую проследить непосредственно за движениями художника. И таким образом сокращается временная дистанция между созданием картины и нашим разглядыванием ее. В этом специфическом смысле все картины абсолютно современны. Отсюда – непосредственность их свидетельствования. Исторический момент в буквальном смысле стоит перед нашими глазами. Сезанн сделал сходное наблюдение с точки зрения художника. «Это всего лишь мгновение мировой жизни! Написать его во всей его реальности и забыть для этого обо всем! Стать этой минутой, быть чувствительной пластинкой... изобразить то, что видишь, забыв обо всем, что было до того...». Что мы сделаем с этим изображенным мгновением, когда оно встанет перед нашими глазами, зависит от того, чего мы ждем от искусства, а это, в свою очередь, зависит сегодня от нашего прежнего опыта переживания смысла картин, увиденных на репродукциях.

Не говорим мы и о том, что искусство может быть понятно самопроизвольно. Мы не утверждаем, будто вырезать из журнала репродукцию древнегреческого бюста, поскольку она созвучна некоему нашему личному опыту, и прикрепить на стенку рядом с другими разнородными картинками – это постичь смысл самого бюста.

Идея невинности имеет две стороны. Отказываясь вступать в заговор, можно остаться непричастным к этому заговору. Но оставаться невинным может еще означать и оставаться невежественным. И вопрос здесь не в выборе между невинностью и знанием (или между природой и культурой), но между тотальным подходом к искусству, стремящимся связать его со всеми аспектами нашего опыта, и эзотерическим подходом немногочисленных узкоспециализированных экспертов, служителей ностальгии угасающего правящего класса (уступающего место не пролетариату, а новой власти корпораций и государства.) Настоящий вопрос звучит так: кому принадлежит значение искусства прошлого? Тем, кто может приложить его к собственной жизни? Или культурной иерархии и специалистам по раритетам?

Визуальные искусства всегда существовали в некотором заповедном пространстве. Первоначально эта заповедность имела магическую или священную природу. Но, кроме того, она была и просто физической: это было место – пещера, здание, в котором (или для которого) писалась картина. Переживание искусства (первоначально бывшее переживанием ритуала) было отделено от остальной жизни именно для того, чтобы над жизнью властвовать. В дальнейшем эта изолированность приобрела социальный характер. Искусство вошло в культуру правящего класса, а физически оно оказалось изолировано, заключено в их дворцы и дома. На протяжении всей этой истории авторитет искусства был неотделим от авторитета заповедного пространства.

Что сделали современные средства воспроизводства изображений, так это разрушили власть искусства и изъяли его (или, вернее, изъяли образы, которые теперь воспроизводятся) из рамок всякой заповедности. Впервые за все времена образы искусства стали мимолетными, вездесущими, нематериальными, доступными, ничего не стоящими, свободными. Они окружают нас так же, как окружает язык. Они вошли в поток жизни, над которым больше сами по себе не имеют власти.

Однако очень мало кто осознает происшедшее, поскольку средства воспроизводства изображений практически все время используются для того, чтобы поддерживать иллюзию, будто ничего не изменилось, за тем исключением, что теперь благодаря репродукции массы могут восхищаться искусством, как когда-то могло восхищаться только образованное меньшинство. Ничего удивительного, что массы остаются незаинтересованными и скептически настроенными.

Если бы новый образный язык использовался иначе, он бы, непосредственно в ходе своего использования, создал новый вид силы. С его помощью мы могли бы точнее описывать свой опыт в тех сферах, которые неадекватно описываются словами. (Зрение первично по отношению к словам.) И речь идет не только о личном опыте, но также и о важнейшем историческом опыте наших отношений с прошлым, то есть об опыте поиска смысла нашей жизни и о попытках понять историю, действующей силой которой мы можем стать.

Искусство прошлого уже не существует в том виде, в каком существовало когда-то. Его власть утеряна. Его место занял язык изображений. Что имеет значение сегодня, так это – кто использует новый язык и в каких целях. Это касается проблемы авторских прав на воспроизведение, права собственности издательств, общей политики художественных галерей и музеев. Обычно это все преподносится как вопросы узкоспециальные. Одной из целей данного эссе было показать: то, что действительно поставлено на карту, значительно более существенно. Народ или класс, отрезанный от своего собственного прошлого, в значительно меньшей степени свободен выбирать и действовать как народ или класс, чем те, кто способен найти свое место в истории. По этой причине (и только по этой причине) вопрос об искусстве прошлого стал теперь вопросом политическим.

Многие идеи, изложенные в этом эссе, позаимствованы из другого, написанного сорока годами ранее немецким критиком и философом Вальтером Беньямином.

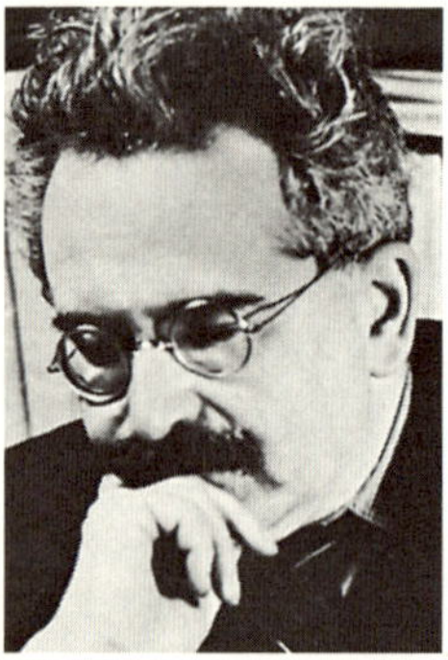

Его эссе называется «ПРОИЗВЕДЕНИЕ ИСКУССТВА В ЭПОХУ ЕГО ТЕХНИЧЕСКОЙ ВОСПРОИЗВОДИМОСТИ». По-русски его можно прочитать в сборнике избранных эссе В. Беньямина «ПРОИЗВЕДЕНИЕ ИСКУССТВА В ЭПОХУ ЕГО ТЕХНИЧЕСКОЙ ВОСПРОИЗВОДИМОСТИ» (Москва: Медиум, 1996).

2

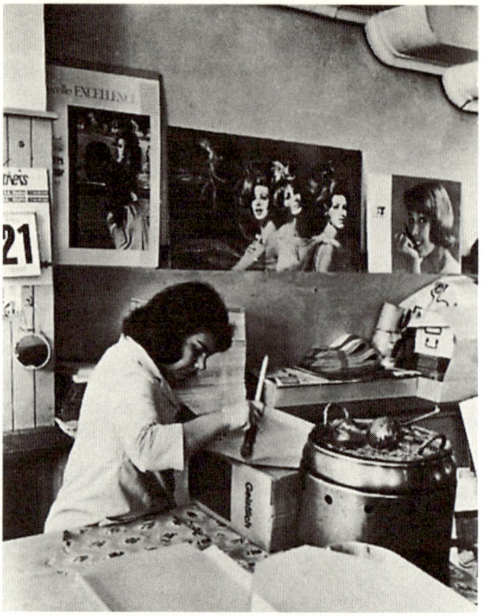
21

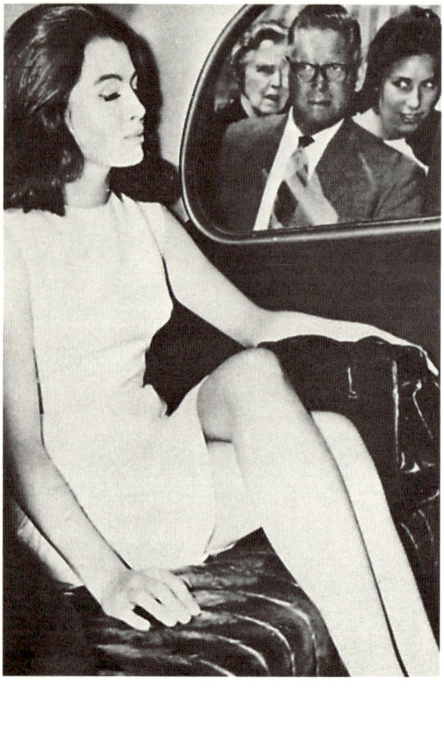

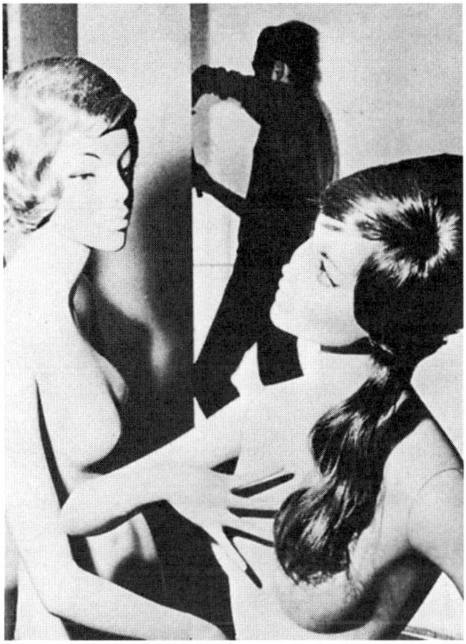

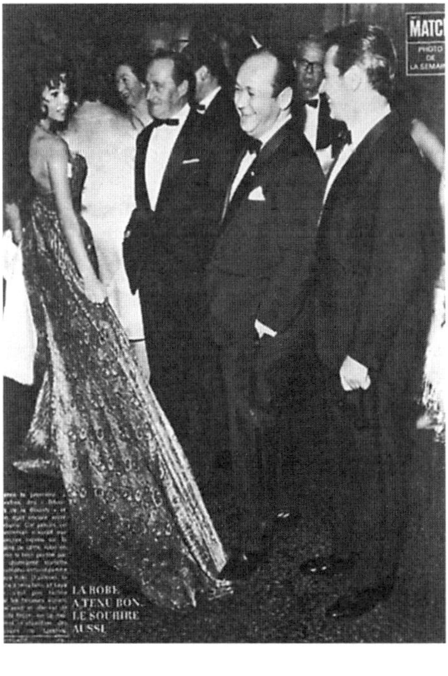
MATC
PHOTO
DE
LA SEMA
LA ROBE
A TENU BON,
LE SOURIRE
AUSSI

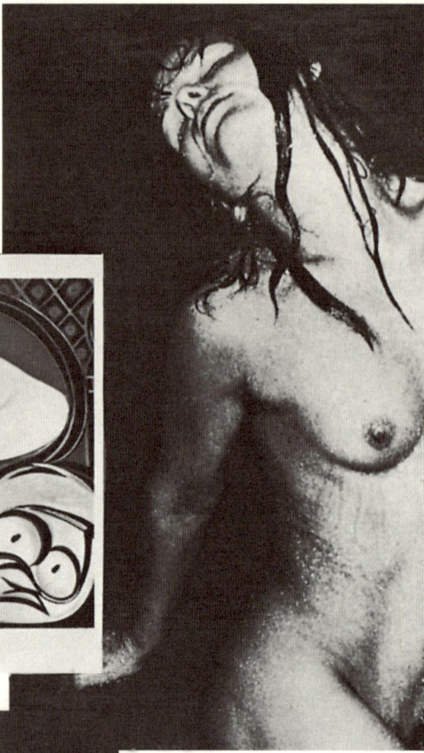
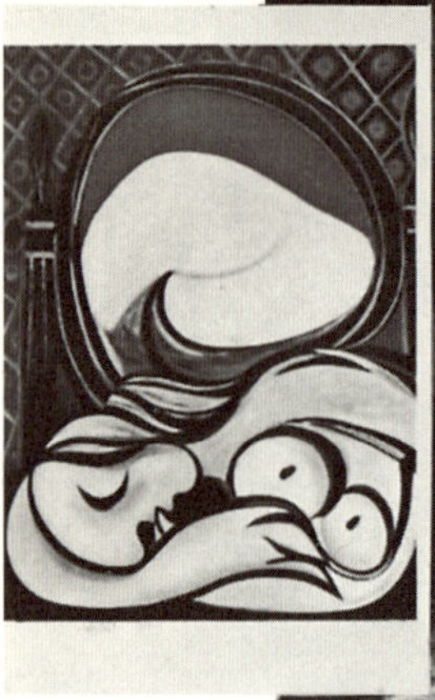
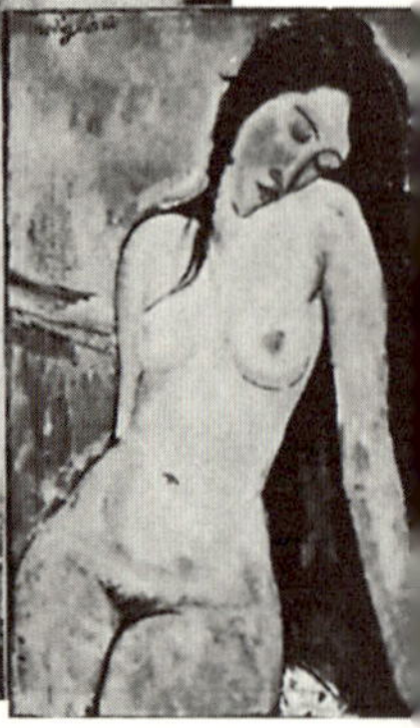
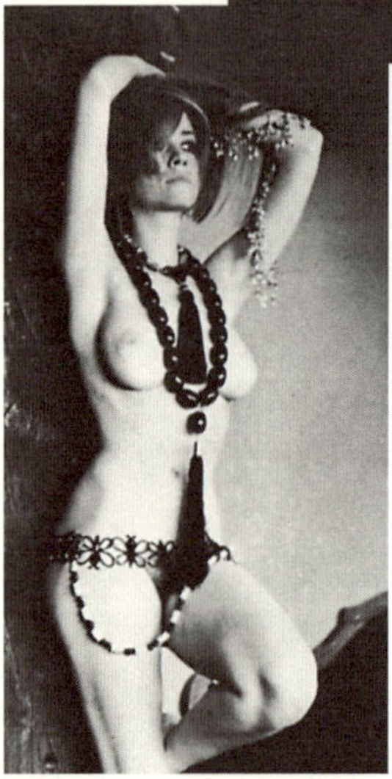
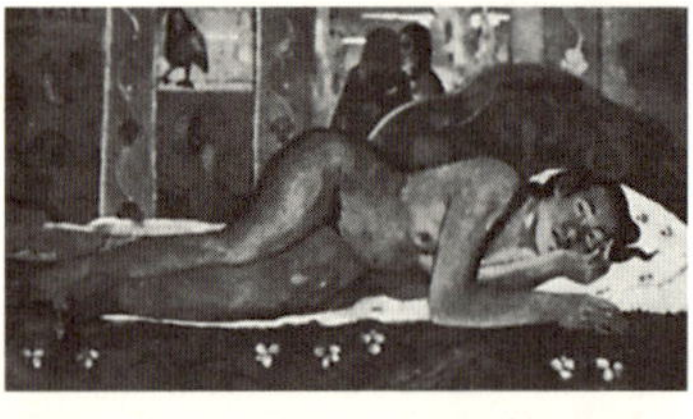
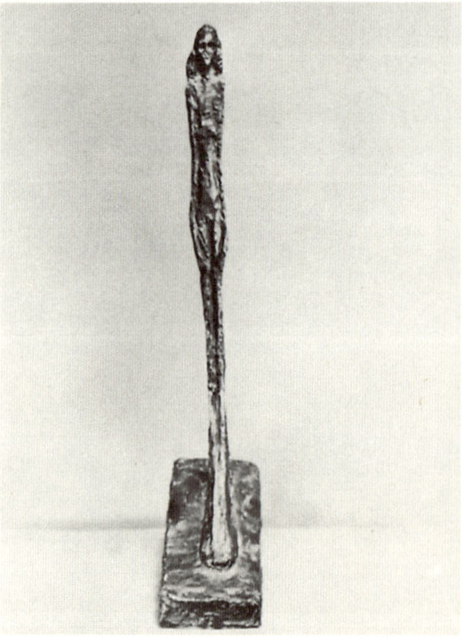

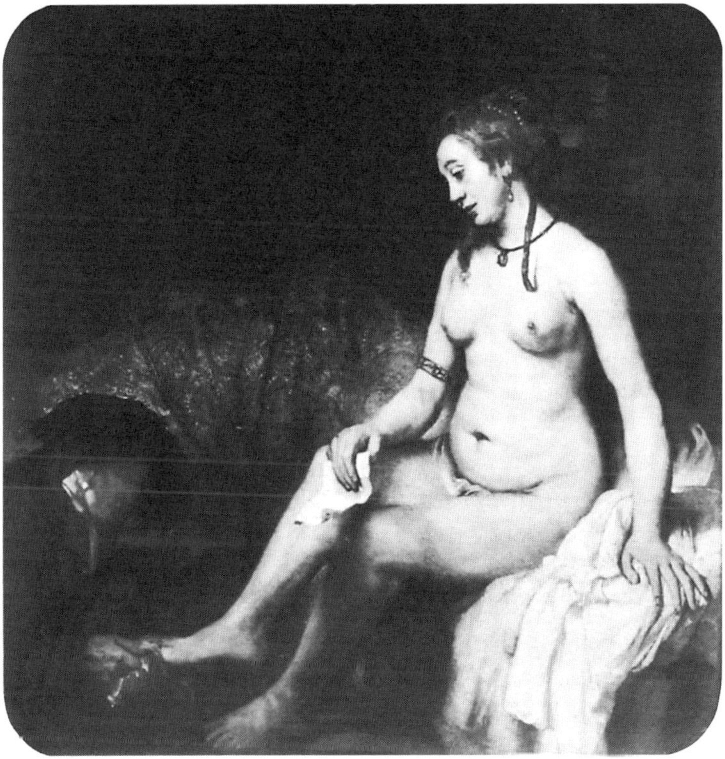

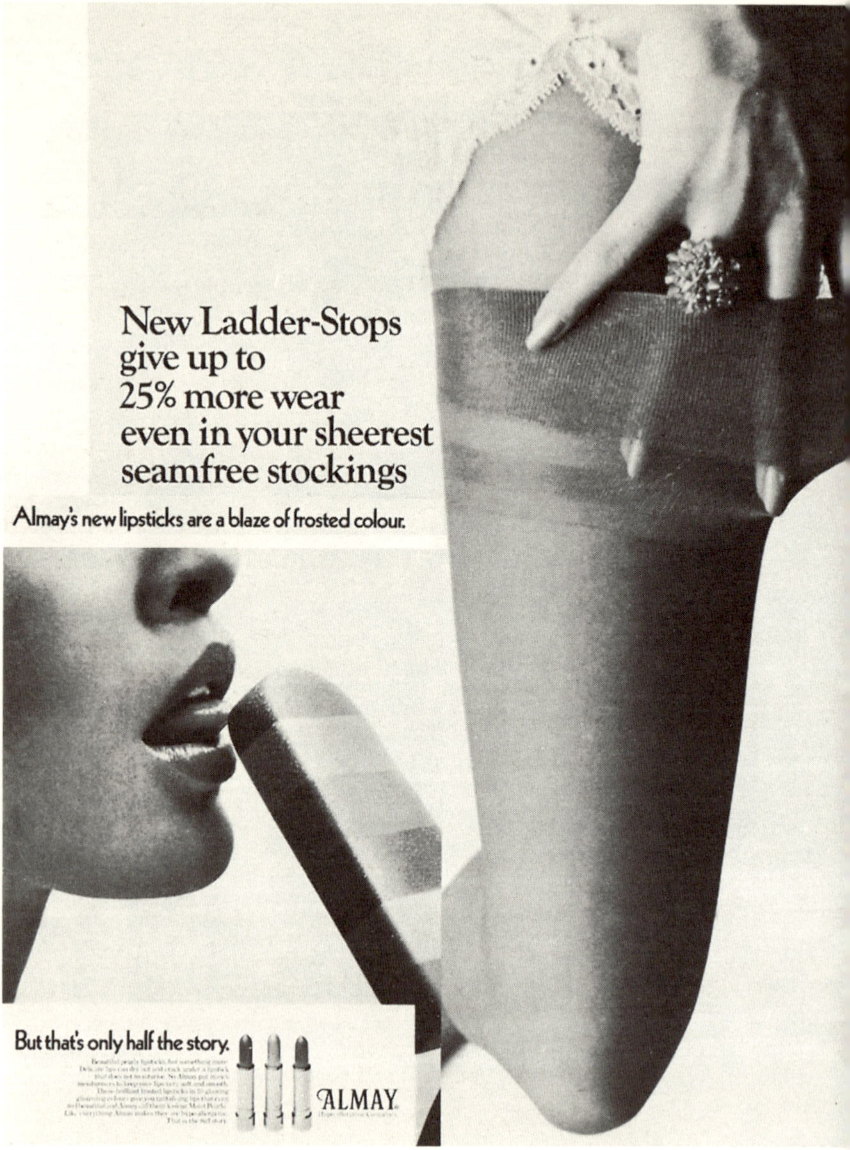
New Ladder-Stops
give up to
25% more wear
even in your sheerest
seamfree stockings
Almay's new lipsticks are a blaze of frosted colour.
But that's only half the story.
ALMAY

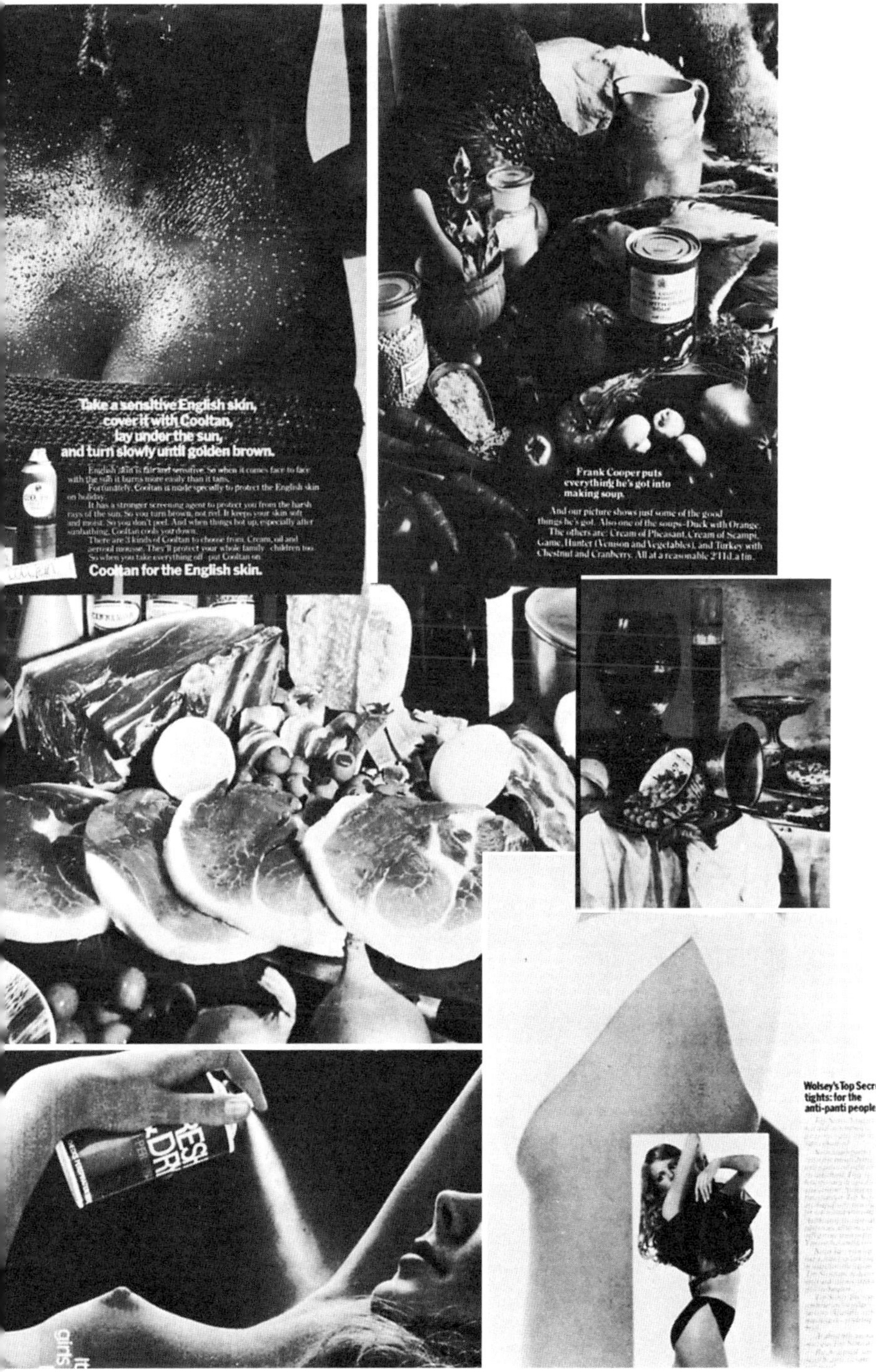
Take a sensitive English skin,
cover it with Cooltan,
lay under the sun,
and turn slowly until golden brown.
English skin is fair and sensitive. So when it comes face to face with the sun it burns more easily than it tans.
Fortunately, Cooltan is made specially to protect the English skin on holiday.
It has a stronger screening agent to protect you from the harsh rays of the sun. So you turn brown, not red. It keeps your skin soft and moist. So you don't peel. And when things hot up, especially after sunbathing, Cooltan cools you down.
There are 3 kinds of Cooltan to choose from. Cream, oil and aerosol mousse. They'll protect your whole family children too.
So when you take everything off put Cooltan on.
Cooltan for the English skin.
Frank Cooper puts everything he's got into making soup.
And our picture shows just some of the good things he's got. Also one of the soups–Duck with Orange.
The others are: Cream of Pheasant, Cream of Scampi, Game, Hunter (Venison and Vegetables), and Turkey with Chestnut and Cranberry. All at a reasonable 2/11d. a tin.
Wolsey's Top Secret tights: for the anti-panti people.

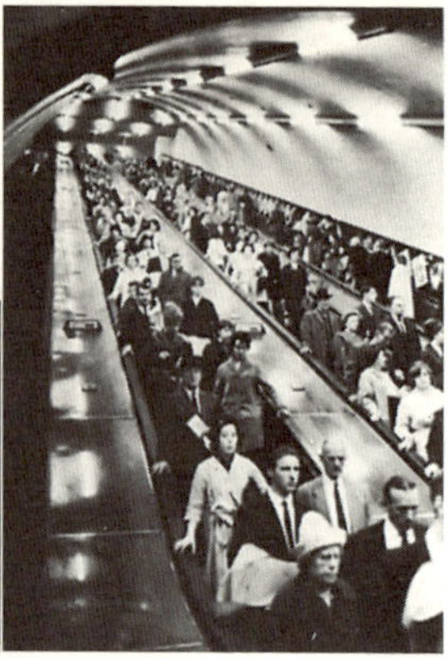

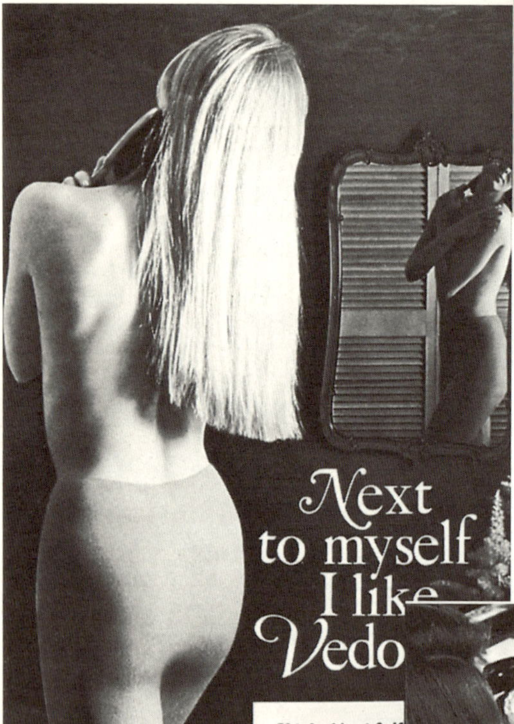
Next
to myself
I lik
Vedo
Obtainable at Self

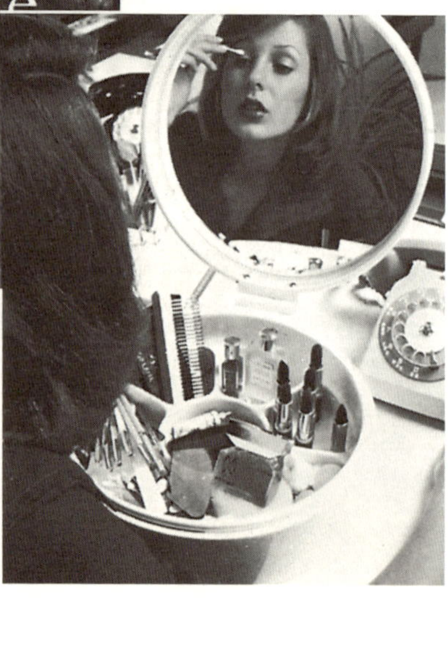

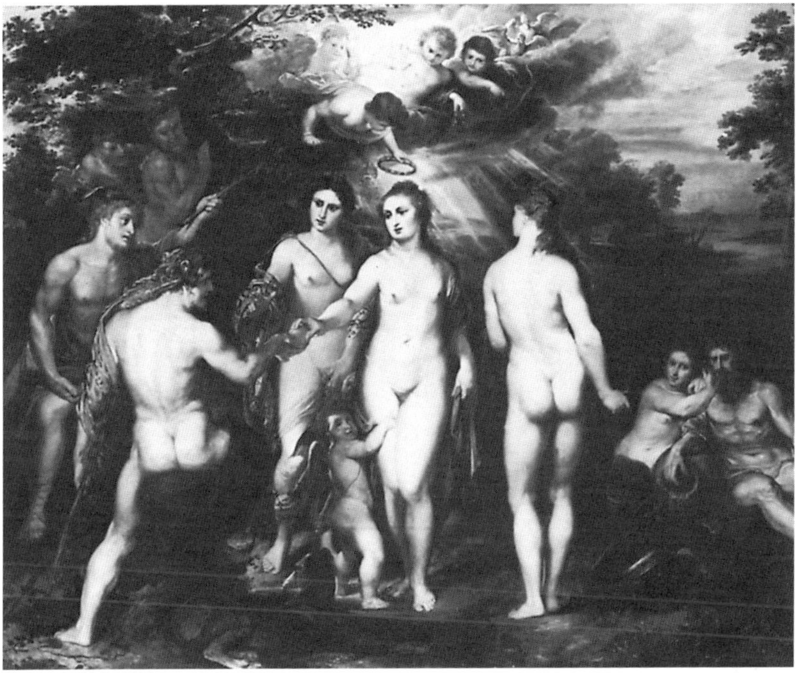

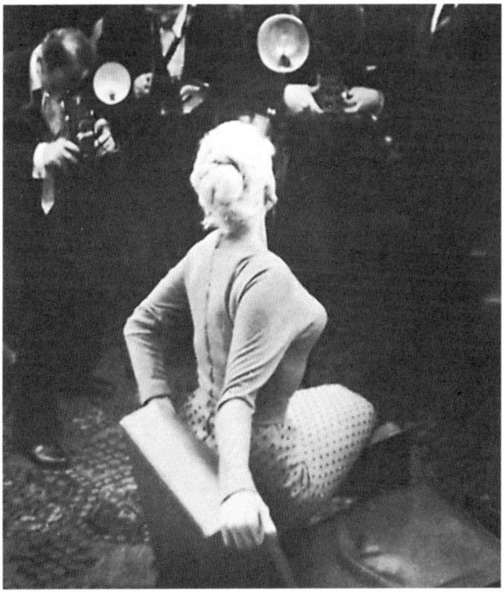

3

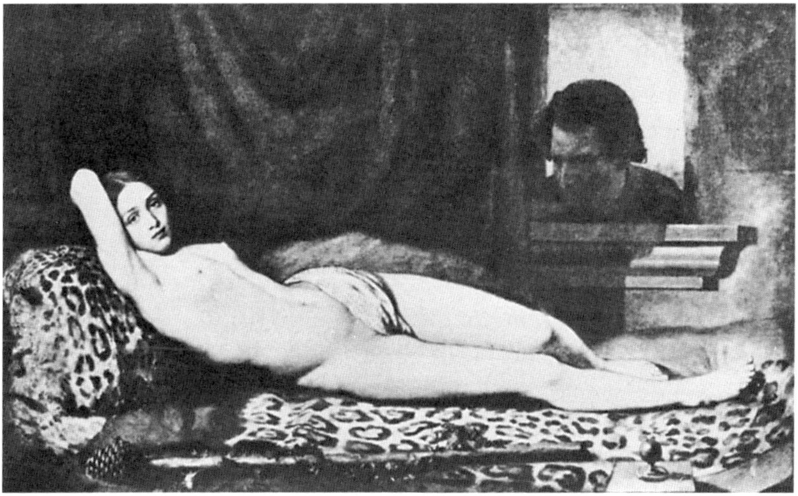

ОБНАЖЕННАЯ НА ШКУРЕ ПАНТЕРЫ. ТРЮТА. 1824–1848

Согласно традиции и обычаю, уже обсуждаемым, но еще не преодоленным, характер присутствия женщины в социуме отличается от характера присутствия мужчины. Присутствие мужчины держится на обещании силы, которую он воплощает. Если это обещание внушительное и убедительное, то и присутствие его заметное. Если же оно скромное или неубедительное, то и место мужчина занимает соответствующее. Обещанная сила может быть моральной, физической, эмоциональной, экономической, социальной, сексуальной, но в любом случае ее объект внеположен самому мужчине. Мужское присутствие говорит о том, *что* он может сделать тебе или для тебя. Это присутствие может быть мистификацией – в том смысле, что мужчина может лишь делать вид, что он способен на что-то, на что в действительности он не способен. Но в любом случае это претензия на силу, которая может быть применена в отношении кого-то другого.

Напротив, характер присутствия женщины выражает ее собственное отношение к себе и определяет, что с нею может или не может быть сделано. Ее присутствие выражается в ее жестах, голосе, мнениях, высказываниях, одежде, избираемом окружении, вкусе; на самом деле буквально все, что она делает, влияет на характер ее присутствия. Присутствовать настолько свойственно женщине, что мужчины склонны воспринимать ее присутствие как некую, можно сказать, физическую эманацию, своего рода тепло, или запах, или ауру.

Родиться женщиной значило родиться в установленном и замкнутом пространстве, под опеку мужчины. Характер женского присутствия в обществе сформировался вследствие навыка женщин жить под такой опекой и в таком ограниченном пространстве. Но за это женщине пришлось поплатиться раздвоением личности. Женщина должна постоянно наблюдать за собой. Она практически все время носит с собой образ самой себя. Идет ли она по комнате или плачет о смерти своего отца, она не может не представлять себя идущей или плачущей. С самого раннего детства ее учили и убеждали все время следить за собой.

И так она привыкает считать *наблюдающего* и *наблюдаемого* в себе двумя обязательными, но всегда отдельными составляющими своей личности.

Она должна все время следить за тем, кто она и что делает, поскольку то, как ее видят окружающие, а в конечном счете то, как ее видят мужчины, имеет решающее значение для того, что обычно считается удачей в женской жизни. Ее переживание себя вытесняется переживанием того, как она оценивается другими.

Прежде чем начать общаться с женщиной, мужчины ее рассматривают. Следовательно, то, какой женщину увидят, может определить то, как с ней будут общаться. Чтобы приобрести какой-то контроль над этим процессом, женщина вынуждена его интериоризировать. Часть женской личности, играющая роль наблюдателя, строит отношения с наблюдаемой частью, чтобы показать окружающим, как следует обращаться с ее личностью в целом. В этом показательном общении с самой собой и состоит ее присутствие. Характер женского присутствия регулирует, что допустимо, а что недопустимо в ее присутствии. В любом ее действии (какой бы ни была его непосредственная цель и мотивировка) также прочитывается указание на то, как женщина хочет, чтобы с ней обращались. Если женщина бросает стакан на пол, она таким образом показывает, как относится к собственному гневу, а значит, как хотела бы, чтобы к нему относились окружающие. Если то же самое делает мужчина, его действие прочитывается просто как выражение его ярости. Если женщина хорошо шутит, то она так демонстрирует свое отношение к шутнику внутри нее, а соответственно, то, как она хочет, чтобы к ней (в роли шутящей женщины) относились окружающие. Только мужчина может просто пошутить, ради самой шутки.

Можно сказать все то же самое проще: *мужчины действуют*, а *женщины выглядят*. Мужчины смотрят на женщин. Женщины смотрят на то, как на них смотрят. Это в большинстве случаев определяет не только отношение мужчин к женщинам, но также и отношение женщин к самим себе. Наблюдатель внутри женщины – мужчина, а наблюдаемый – женщина. Таким образом, она превращает себя в объект, в объект видения – в зрелище.

В одной из категорий европейской масляной живописи женщины были основным, постоянно повторяющимся сюжетом. Речь идет об изображении обнаженной натуры. Обнаженные фигуры европейской живописи помогут нам выявить некоторые условности и критерии, в рамках которых женщины виделись и расценивались как зрелище, предмет рассмотрения.

Первые обнаженные фигуры в этой традиции – изображения Адама и Евы. Стоит вспомнить их историю, как она изложена в Книге Бытия:

> «И увидела жена, что дерево хорошо для пищи и что оно приятно для глаз и вожделенно, потому что дает знание; и взяла плодов его и ела; и дала также мужу своему, и он ел. И открылись глаза у них обоих, и узнали они, что наги, и сшили смоковные листья, и сделали себе опоясания…
>
> И воззвал Господь Бог к Адаму и сказал ему: где ты?
>
> Он сказал: голос Твой я услышал в раю, и убоялся, потому что я наг, и скрылся…
>
> И сказал Господь Бог жене: умножая умножу скорбь твою в беременности твоей; в болезни будешь рождать детей; и к мужу твоему влечение твое, и он будет господствовать над тобою».

Что поражает в этой истории? Они осознали, что они наги, поскольку, съев яблоко, каждый увидел другого в ином свете. Нагота возникла в сознании зрителя.

Во-вторых, обращает на себя внимание то, что женщина обвиняется в произошедшем и наказывается подчинением мужчине. В отношении женщины мужчина становится представителем Бога.

В средневековой традиции эта история часто иллюстрировалась сцена за сценой, как в комиксе.

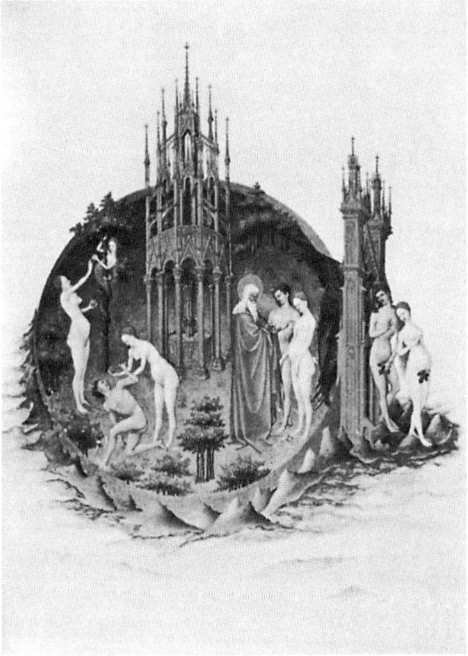

ГРЕХОПАДЕНИЕ И ИЗГНАНИЕ ИЗ РАЯ.
ПОЛЬ ДЕ ЛИМБУРГ.
НАЧАЛО XV ВЕКА

АДАМ И ЕВА.
МАБЮЗ.
НАЧАЛО XVI ВЕКА

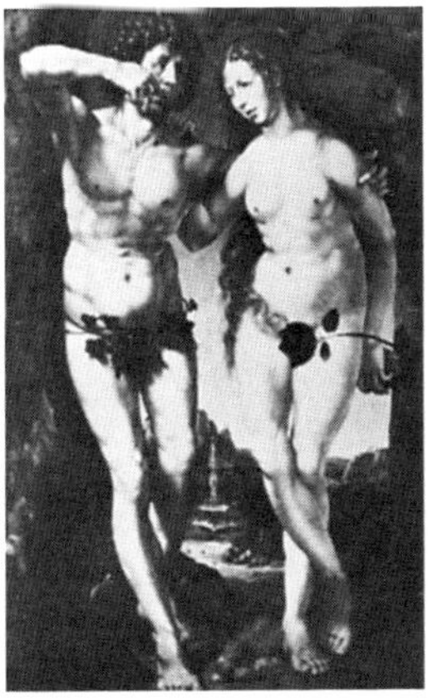

В эпоху Возрождения повествовательная последовательность исчезла и единственным изображаемым моментом стал момент стыда. Пара держит большие фиговые листы и прикрывается руками. Но теперь они стыдятся не столько друг друга, сколько зрителя.

Позднее стыд стал уже своего рода игрой на публику.

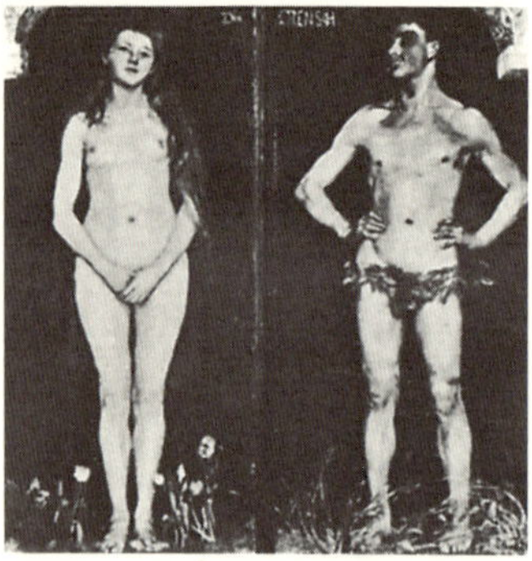

ПАРА. МАКС СЛЕФОГТ. 1868–1932

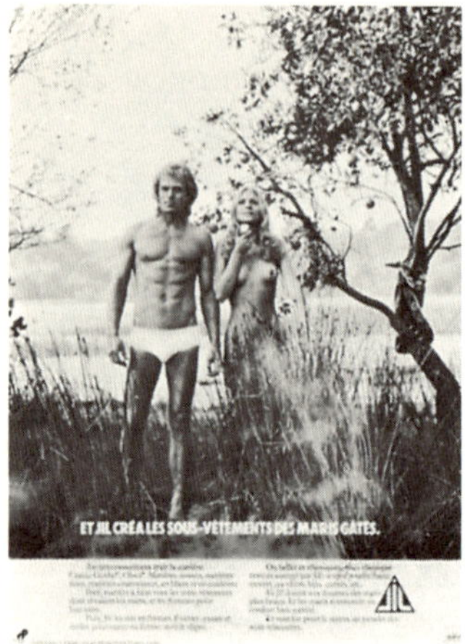

РЕКЛАМА НИЖНЕГО БЕЛЬЯ

Когда живописная традиция сделалась более светской, обнаженную натуру стали изображать и в рамках иных тем. Но во всех случаях сохраняется впечатление, будто предмет изображения – женщина – осознает, что на нее смотрит зритель.

Она обнажена не сама по себе.

Она обнажена в глазах зрителя.

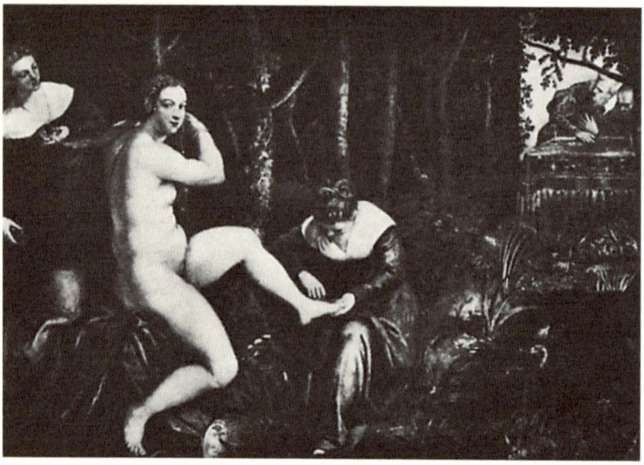

СУСАННА И СТАРЦЫ. ТИНТОРЕТТО

Нередко (как в случае с излюбленным сюжетом «Сусанна и старцы») это является и непосредственным сюжетом картины. Мы вместе со старцами подглядываем за тем, как Сусанна купается. Она оглядывается на нас, смотрящих на нее.

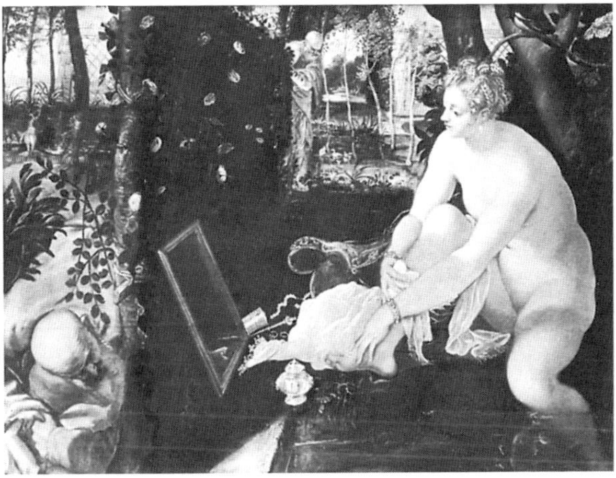

СУСАННА
И СТАРЦЫ.
ТИНТОРЕТТО.
1518–1594

В другой версии того же сюжета у Тинторетто Сусанна смотрит на себя в зеркало, таким образом присоединяясь к собственным зрителям.

Зеркало часто использовалось как символ женского тщеславия. Впрочем, в основном такого рода морализаторство – чистое лицемерие.

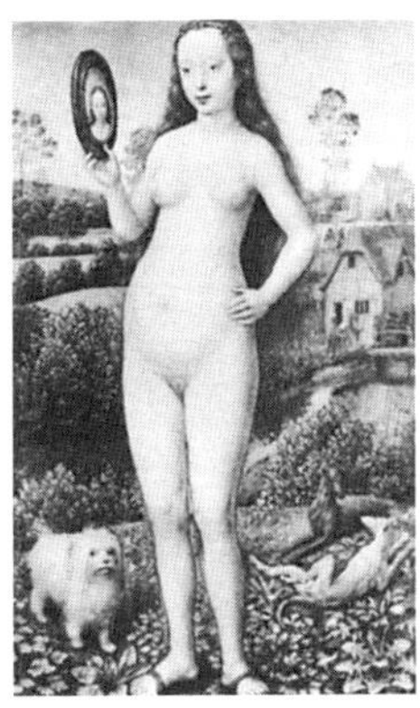

ЗЕМНОЕ ТЩЕСЛАВИЕ
И БОЖЕСТВЕННОЕ ИСКУПЛЕНИЕ.
МЕМЛИНГ.
1435–1494

Вы изображаете обнаженную женщину, потому что вам нравится смотреть на нее, вы даете ей в руку зеркало и называете картину «Земное тщеславие», таким образом порицая женщину, наготу которой вы изобразили ради собственного удовольствия.

Реальная функция зеркала была иной. Оно было нужно для того, чтобы женщина сама санкционировала отношение к себе как – главным образом и в первую очередь – к зрелищу.

Суд Париса – другая тема, развивающая ту же идею мужчины (или мужчин), смотрящего (смотрящих) на обнаженных женщин.

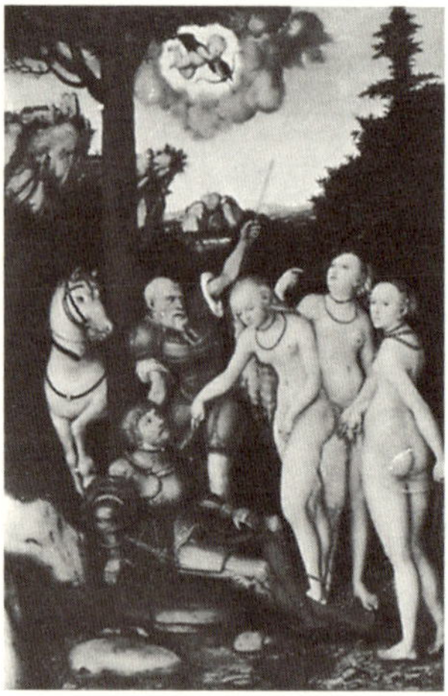

СУД ПАРИСА.
КРАНАХ.
1472–1553

Но здесь оказывается добавлен дополнительный элемент. Элемент оценки. Парис преподносит яблоко женщине, которую находит самой красивой. Таким образом, Красота становится предметом соревнования. (Сегодня Суд Париса превратился в Конкурс красоты.) Те, кого не признали красивыми, некрасивы. Те, кого признали, получают приз.

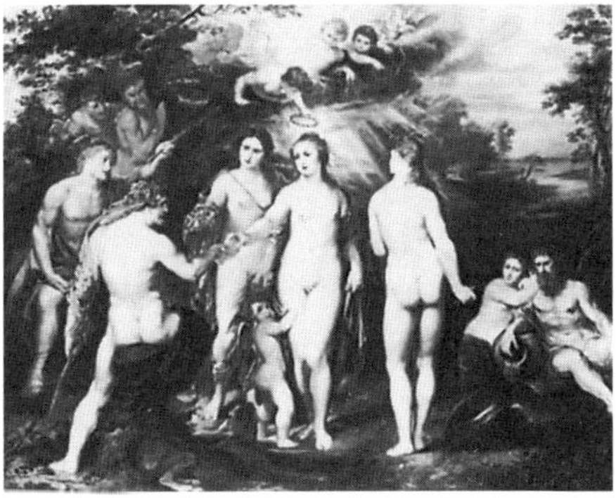

СУД ПАРИСА.
РУБЕНС.
1577–1640

Приз – это не что иное, как стать собственностью судьи, быть ему доступной. Карл II сделал Лели тайный заказ. Мы видим крайне характерное для данной традиции изображение: номинально это может быть Венера и Купидон. Фактически – это портрет одной из любовниц короля, Нелль Гвин. Она пассивно смотрит на зрителя, рассматривающего ее обнаженной.

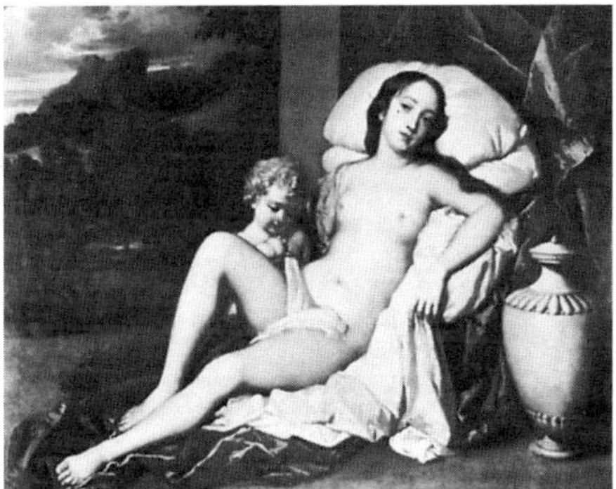

НЕЛЛЬ ГВИН.
ЛЕЛИ.
1618–1680

Однако ее нагота не является выражением ее собственных чувств; это знак ее подчинения чувствам и желаниям владельца. (Владельца и картины, и женщины.) Картина, когда король показывал ее кому-нибудь, демонстрировала это подчинение – и его гости ему завидовали.

Следует отметить, что в других, не европейских, традициях – в индийском, в персидском, в африканском искусстве – нагота не бывает такой пассивной. И если в рамках этих традиций предметом изображения становится сексуальное влечение, то, скорее всего, здесь будет показано активное сексуальное взаимодействие между двумя людьми: женщина не менее активна, чем мужчина, действия участников захватывают их обоих.

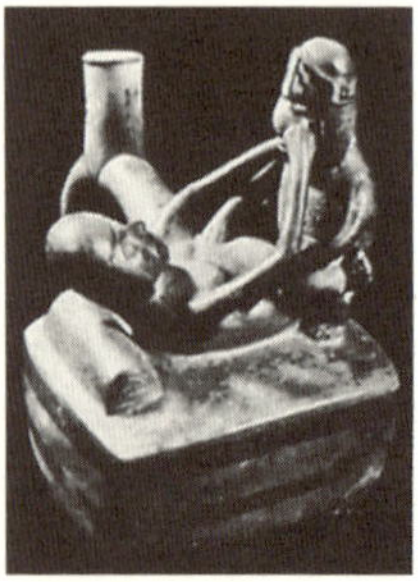
КЕРАМИКА МОЧЕ

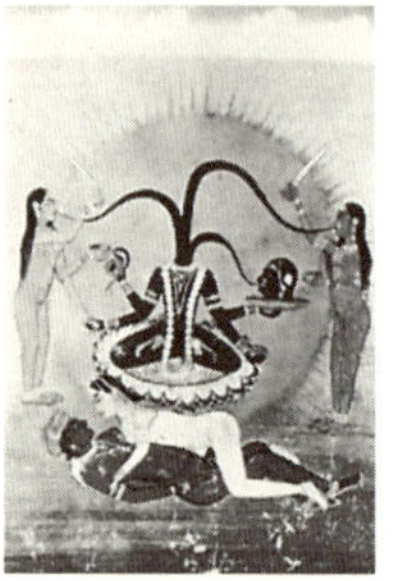
РАДЖАСТАН. XVIII ВЕК

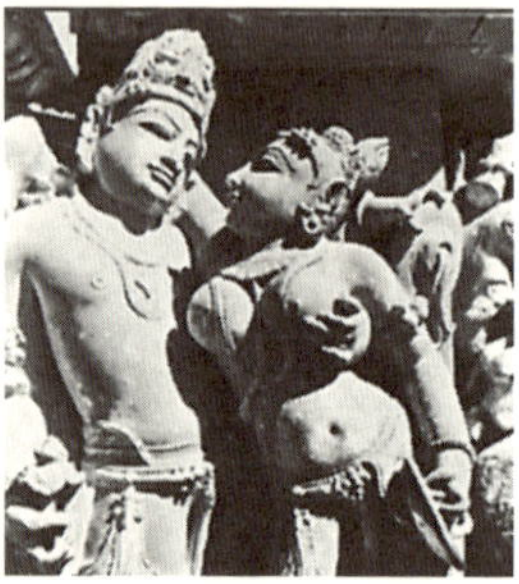
ВИШНУ И ЛАКШМИ. XI ВЕК

Теперь мы можем рассмотреть разницу между голым телом и обнаженной натурой в европейской традиции. В своей книге о наготе Кеннет Кларк доказывает, что голое тело просто лишено одежды, в то время как обнаженная натура – это форма искусства. Согласно Кларку нагота – это не отправная точка для создания картины, а способ видения, которым пользуется художник. В некоторой степени это правда, но такой способ видения не ограничивается исключительно живописью: существует, например, обнаженная модель в фотографии. Что правда, так это

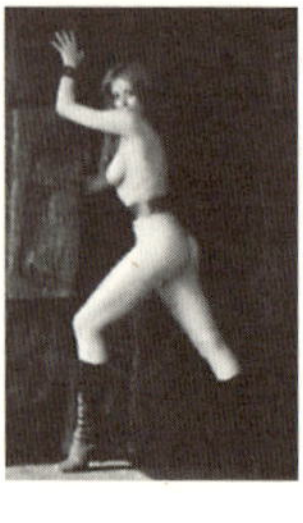

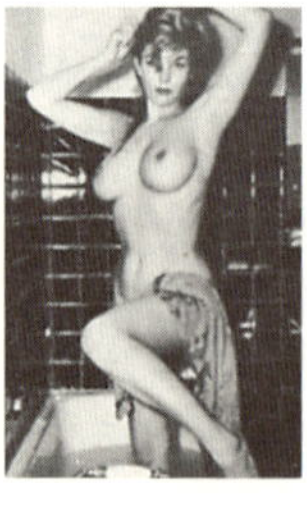

то, что обнаженная натура всегда подчиняется определенного рода условностям, и влиянием своим эти условности обязаны вполне определенной художественной традиции.

Что означают эти условности? Что обозначает собой нагота? Недостаточно ответить на эти вопросы просто в искусствоведческих терминах, поскольку вполне очевидно, что нагота имеет отношение также и к переживаемой сексуальности.

Быть голым – это быть самим собой.

Быть обнаженным – это быть увиденным голым со стороны и в то же время не осознавать свою наготу самому. Голое тело, чтобы стать обнаженным, должно быть увидено как объект. Голое тело открывает себя. Обнаженная модель выставлена на обозрение.

Быть голым – значит оставаться без всякой маски.

Быть на всеобщем обозрении – значит превратить поверхность своей собственной кожи, волоски своего собственного тела в маску, которую уже невозможно снять. Обнаженная натура не имеет возможности стать голым телом. Обнаженность – вид одежды.

На среднестатистической европейской картине, изображающей обнаженную модель, никогда нельзя увидеть ее главного героя. Главный герой – зритель, стоящий перед картиной, и предполагается, что он мужчина. Все обращено к нему. Все должно выглядеть результатом его присутствия. Это для него фигуры на картине обрели свою наготу. Но он, по определению, посторонний, и вся его одежда на нем.

Рассмотрим «Аллегорию с Венерой и Амуром» Бронзино.

Сложная символика, стоящая за этой картиной, не будет нас сейчас занимать, поскольку она не влияет на ее сексуальный смысл, который мы воспринимаем в первую очередь. Прежде всего остального это полотно – сексуальная провокация.

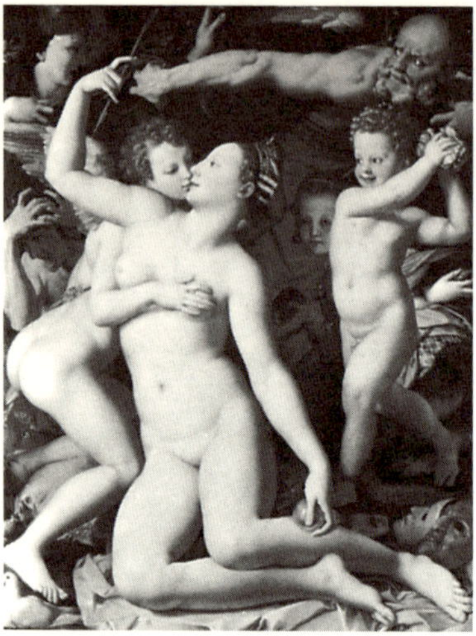

ВЕНЕРА, КУПИДОН, БЕЗРАССУДСТВО И ВРЕМЯ. БРОНЗИНО. 1503–1572

Эта картина была подарена королю Франции Великим герцогом Флорентийским. Опирающийся коленями на подушку и целующий женщину мальчик – это Купидон. Она – Венера. Но ее поза не имеет никакого отношения к их поцелую. Эта поза придана ее телу для того, чтобы его лучше мог рассмотреть глядящий на картину мужчина. Картина написана таким образом, чтобы будить именно его сексуальность. Она не имеет никакого отношения к ее сексуальности. (Здесь, как и в европейской традиции в целом, той же цели служит правило, согласно которому на женском теле не изображаются волосы. Волосы ассоциируются с сексуальной силой, со страстью. Женская страсть должна быть минимизирована, чтобы зритель мог почувствовать себя монопольным обладателем сексуальной силы). Женщина присутствует здесь для того, чтобы удовлетворять мужской аппетит, а не для того, чтобы выказывать собственный.

Сравните выражения лиц этих женщин:
одна из них изображена на известной картине Энгра, вторая – сфотографирована для мужского журнала.

БОЛЬШАЯ ОДАЛИСКА.
ЭНГР.
1780–1867

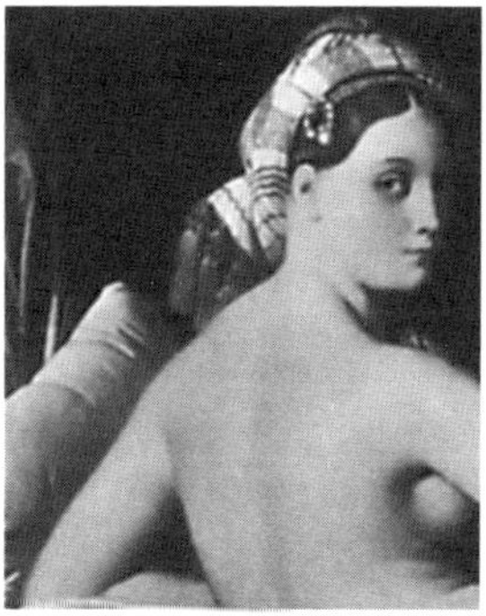

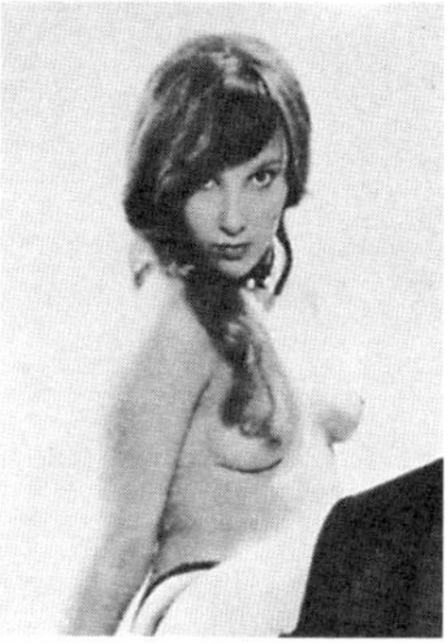

Не кажутся ли вам их лица поразительно схожими? И там и там женщина глядит с умело просчитанным очарованием на мужчину, который, как ей представляется, смотрит на нее, хотя она его и не знает. Она предлагает свою женственность как предмет рассмотрения.

Это правда, что порой такого рода картины изображают еще и мужчину-любовника.

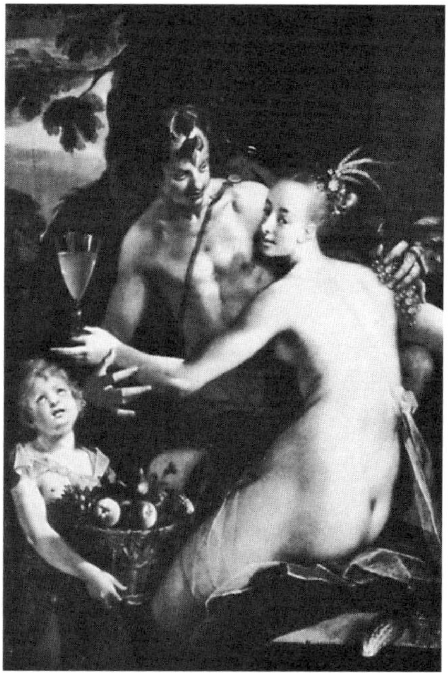

ВАКХ, ЦЕРЕРА И КУПИДОН.
ФОН ААХЕН.
1552–1615

Однако внимание женщины редко направлено на него. Очень часто она смотрит мимо него или вовне, на того, кто считает себя ее настоящим любовником: на зрителя-владельца.

Существовала и отдельная категория частных порнографических картин (особенно в XVIII веке), на которых изображались пары, занимающиеся любовью. Но даже в отношении таких картин очевиден факт, что зритель-владелец в своих фантазиях призван вытеснить изображенного там мужчину – или идентифицироваться с ним. И напротив, изображение двух любовников в неевропейской традиции несет в себе идею, что занимающихся любовью – великое множество. «У нас тысяча рук и тысяча ног, и мы никогда не будем одиноки».

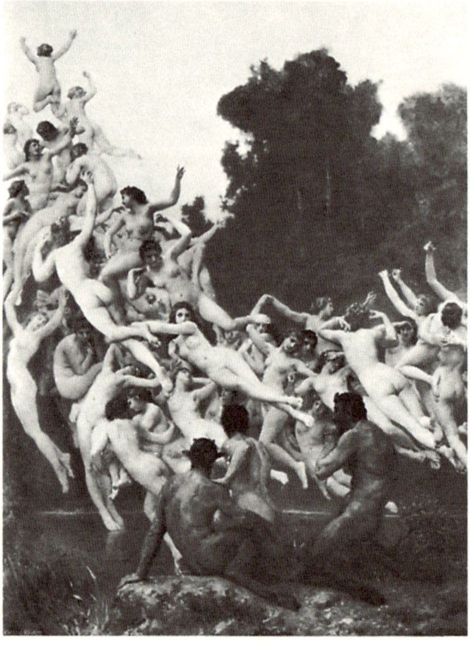

ОРЕАДЫ.
БУГРО.
1825–1905

Практически вся постренессансная европейская живопись эротического характера прямолинейна (в прямом и переносном смысле), поскольку главный сексуальный герой этой живописи – зритель-владелец, глядящий на нее.

Абсурдность этой лести мужчин самим себе достигла вершины в монументальной академической живописи XIX века. Государственные мужи и деловые люди вели споры о политике и бизнесе под картинами вроде «Ореад» Бугро. Когда кто-то из них чувствовал, что его побеждают, он поднимал глаза, ища утешения. То, что он видел, напоминало ему о том, что он – мужчина.

В европейской традиции масляной живописи существует ряд картин, представляющих собой исключение из этого правила; к ним приложимо очень немногое из сказанного выше. На самом деле тут перед нами уже не обнаженная модель, эти картины выходят за пределы описанной формы искусства; это картины, изображающие любимых женщин, более или менее обнаженных. На сотни тысяч портретов обнаженных моделей, составляющих традицию, приходится не больше сотни таких исключений. В каждом из этих портретов личное видение художником женщины, которая ему позирует, оказывается настолько сильным, что уже не учитывает зрителя. Видение художника рождает прочнейшую связь между ним и женщиной на картине. Художник и модель становятся неразделимы – словно высечены из одного камня. Зритель может быть свидетелем их отношений, но не более того: его заставляют осознать, что он тут посторонний. Зритель не может убедить себя, что женщина на картине обнажена для него. Он не может превратить ее в обнаженную модель. То, как художник нарисовал ее, включает ее волю и ее намерения в саму структуру образа, в выражение ее лица, в ее позу.

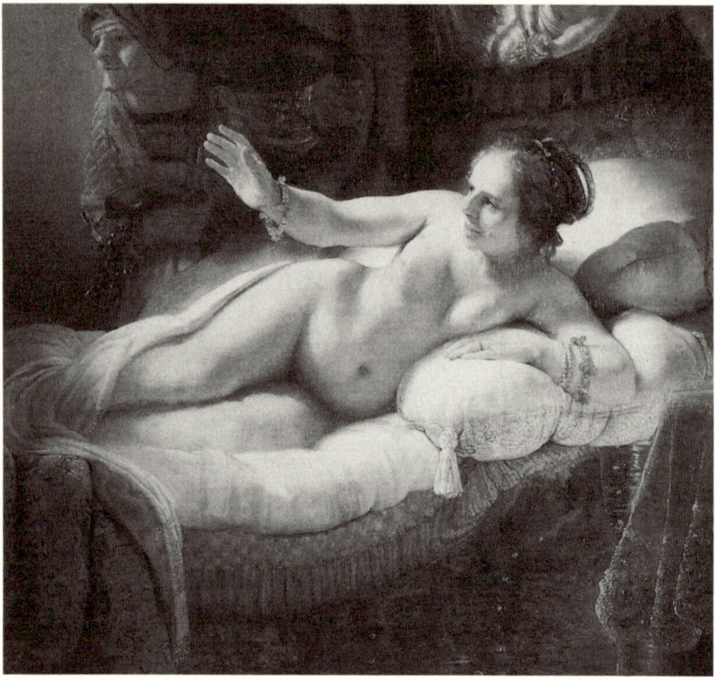

ДАНАЯ. РЕМБРАНДТ. 1606–1669

Типичное и исключительное в рамках традиции может быть описано с помощью антиномии «голое тело» vs «обнаженная модель», но сама проблема изображения наготы не так проста, как может сперва показаться.

Какова сексуальная функция наготы в реальности? Одежда мешает контакту и сковывает движения. Но все-таки нагота имеет положительный визуальный смысл и сама по себе: мы хотим *видеть* чужую наготу. Другой позволяет нам себя видеть – и мы хватаемся за эту возможность, порой совершенно независимо от того, происходит это в первый раз или в сотый. Что для нас значит вид другого человека? Как этот момент полной обнаженности влияет на наши чувства?

Чужая нагота – это доказательство, которое вызывает очень сильное чувство облегчения. Она такая же женщина, как и любая другая. Или: он такой же мужчина, как и любой другой. Мы поражены изумительной простотой знакомого сексуального механизма.

Разумеется, на уровне сознания мы не ожидали, что все будет по-другому: к подспудному ожиданию чего-то иного могли привести скорее бессознательные гомосексуальные влечения (или бессознательные гетеросексуальные влечения, если рассматривать гомосексуальную пару). Но «облегчение», о котором шла речь, можно объяснить без обращения к бессознательному.

Мы и не ожидали увидеть их иными, но сила и сложность наших чувств порождают ощущение уникальности, которое рассеивается при виде другого, каков он есть. Он больше похож на остальных людей его пола, чем отличается от них. В этом открывается нам теплая и дружественная (в противовес холодной и безличной) анонимность наготы.

Можно сказать по-другому: обнажение привносит с собой элемент банальности (но этот элемент существует только потому, что мы нуждаемся в нем).

Вплоть до самого этого мгновения другой остается для нас в той или иной степени тайной. Этикетная скромность не является исключительно пуританством или сентиментальностью: есть смысл в том, чтобы утрата тайны была значимым событием. И объяснение этой утраты может быть во многом именно визуальным, поскольку речь здесь идет о смене фокуса восприятия. С глаз, рта, плеч, рук (которым свойственна такая тонкость экспрессии, что личность, выражаемая ими, предстает как крайне многогранная) восприятие переключается на собственно сексуальные части тела, устройство которых наводит на мысль о чрезвычайно манящем, но одном-единственном процессе. Другой сводится к первичным сексуальным категориям (или расширяется до них): мужчина или женщина. Наше облегчение – это облегчение от того, что мы обнаружили под одеждой не вызывающую вопросов реальность, прямым запросам которой наше, до того момента крайне запутанное, сознание теперь должно соответствовать.

Мы нуждаемся в банальности, которая обнаруживается в момент обнажения, потому что она дает нам чувство реальности. Но не только. Эта реальность, обещая хорошо знакомый, общеизвестный механизм секса, дает нам в то же время возможность испытать общую на двоих субъективность секса.

Утрата тайны происходит одновременно с обретением способов создания общей тайны. Последовательность тут следующая: субъективное – объективное – субъективное, возведенное во вторую степень.

Теперь можно понять, в чем заключается сложность, возникающая при создании статичного образа человеческой наготы. В живом сексуальном опыте нагота – это скорее процесс, чем состояние. Если изолировать из этого процесса отдельный момент, то получившийся образ будет казаться банальным, и его банальность произведет леденящее впечатление, вместо того чтобы служить мостом между двумя очень глубокими и поэтичными состояниями. По этой причине выразительные фотографии обнаженных женщин встречаются еще реже, чем картины. Простое решение для фотографа – это превратить фигуру в обнаженную модель, которая, обобщая и зрелище, и зрителя, и лишая сексуальность конкретности, превращает желание в фантазию.

Давайте рассмотрим одно исключение из описанной традиции изображения наготы. Это картина Рубенса,

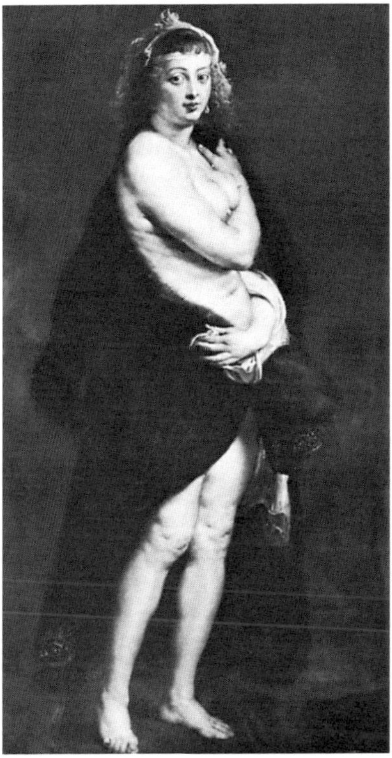

ШУБКА.
ПОРТРЕТ ЕЛЕНЫ ФОУРМЕН.
РУБЕНС.
1577–1640

портрет его юной второй жены, на которой он женился, уже будучи пожилым человеком.

Мы видим ее в движении: она поворачивается, шубка готова вот-вот упасть с ее плеч. Совершенно очевидно, что в такой позе она простоит не более секунды. В определенном смысле этот ее образ в своей мгновенности подобен фотографии. Но если смотреть глубже, картина «заключает» в себе время и его переживание. Легко можно представить, что за секунду до того как эта женщина накинула себе на плечи шубку, она была полностью обнажена. Последовательность, ведущая к моменту полной обнаженности или от него, оказывается преодолена. Изображенная женщина может принадлежать к любому из моментов этой последовательности или ко всем сразу.

Ее тело встает перед нами не как непосредственное зрелище, а как переживание – переживание художника. Почему? Есть этому поверхностные, несистемные объяснения: ее растрепанные волосы, ее взгляд, направленный на художника, умиление, с которым прописана чрезвычайная нежность ее кожи. Но глубинная причина вполне формальна. Ее внешность была в буквальном смысле переработана субъективным восприятием художника. Верхняя часть ее тела и ее ноги не могут встретиться под накинутой шубкой. Они смещены друг относительно друга примерно на девять дюймов.

Вероятно, Рубенс не планировал эту диспропорцию, а зритель может ее и не осознать. Сама по себе она несущественна. Важен эффект, который она производит. Она создает ощущение невероятной динамики. Тело находит свое единство уже не в самом себе, а в переживании художника. Точнее, указанная диспропорция позволяет верхней и нижней частям тела вращаться отдельно друг от друга и в разных направлениях, вокруг скрытого сексуального центра: торс движется вправо, а ноги влево. В то же время скрытый сексуальный центр связан посредством темной шубки с окружающей фигуру темнотой – и таким образом фигура оказывается двигающейся и вокруг темноты, и в темноте, а темнота, в свою очередь, становится метафорой ее пола.

Помимо необходимости преодолеть границы единственного мгновения и допустить вторжение субъективности, есть еще один элемент, обязательный, как мы видели, для любого выдающегося изображения наготы. Это элемент банальности, которая должна быть явной, но не отталкивающей. Это то, что проводит грань между вуайеристом и любовником. Здесь такая банальность обнаруживается в том, как маниакально Рубенс выписывает мягкость полного тела Елены, разбивающую всякие условности идеальной формы и говорящую (ему) о ее неповторимости.

Обнаженная натура в европейской живописи обычно преподносится как восхитительное выражение духа европейского гуманизма. Этот дух был неотделим от индивидуализма. И без развития предельно осознанного индивидуализма исключения из этой традиции (чрезвычайно личностные изображения обнаженных) не могли быть созданы. Однако традиция заключала в себе конфликт, который не мог разрешиться сам по себе. Несколько художников интуитивно осознали этот конфликт и разрешили его собственными методами, но их решения не могли быть усвоены культурной традицией в рамках ее методов и понятий.

Конфликт этот может быть описан очень просто. Это конфликт между индивидуализмом художника, мысли-

ХУДОЖНИК, РИСУЮЩИЙ ЛЕЖАЩУЮ ЖЕНЩИНУ. ДЮРЕР. 1471–1528

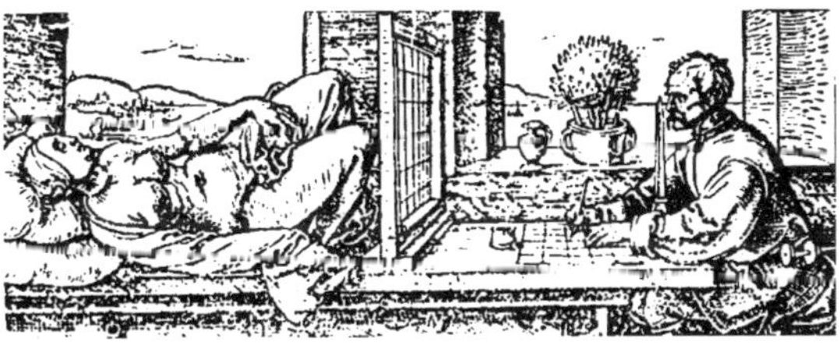

ГРАВЮРА НА ДЕРЕВЕ. ДЮРЕР. 1471–1528

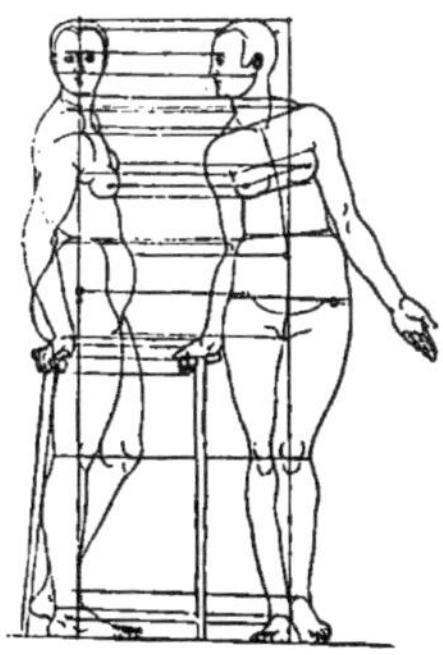

теля, покровителя, владельца – и тем, кто является объектом действия, то есть женщиной, к которой относятся как к вещи или как к абстракции.

Дюрер считал, что идеальная обнаженная фигура может быть создана, если соединить вместе лицо от одного тела, грудь от другого, ноги от третьего, плечи от четвертого, руки от пятого и так далее.

Результат должен был прославлять Человека. Но само это упражнение предполагало изрядное равнодушие к тому, кем является каждый отдельный человек.

В европейской традиции художниками и зрителями-владельцами обычно были мужчины, а теми, к кому относились как к объектам, – обычно женщины. Это неравноправие отношений настолько укоренено в нашей культуре, что до сих пор структурирует сознание многих женщин. Они обходятся с собой так, как с ними обходятся мужчины. Они, подобно мужчинам, наблюдают собственную женственность.

В современном искусстве обнаженность стала категорией менее важной. Сами художники начали смотреть на нее критически. В этом отношении (как и во многих других) поворотной фигурой был Мане. Если сравнить его «Олимпию» с оригиналом Тициана, то увидишь женщину, исполняющую традиционную роль, но исполняющую ее уже с некоторым вызовом.

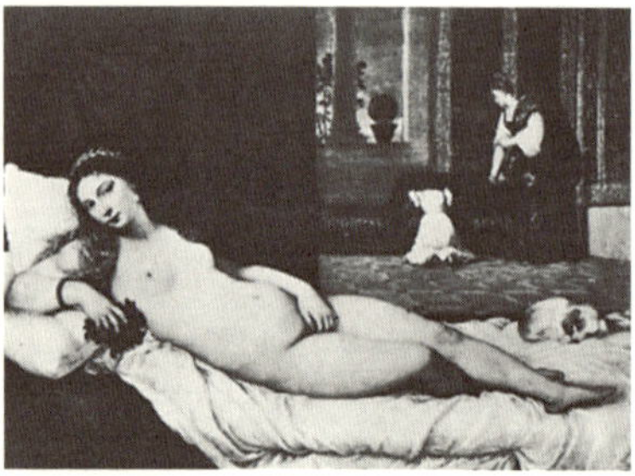

ВЕНЕРА УРБИНСКАЯ. ТИЦИАН. 1487–1576

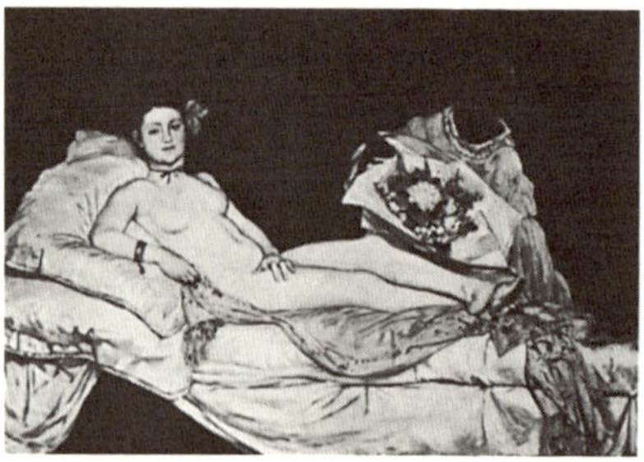

ОЛИМПИЯ. МАНЕ. 1832–1883

Идеал был разбит. Но его практически нечем было заменить, кроме «реализма» проститутки, ставшей самым характерным женским образом для авангарда начала XX века (Тулуз-Лотрек, Пикассо, Руо, немецкие экспрессионисты и т. д.) В академической же живописи традиция продолжала свое существование.

Сегодня установки и ценности, формировавшие эту традицию, выражают себя при помощи информационных средств, имеющих куда больший охват, – рекламы, журналистики, телевидения.

Но собственно способ видеть женщину и характер использования женских образов не изменились. Женщины изображаются совершенно иначе, чем мужчины, и не потому, что женственность отличается от мужественности, а потому, что «идеальный» зритель всегда мыслится как мужчина и женский образ создается так, чтобы польстить мужчине. Если у вас есть хоть какие-то сомнения в этом, проведите следующий эксперимент. Выберите одно из традиционных женских изображений, приведенных в нашей книге. И превратите эту женщину в мужчину. Можете сделать это в воображении, а можете подрисовать прямо на репродукции. Вы увидите, что такая трансформация воспринимается как насилие. Не по отношению к изображению, а по отношению к ожиданиям предполагаемого зрителя.

4

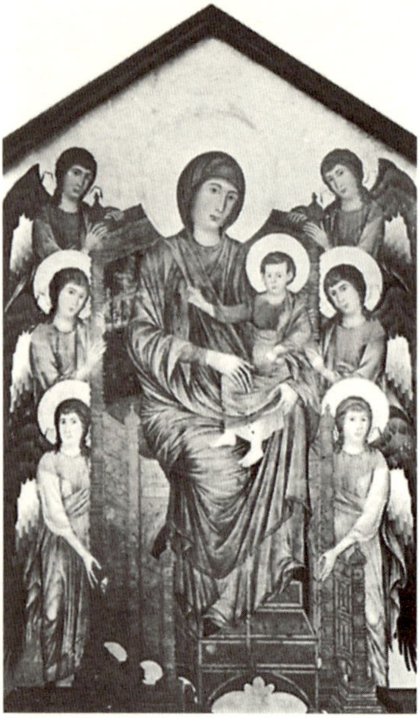

ЧИМАБУЭ. ОК. 1240–1302(?)

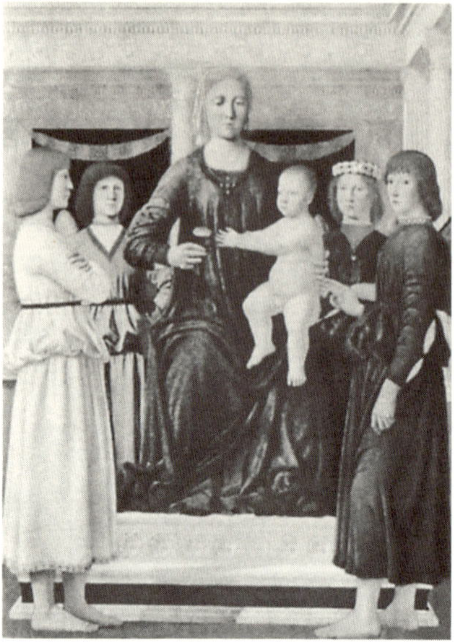

ПЬЕРО ДЕЛЛА ФРАНЧЕСКА. 1410/20–1492

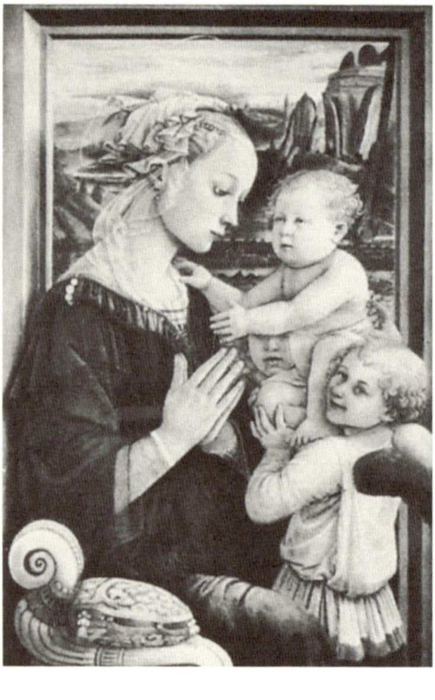

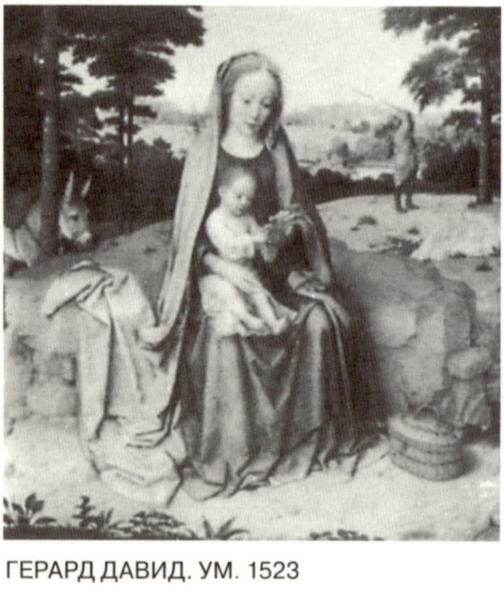

ГЕРАРД ДАВИД. УМ. 1523

ФРА ФИЛИППО ЛИППИ. 1457/8–1504

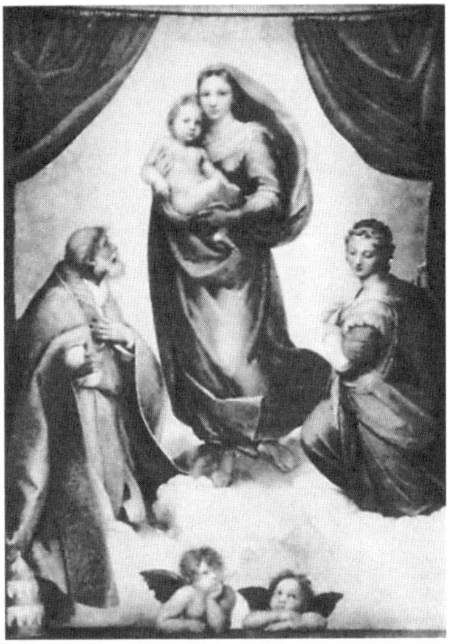

РАФАЭЛЬ. 1483–1520

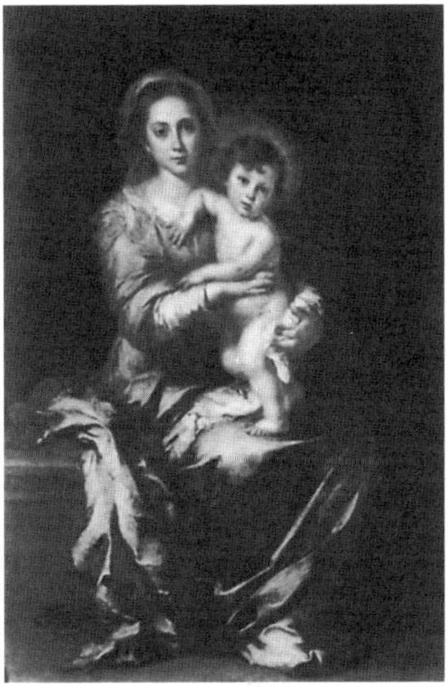

МУРИЛЬО. 1617–1682

ФОРД МЭДОКС БРАУН. 1821–1893

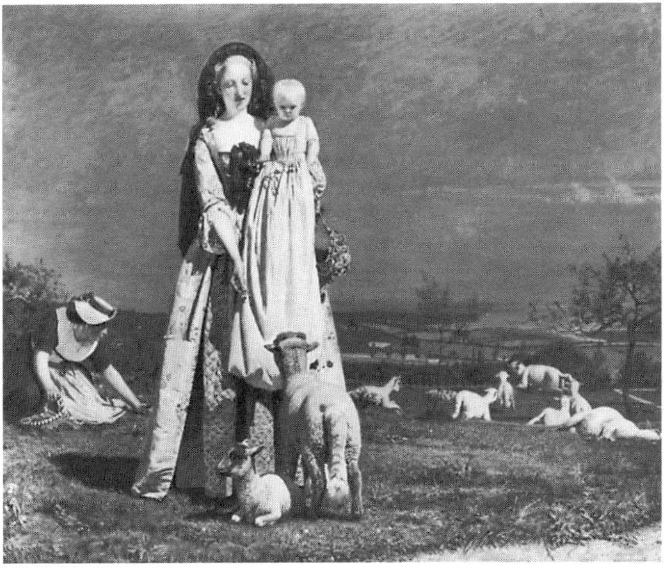

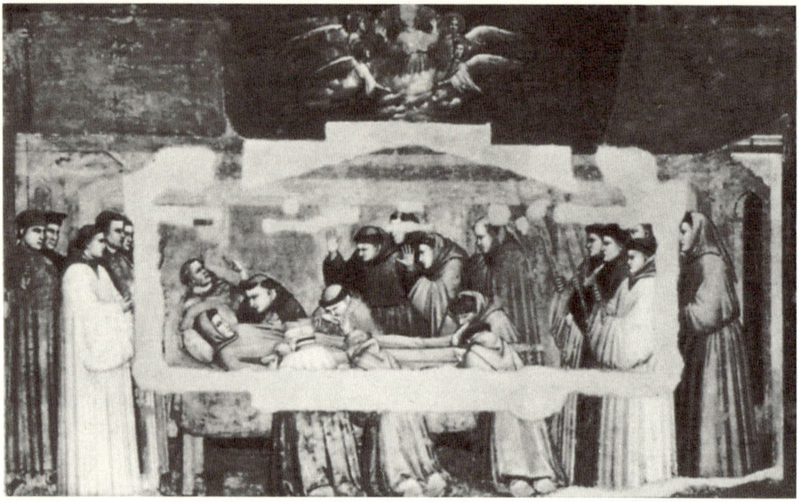

ДЖОТТО. 1266/7–1337

ПИТЕР БРЕЙГЕЛЬ. 1525–1569

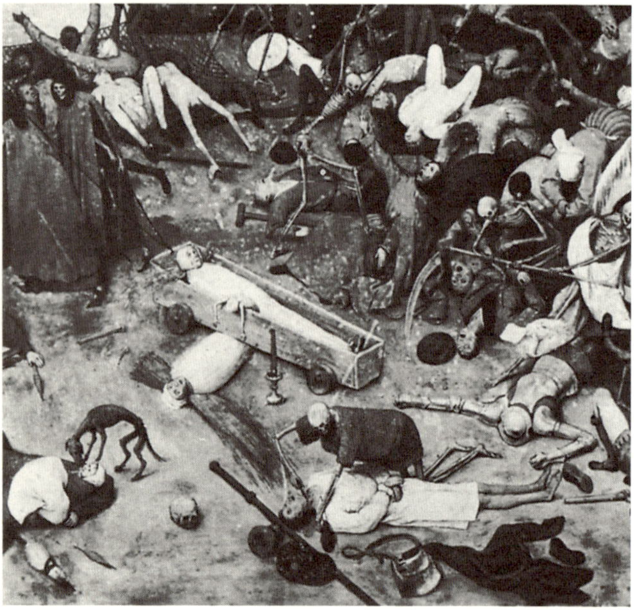

ХАНС БАЛЬДУНГ ГРИН.
1483–1545

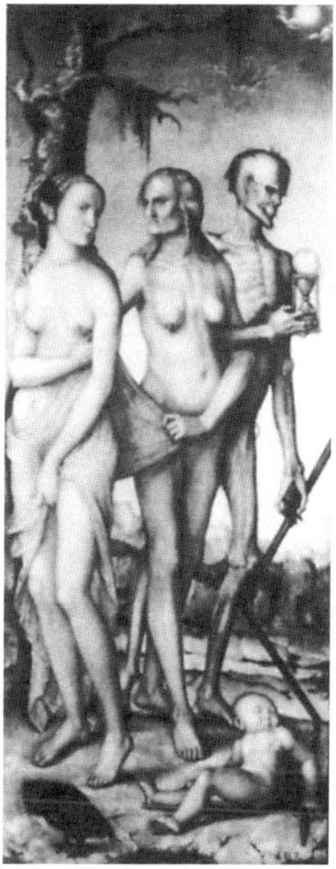

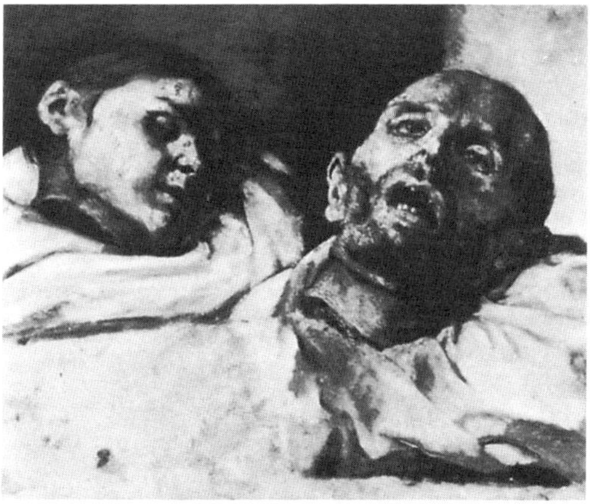

ЖЕРИКО. 1791–1824

ЭДУАРД МАНЕ. 1832–1883

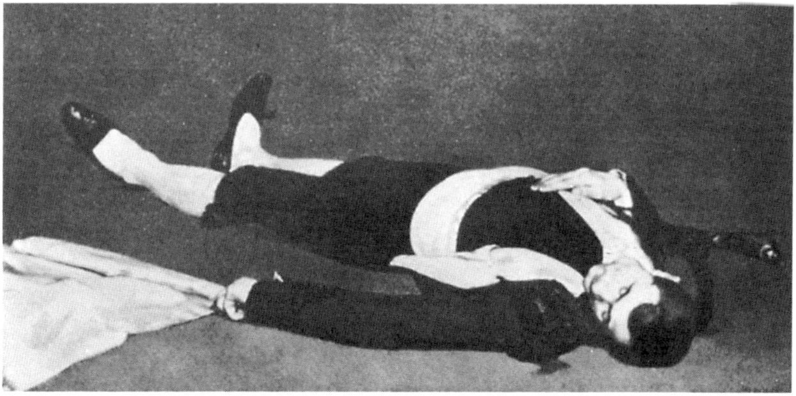

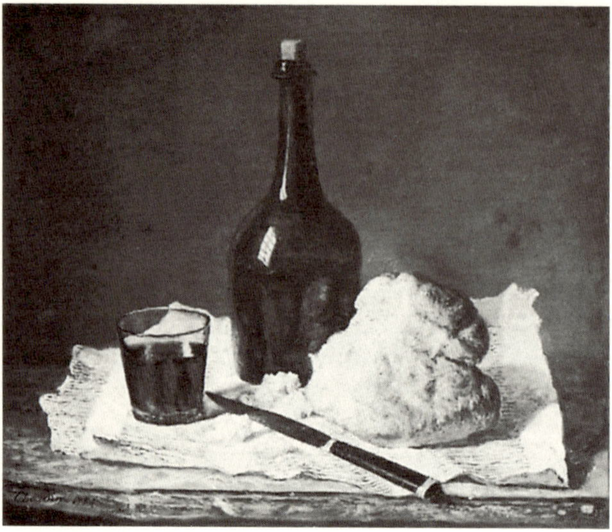

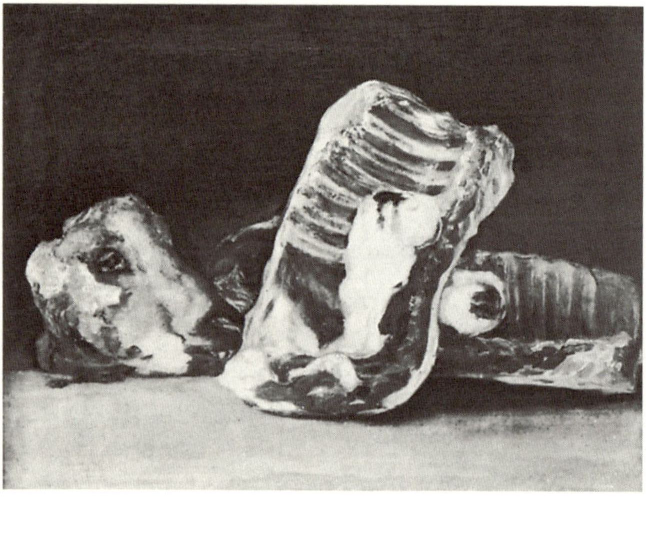

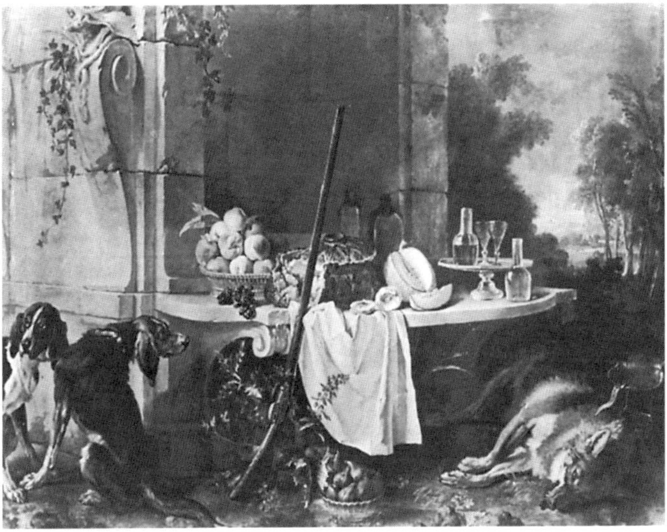

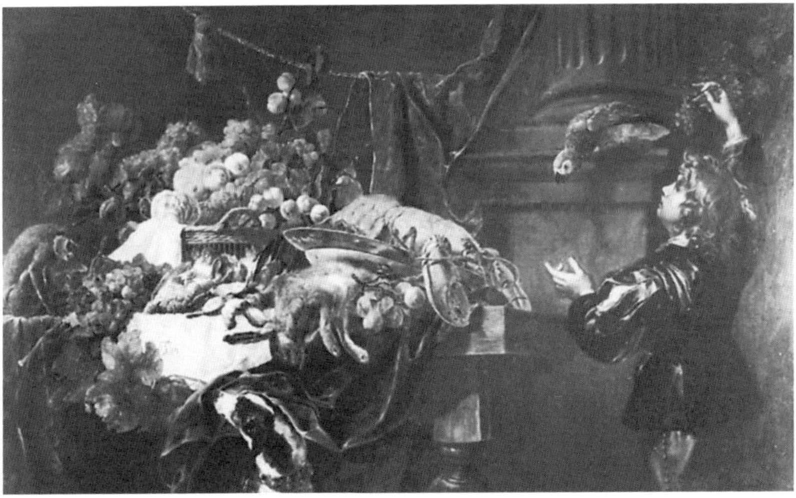

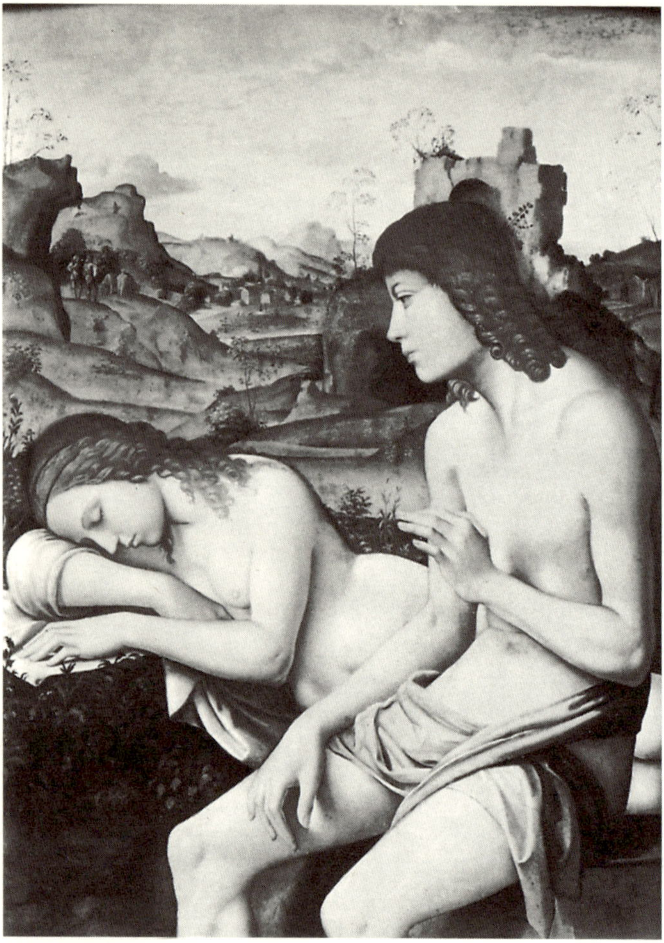

ДАФНИС И ХЛОЯ. XV ВЕК

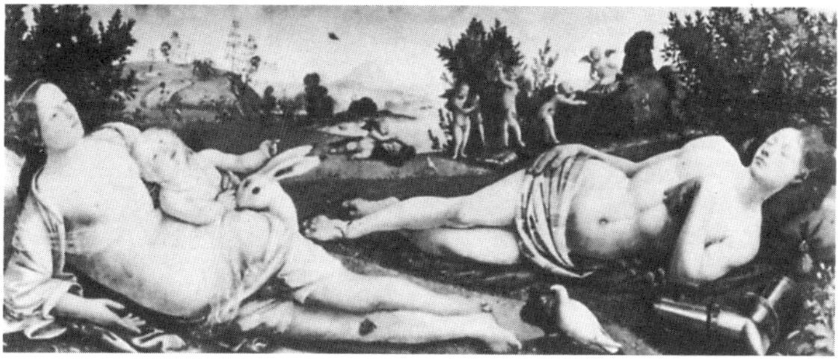

ВЕНЕРА И МАРС. XV ВЕК

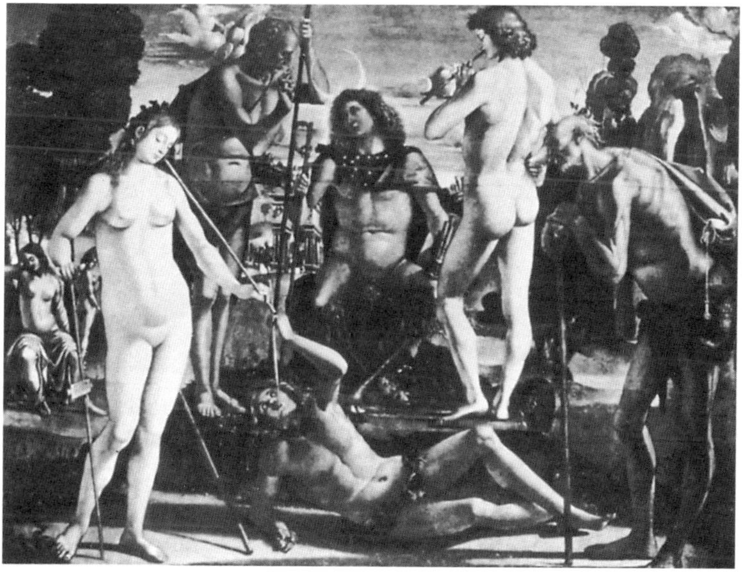

ПАН. XV ВЕК

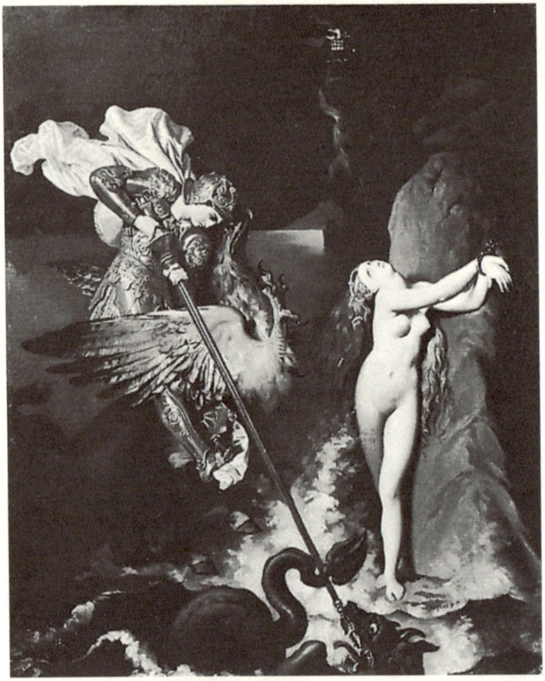

РУДЖЕРО
И АНЖЕЛИКА.
XIX ВЕК

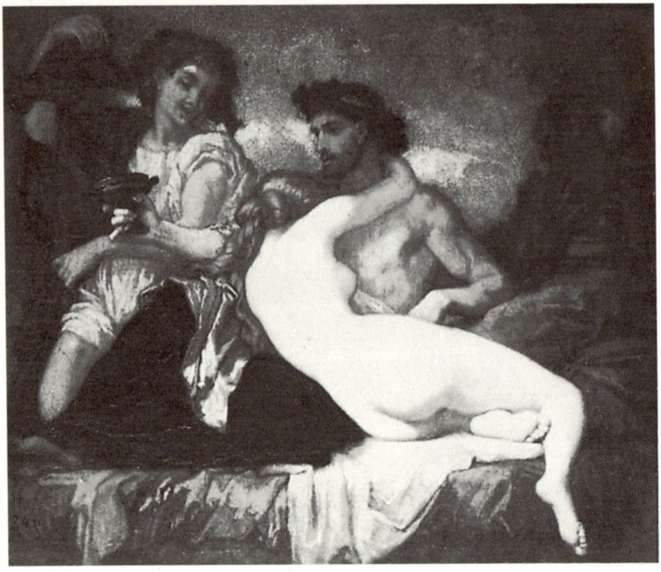

РИМСКИЙ ПИР. XIX ВЕК

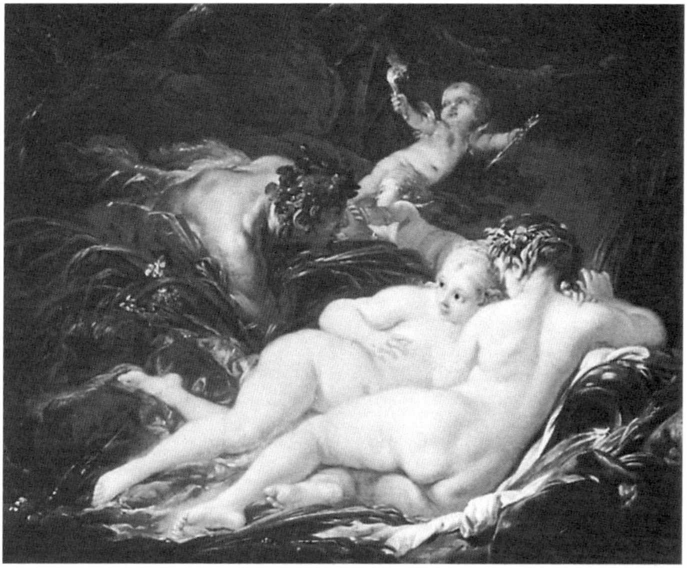

ПАН И СИРИНГА.
XVIII ВЕК

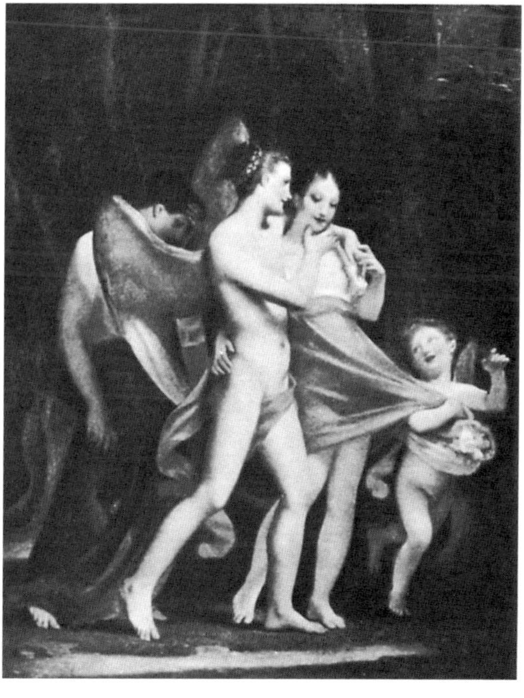

ЛЮБОВЬ, ИСКУШАЮЩАЯ
НЕВИННОСТЬ,
НАСЛАЖДЕНИЕ,
УВЛЕКАЮЩЕЕ ЕЕ,
И СЛЕДУЮЩЕЕ ЗА НИМИ
РАСКАЯНИЕ. XVIII ВЕК

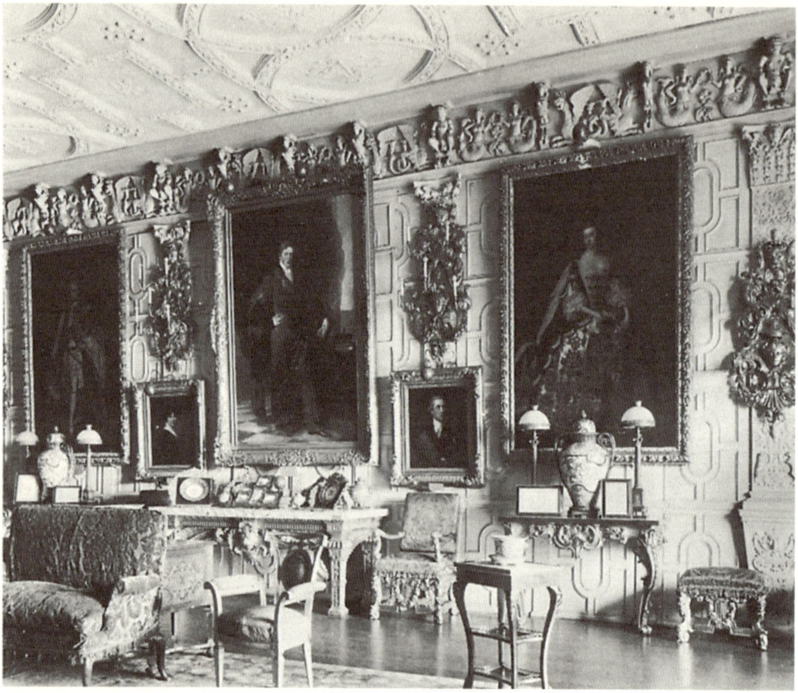

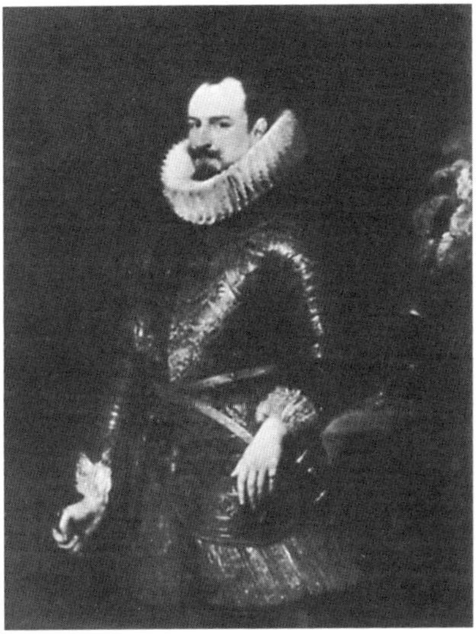

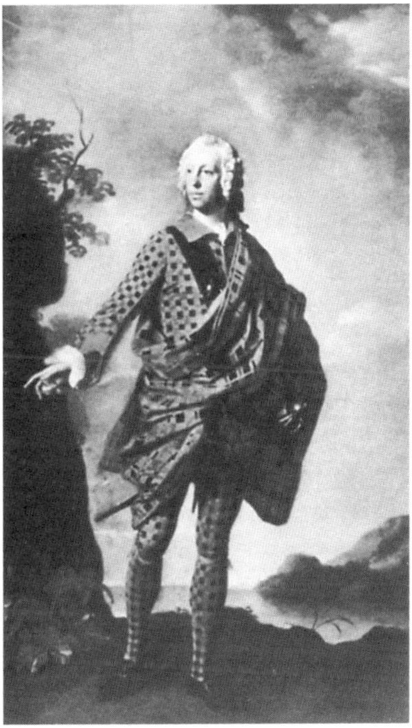

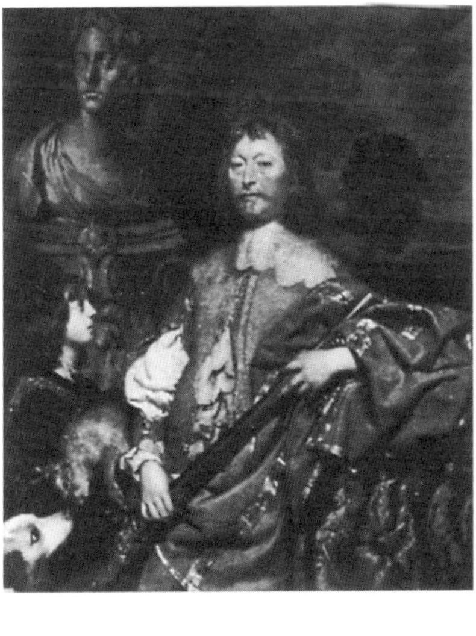

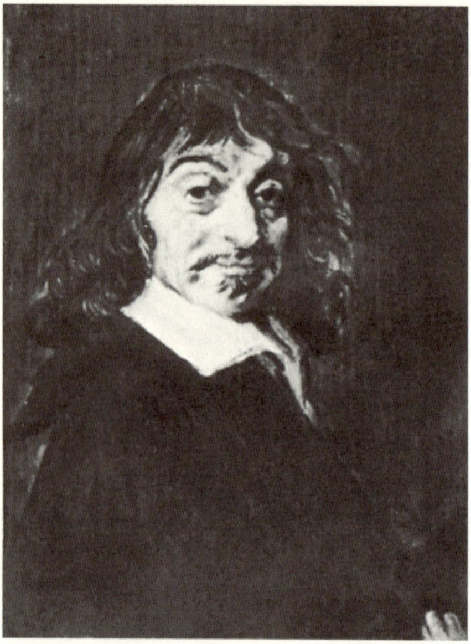

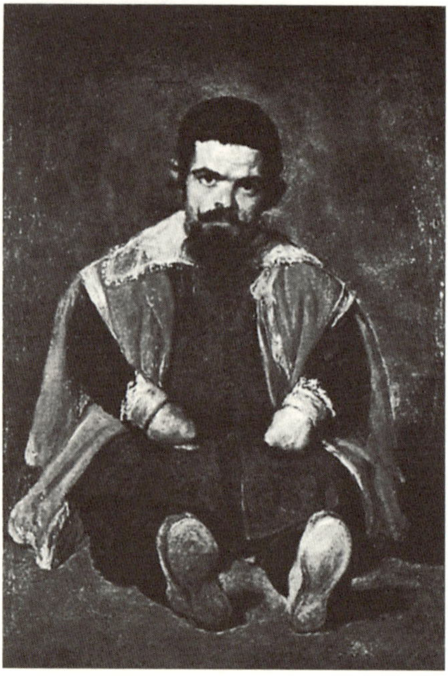

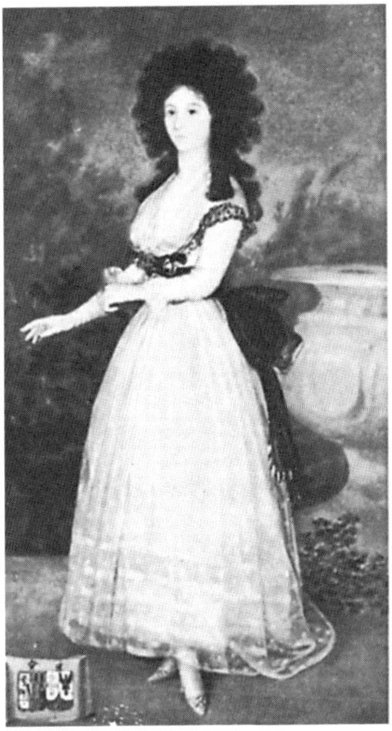

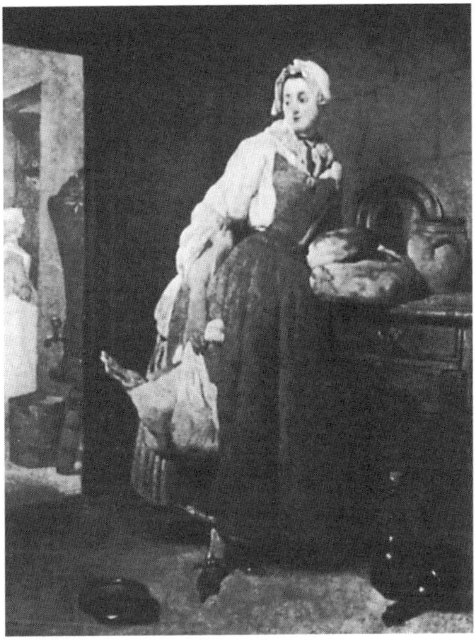

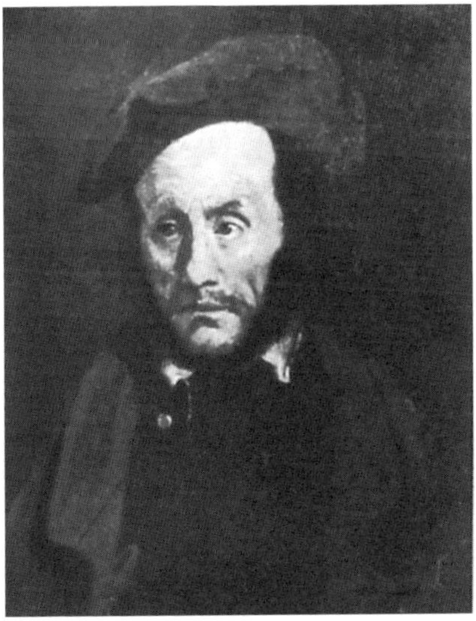

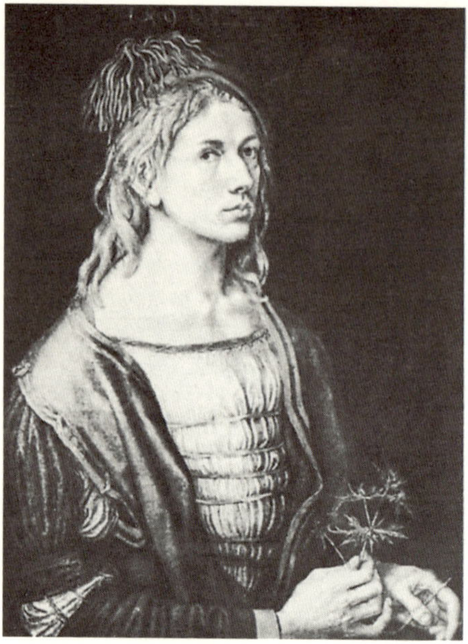

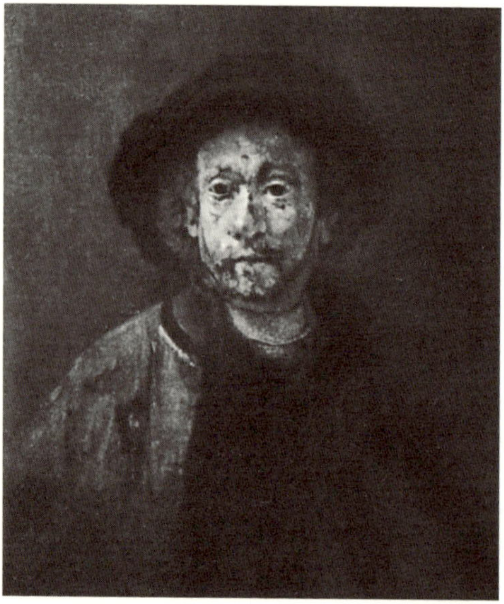

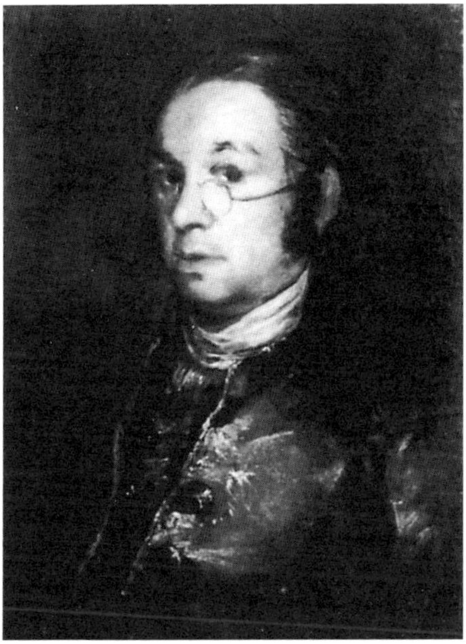

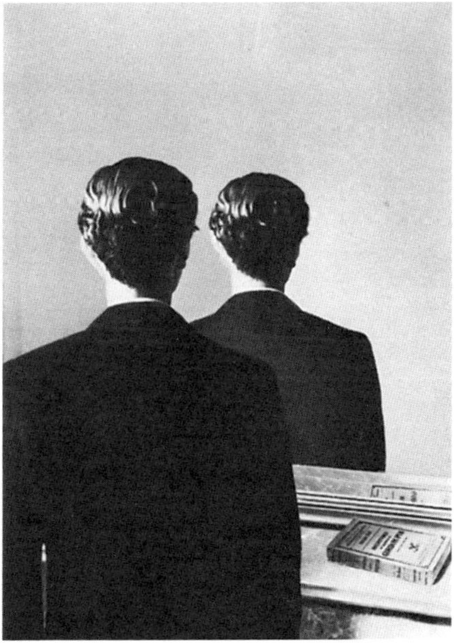

5

Масляная живопись часто изображает вещи. Вещи, которые в реальности можно купить. Приобрести нарисованную, помещенную на холст вещь – это почти то же, что приобрести ее саму и поместить ее у себя дома. Покупая живописное полотно, вы покупаете возможность видеть вещь, на нем изображенную.

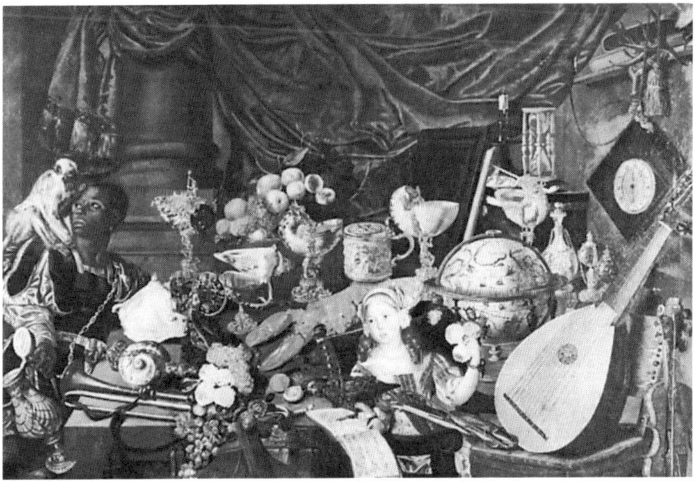

СОКРОВИЩА ПАСТОНОВ В ОКСНИД-ХОЛЛ. ФЛАМАНДСКАЯ ШКОЛА. ОК. 1665

Эта аналогия между *обладанием* и тем способом видеть, который укоренен в традиции масляной живописи, обычно игнорируется искусствоведами. Знаменательно, что ближе всех к пониманию ее подошел антрополог.

Леви-Стросс пишет:

> Что, по-моему, является весьма специфической чертой искусства Запада, так это его жадное и честолюбивое стремление захватить вещь в пользу владельца картины или даже ее зрителя.[3]

Если это правда (хотя, быть может, исторический диапазон, в рамках которго Леви-Стросс делает свое обобщение, и шире, чем следует), то данная тенденция достигла своего апогея как раз в эпоху классической масляной живописи.

Термин *масляная живопись* подразумевает не только технику. Им обозначается определенная форма искусства. Техника смешения пигментов с маслом существовала уже в античности. Но масляная живопись как форма искусства родилась только тогда, когда возникла потребность развить и усовершенствовать эту технику (что вскоре привело к использованию холста вместо деревянной основы), для того чтобы выразить особый взгляд на жизнь, которому техники темперной и фресковой живописи не соответствовали. Когда масляными красками впервые стали писать (в начале XV века в Северной Европе) картины нового характера, этот характер в определенной степени подавлялся сохранявшимися в искусстве средневековыми условностями. Собственные нормы, собственный способ видеть мир масляная живопись установила лишь к XVI веку.

Аналогично невозможно определить, когда именно пришел конец эпохи масляной живописи. Масляная живопись продолжает существовать и сегодня. Однако основы ее традиционного мировидения были подорваны импрессионизмом и низвергнуты кубизмом. Примерно в то же время место масляной живописи как главного источника визуальных образов заняла фотография. Таким об-

---

[3] Lévi-Strauss, Claude. CONVERSATIONS WITH CHARLES CHARBONNIER. – London: J.Cape, 1969.

разом, эпоху традиционной масляной живописи можно приблизительно ограничить периодом 1500–1900 годов.

Тем не менее, эта традиция по-прежнему формирует многие наши культурные представления. Именно она определяет наше понимание изобразительного сходства. Ее нормы все так же влияют на то, как мы видим пейзажи, женщин, еду, сановников, мифологию. Она же снабдила нас архетипом «гениального художника». А история этой традиции, как она обычно преподается, учит нас тому, что искусство процветает, если среди сограждан есть должное количество любителей искусства.

Что значит «любить искусство»?

Рассмотрим картину, принадлежащую к той традиции, предметом изображения которой были как раз любители искусства.

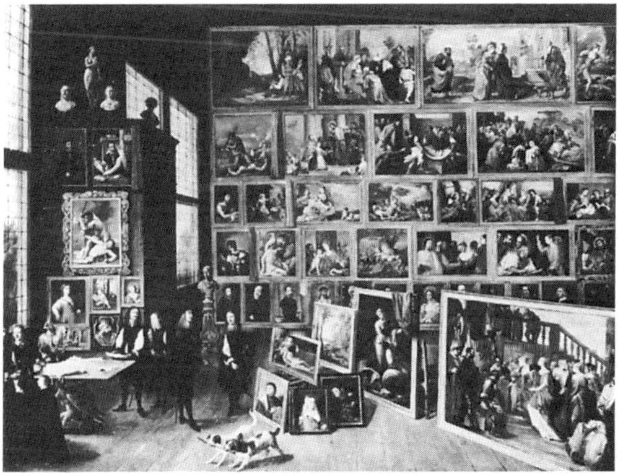

ЭРЦГЕРЦОГ ЛЕОПОЛЬД-ВИЛЬГЕЛЬМ В СВОЕЙ КАРТИННОЙ ГАЛЕРЕЕ. ТЕНИРС (1582-1649)

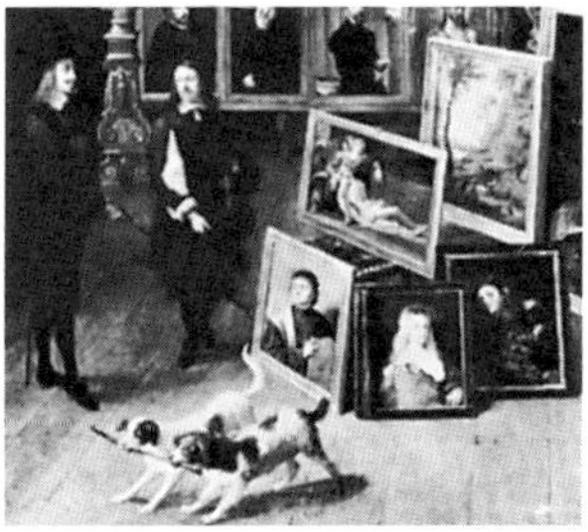

Кого мы на ней видим?

Одного из тех людей XVII века, для которых художники писали свои картины.

Что это за картины?

Прежде всего это вещи, которые можно купить и которыми можно обладать. Абсолютно уникальные вещи. Музыкой и стихами меценат не может быть окружен так, как он окружен картинами.

Создается впечатление, что коллекционер живет в доме, построенном из картин. В чем их преимущество перед стенами из камня и дерева?

Они демонстрируют своему владельцу то, чем он может обладать.

Обратимся к Леви-Строссу: он пишет о том, как коллекция живописи способна подпитывать гордость и самолюбие владельца:

> Для художников эпохи Возрождения живопись, возможно, и была инструментом познания, но кроме этого она была еще и инструментом обладания, и не стоит забывать, имея дело с ренессансной живописью, что она существовала лишь благодаря огромным богатствам, скопленным во Флоренции и в других городах, и что богатые итальянские купцы смотрели на художников как на людей, способных подтвердить, что это они владеют всем, что в мире есть прекрасного и желанного. Картины во флорентийском дворце представляли собой такой микрокосм, в котором их хозяин благодаря своим художникам воссоздавал — в прямой доступности и в максимально реальной форме — все то, что ему в мире нравилось.

В любые времена искусство склонно обслуживать идеологию правящего класса. Если бы мы просто сказали, что европейское искусство в 1500–1900 годах служило интересам сменявших друг друга правящих классов (все они так или иначе опирались на новую мощь капитала), то мы не сказали бы ничего особенно нового. Но здесь выдвигается несколько более конкретный тезис, а именно: способ видеть мир, обусловленный новым отношени-

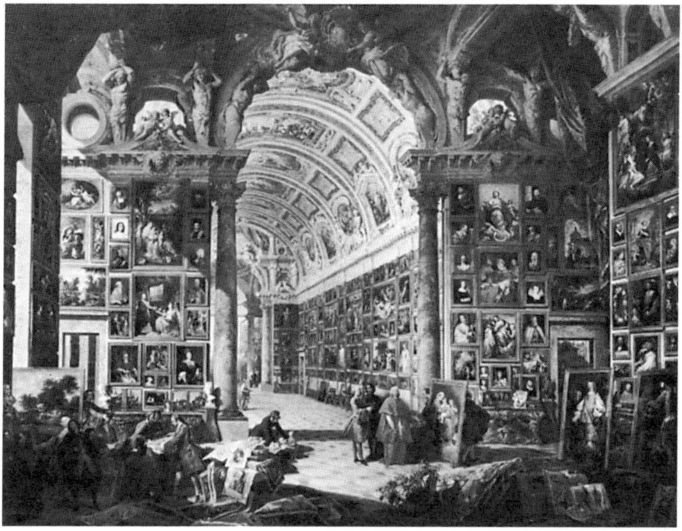

КАРТИННАЯ ГАЛЕРЕЯ КАРДИНАЛА ВАЛЕНТИ ГОНЗАГИ. ПАНИНИ. 1692–1765/8

ем к собственности и обмену, нашел свое визуальное выражение в масляной живописи – и в любой другой форме визуального искусства это было бы невозможно.

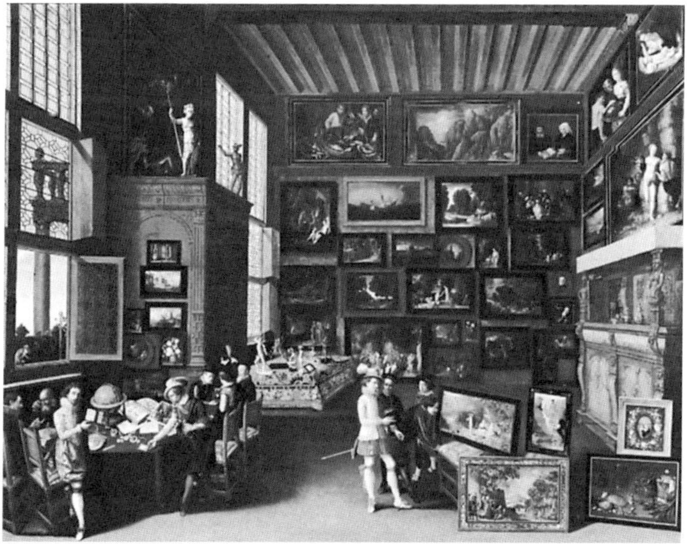

КАРТИННАЯ ГАЛЕРЕЯ. ФЛАНДРИЯ. XVII ВЕК

Масляная живопись сделала с видимым миром то, что капитал сделал с социальными отношениями. Все оказалось сведено к соизмеримости вещей. Все стало подлежать обмену, потому что все стало предметом потребления. Вся реальность была механически измерена исходя из ее материальной природы. Душа – благодаря картезианской системе – сохранилась как отдельная категория. Масляная живопись могла что-то говорить душе – при посредстве того, к чему она отсылала, но никак не тем, как она это изображала. Масляная живопись выражала идею полной овнешненности.

Несложно вспомнить примеры картин, опровергающих это утверждение. Работы Рембрандта, Эль Греко, Джорджоне, Вермеера, Тернера и др. Однако если рассмотреть их полотна на фоне традиции в целом, обнаружится, что это были исключения совершенно особого рода.

Традиция – это сотни тысяч полотен и этюдов по всей Европе. Многие из них не сохранились. Из тех, что дошли до нас, очень малая часть всерьез считается сегодня произведениями искусства, а среди них столь же немногочисленны те картины, что бесконечно воспроизводятся и преподносятся как работы «мастеров».

Посетители музеев и галерей нередко бывают подавлены количеством выставленных там работ – и собственной постыдной, как им кажется, неспособностью сосредоточиться больше чем на двух-трех картинах. В действительности это вполне нормальная реакция. История искусства так и не смогла разобраться, в каких отношениях находятся выдающиеся творения европейской традиции и ее среднестатистический продукт. Отсылка к гениальности сама по себе не является удовлетворительным ответом. Эта неразбериха, разумеется, сохраняется и на стенах картинных галерей. Шедевры окружены здесь третьестепенными полотнами; в таком расположении нет ни понимания, ни тем более объяснения фундаментальной разницы между ними.

Уровень одаренности художников очень различается в искусстве любой культуры. Но ни в одной другой культуре этот разрыв между «шедевром» и средней работой не был так велик, как в традиции масляной живописи. Здесь это различие сопряжено не только с мастерством художника и его воображением, но и с вопросами морали. Обычная картина (особенно после XVII века) создавалась с известной долей цинизма, иными словами: те ценности, которые она номинально выражала, были для художника менее важны, чем необходимость выполнить заказ или продать свою продукцию. «Топорность» работы тут не следствие необразованности или провинциальности ее создателя; это следствие того, что требования рынка оказывались важнее, чем требования искусства. Период масляной живописи совпадает с эпохой развития открытого художественного рынка. В этом-то противоречии между рынком и искусством и следует искать причину рассматриваемого контраста (антагонизма) между полотнами выдающимися и обычными.

Помня о том, что существуют выдающиеся произведения, к которым мы вернемся позже, сперва опишем в общих чертах, что из себя представляла традиция.

Что отличает масляную живопись от любых других видов живописи, так это ее способность передавать осязаемость, текстуру, блеск, плотность того, что она изображает. Для масляной живописи реальное – это то, что можно потрогать руками. Ее возможности в создании иллюзий куда более значительны, чем у скульптуры, хотя изображение на холсте двумерное – ведь масляная живопись предлагает зрителю предметы, имеющие цвет, текстуру и температуру, занимающие место в пространстве и (что подразумевается) заполняющие собой весь мир.

Картина Гольбейна «Послы» (1533) стоит у истоков этой традиции, и, как часто бывает с работами, открывающими новый период, она не маскирует своей природы. То, как она написана, открыто показывает нам, о чем она. Так как же она написана?

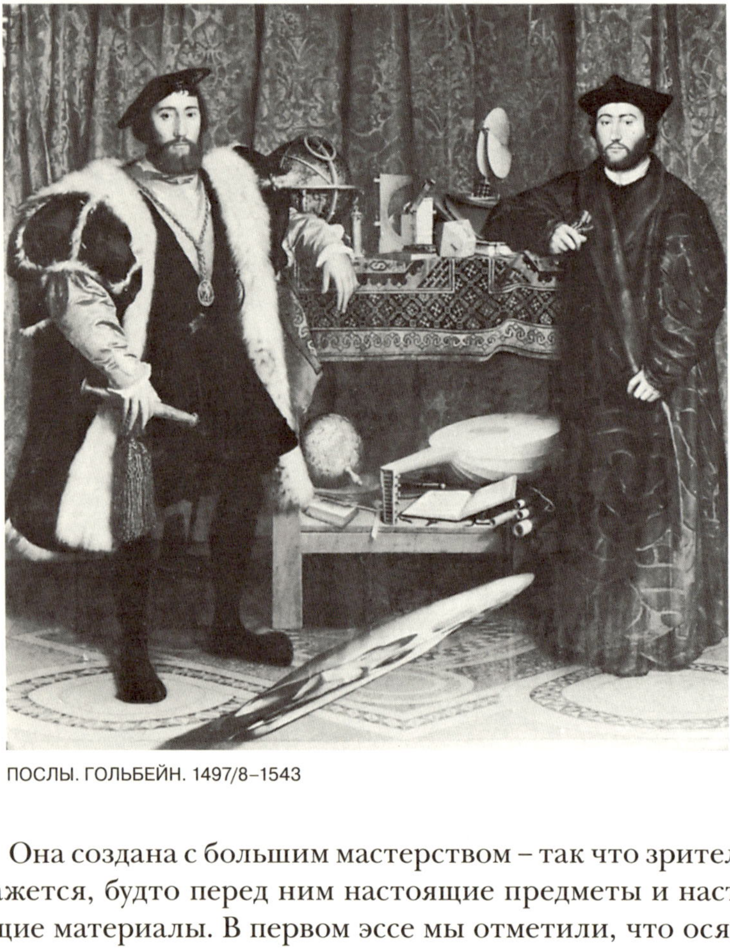

ПОСЛЫ. ГОЛЬБЕЙН. 1497/8–1543

Она создана с большим мастерством – так что зрителю кажется, будто перед ним настоящие предметы и настоящие материалы. В первом эссе мы отметили, что осязание сродни ограниченному, статичному зрению. Каждый квадратный сантиметр этого полотна, оставаясь всего лишь изображением, в то же время очень настойчиво обращается к осязанию. Взгляд переходит с меха на шелк, затем на металл, затем на дерево, на бархат, на мрамор, на бумагу, на фетр – и всякий раз то, что воспринимается глазом, тут же переводится (самой живописью) на язык тактильного восприятия. На картине присутствуют двое мужчин и вещи, символизирующие некие идеи, но что здесь преобладает, так это материалы, материя, которой эти мужчины окружены и в которую они одеты.

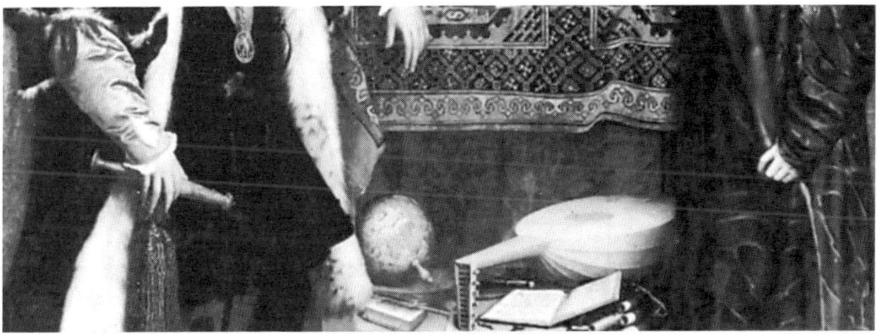

Всё на этой картине, за исключением разве что рук и лиц, говорит нам о том, как искусно оно сделано — ткачами, вышивальщиками, ковровщиками, ювелирами, кожевниками, скорняками, – и о том, как эта кропотливая работа и проистекающий из нее безупречный вид вещей были в конце концов столь же кропотливо воспроизведены Гольбейном – художником.

Такого рода выразительность и стоящее за ней мастерство останутся неизменно ценимы на протяжении всей истории масляной живописи.

В более ранней традиции произведения искусства прославляли богатство. Но тогда богатство было символом установленного социального и божественного порядка.

Масляная живопись прославляет богатство нового толка – динамическое, находящее себе оправдание исключительно в высшей власти денег, то есть в их покупательной способности. Следовательно, живопись должна была найти способ продемонстрировать, как вожделенно все то, что можно купить за деньги. А визуальная желанность того, что может быть куплено, заключается в его осязаемости, в том, как оно ответит на прикосновение, на руку хозяина.

На переднем плане картины Гольбейна изображен загадочный перекошенный овал. Это крайне искаженное изображение черепа: череп, как он мог бы быть увиден в кривом зеркале. Существует несколько теорий относительно того, как он был изображен и почему послы хотели, чтобы он был помещен на полотно. Но все согласны с тем, что это своего рода memento mori – игра со средневековой идеей использовать череп как постоянное напоминание о неизбежности смерти. Для нашего рассуждения существенно, что череп изображен в совершенно иной оптике, нежели все остальные предметы на этой картине. Если бы череп был написан точно так же, как и все прочее, то его метафизический смысл исчез бы; он стал бы предметом среди остальных предметов, просто частью обычного скелета, оставшегося от умершего человека.

Эта проблема сохранялась на протяжении всей эпохи масляной живописи. Когда метафизические символы помещались на холст (к примеру, череп как символ смерти изображался в реалистической манере), их символизм оказывался неубедительным или неестественным на фоне однозначного, статичного материализма используемой живописной техники.

Из-за того же противоречия в рамках данной традиции кажется лицемерной среднестатистическая картина на религиозную тему. Тематика выхолащивается за счет

VANITAS.
ДЕ ПОРТЕР.
1608–1648

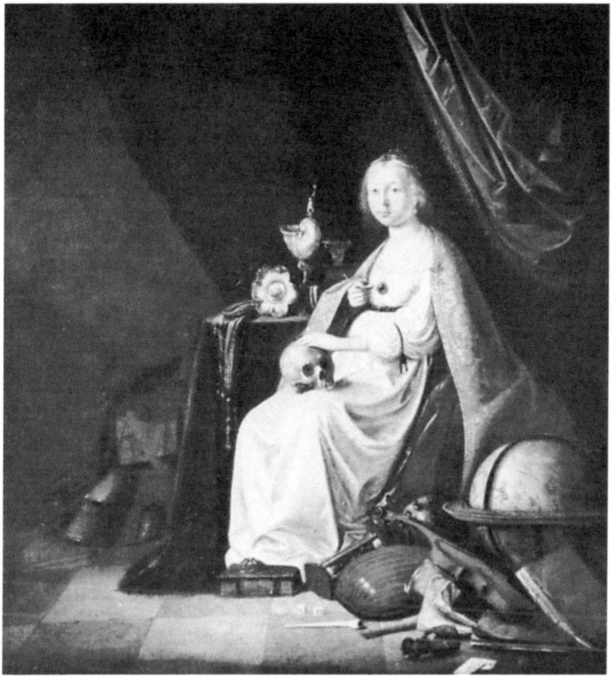

способа изображения предмета. Краска не может освободиться от присущей ей способности воссоздавать осязаемость, доставляющую удовольствие хозяину. Вот, например, три изображения Марии Магдалины.

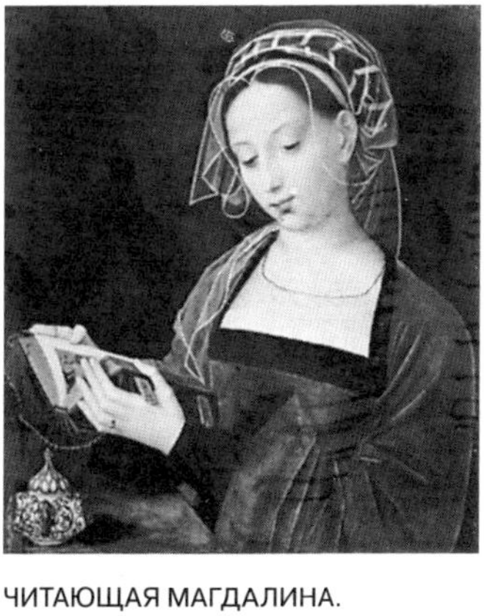

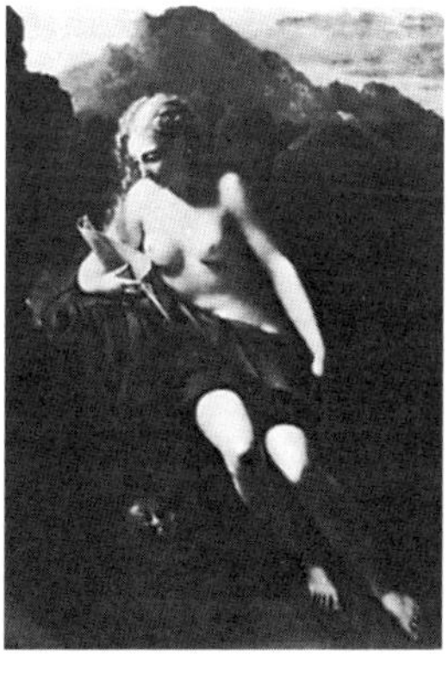

МАРИЯ МАГДАЛИНА. ВАН ДЕР ВЕРФ. 1659–1722

ЧИТАЮЩАЯ МАГДАЛИНА. МАСТЕРСКАЯ АМВРОСИЯ БЕНСОНА. 1519–1550

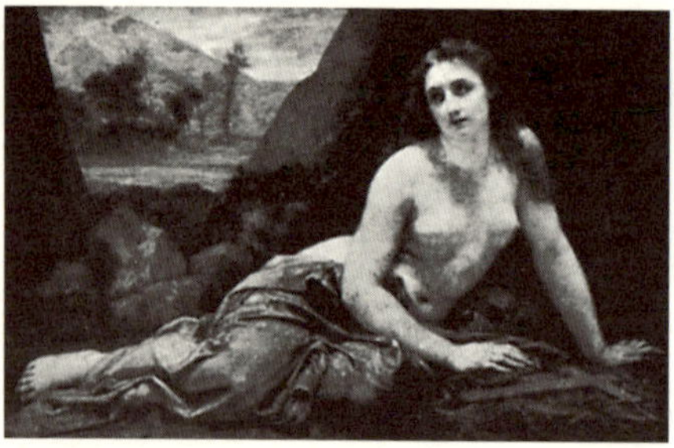

КАЮЩАЯСЯ МАГДАЛИНА. БОДРИ. САЛОН 1859 г.

Вспомним историю Марии Магдалины: она так любила Христа, что раскаялась в своем прошлом и пришла к осознанию смертности плоти и бессмертия души. Однако манера, в которой написаны картины, противоречит сути этой истории: Мария Магдалина на них выглядит так, как будто вызванных раскаянием изменений в ее жизни просто не было. Эта живописная техника оказывается неспособной выразить то самоотречение, к которому, как подразумевается, пришла героиня. Она показана, прежде всего, как доступная и желанная женщина. Она остается покорным объектом живописного метода, призванного соблазнять зрителя.

Интересно отметить здесь исключение в лице Уильяма Блейка. Как рисовальщик и гравер он был обучен в соответствии с законами традиции. Но, создавая свои живописные произведения, Блейк очень редко использовал масляную краску. По-прежнему опираясь на традиционные правила рисунка, Блейк, между тем, делал все, чтобы фигуры на его картинах утратили материальность, стали прозрачными и неотличимыми друг от друга, перестали подчиняться силе тяжести; чтобы они присутствовали, но были неосязаемы, чтобы светились, но было непонятно, из чего они – для того, чтобы они не превратились в вещи.

Это стремление Блейка преодолеть «материальность» масляной живописи вытекает из глубокого понимания ее смысла и ее ограниченности.

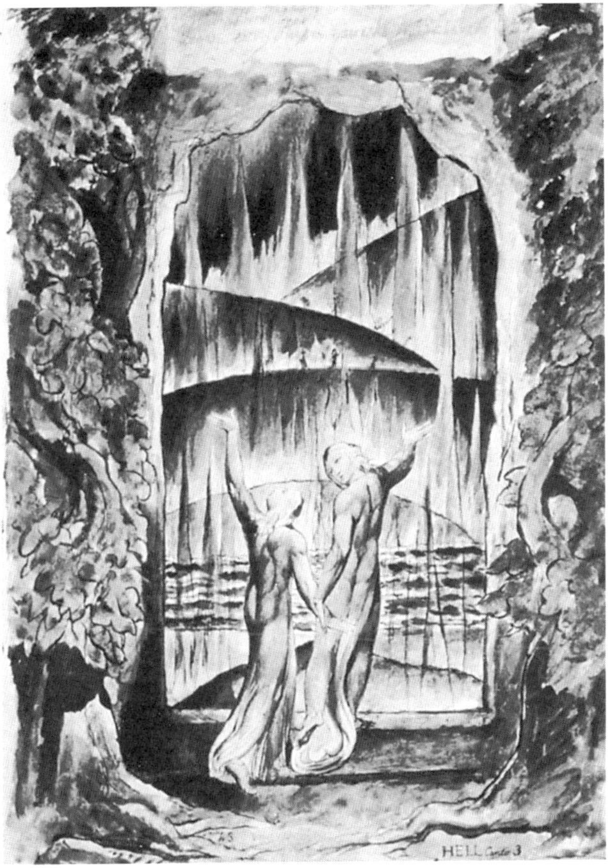

ИЛЛЮСТРАЦИЯ К «БОЖЕСТВЕННОЙ КОМЕДИИ» ДАНТЕ. БЛЕЙК. 1757–1827

Вернемся к нашим послам, к тому, как они представлены здесь как люди. Это будет значить, что мы прочитаем картину по-иному: не в аспекте того, что она изображает в собственных рамках, но в аспекте той реальности, к которой она отсылает.

Изображенные мужчины держатся уверенно и официально, при этом между ними нет ни малейшего напряжения. Но как они смотрят на художника – то есть на нас? Их взгляд и поза говорят о том, что эти люди не ждут признания с нашей стороны. Так, словно их достоинства в

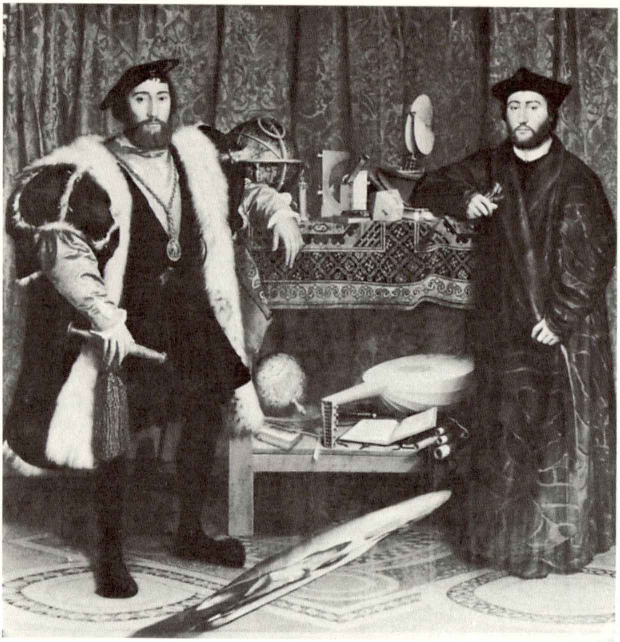

ПОСЛЫ.
ГОЛЬБЕЙН.
1497/8–1543

принципе не могут быть должным образом оценены другими. Они смотрят так, будто перед ними нечто, частью чего они не являются. Нечто, что окружает их, но к чему они не хотят быть причастны. В лучшем случае это может быть толпа, приветствующая их; в худшем – толпа, вторгающаяся к ним.

Каковы отношения таких людей со всем остальным миром?

Предметы на полках должны были сообщить (тем немногим, кто способен понять аллюзии), каково положение в мире изображенных здесь людей. Спустя четыре столетия мы можем проинтерпретировать эту информацию с нашей современной точки зрения.

Стоящие на верхней полке инструменты предназначены для навигации. Это было время, когда открывались морские торговые пути – для работорговли и для перекачки богатств с других континентов в Европу, а позднее – для обеспечения капиталом начинавшейся промышленной революции.

В 1519 году Магеллан, при поддержке Карла V, отправился в кругосветное плавание. Он и его друг-астроном, с которым это путешествие было спланировано, договорились с испанским двором, что им лично достанется двадцать процентов от полученных богатств и право управлять любой из захваченных земель.

Глобус на нижней полке – новый, учитывающий это последнее путешествие Магеллана. Гольбейн также разместил на глобусе название поместья во Франции, принадлежащего послу слева. Рядом с глобусом положены книга по арифметике, псалтырь и лютня. Чтобы колонизировать новую землю, нужно было обратить ее жителей в христианство и научить счетоводству, доказав им таким образом, что европейская цивилизация – самая передовая в мире. В том числе и ее искусство.

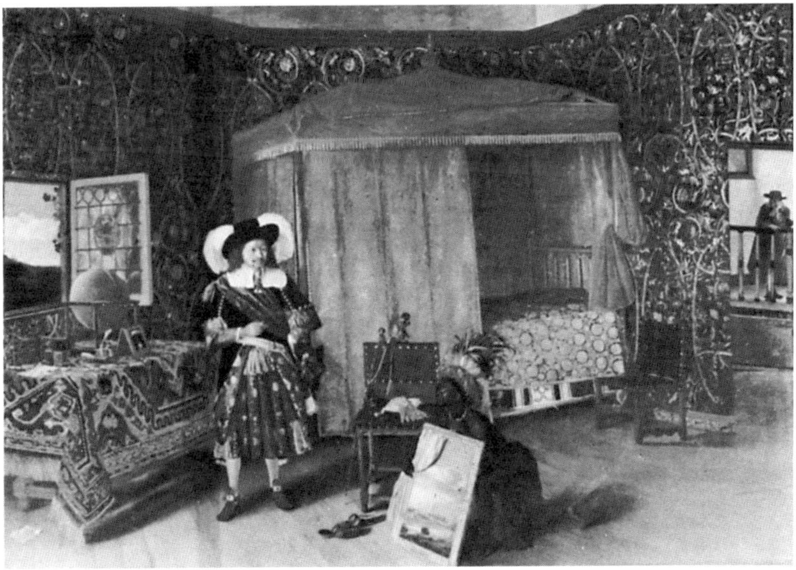

АДМИРАЛ ДЕ РЮЙТЕР В КРЕПОСТИ ЭЛЬМИНА.
ДЕ ВИТТЕ. 1617–1692

У де Витте африканец, стоя на коленях, показывает своему хозяину написанную маслом картину. На картине изображен замок, возвышающийся над одним из главных центров работорговли в Западной Африке.

Что касается двух послов, то не так важно, участвовали они лично в первых колонизаторских предприятиях или нет: здесь нас интересует позиция по отношению к миру, характерная для всего этого сословия. Наши два посла принадлежали к тому классу, который был уверен: мир только для того и существует, чтобы обустраивать их жизнь в нем. В своей крайней форме эта уверенность реализовалась в отношениях, утвердившихся между захватчиком-колонизатором и жителями захваченных земель.

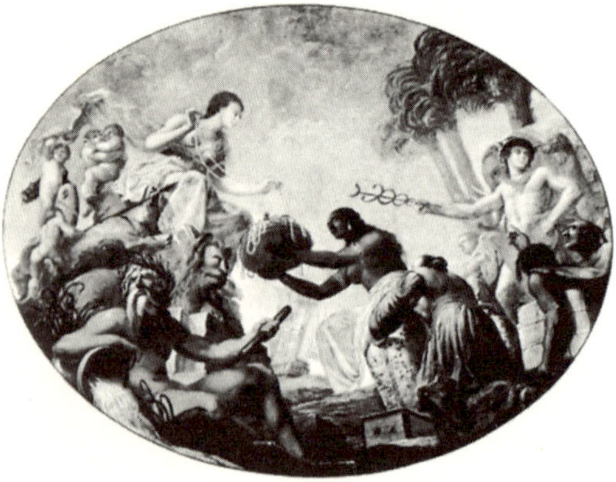

ИНДИЯ ПРИНОСИТ СВОИ ЖЕМЧУГА БРИТАНИИ. XVIII ВЕК

Указанные отношения между поработителем и порабощенным имели тенденцию к самовоспроизводству. Вид другого утверждает каждого из участников в собственной «нечеловеческой» самооценке. Цикличность этих отношений представлена на схеме – равно как и обоюдное одиночество контрагентов. То, как каждая из сторон видит другую, подтверждает ее представление о себе.

Взгляд у послов одновременно надменный и настороженный. Они не ждут никакой взаимности. Они хотят,

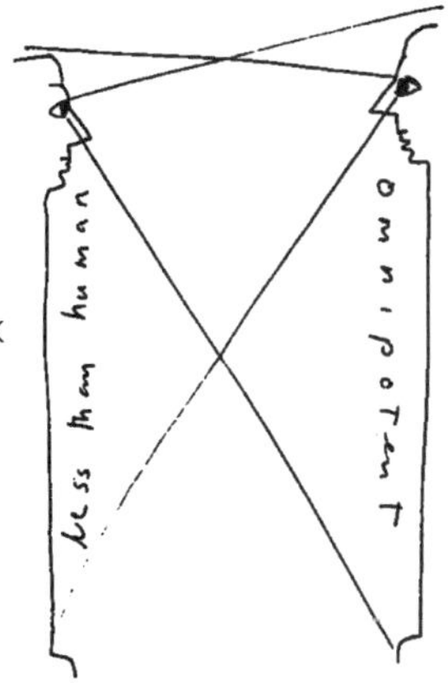

НЕДОЧЕЛОВЕК ВСЕМОГУЩИЙ

чтобы зрители были поражены их бдительностью и недоступностью. Когда-то такое впечатление производило присутствие королей и императоров, но их образы были относительно безличными. Что здесь нового и что вызывает недоумение, так это как раз *индивидуализированное присутствие*, стремящееся, между тем, создать *дистанцию*. Индивидуализм, в конечном счете, утверждает равенство. Однако тут нужно, чтобы равенство нельзя было даже вообразить.

Конфликт вновь кроется в самой живописной технике. Правдоподобие масляной живописи заставляет зрителя поверить в то, что он находится очень близко к изображенным на переднем плане картины предметам (буквально может дотронуться до них). Если же там изображен человек, то такая близость подразумевает определенную степень интимности.

Однако официальный портрет призван, напротив, подчеркивать наличие дистанции. Именно поэтому (а не по причине недостатка мастерства у художника) человек на среднестатистическом портрете, написанном в рамках традиции, выглядел таким скованным и неподвижным. Эта искусственность коренится в самих требованиях к изображению: объект должен быть одновременно

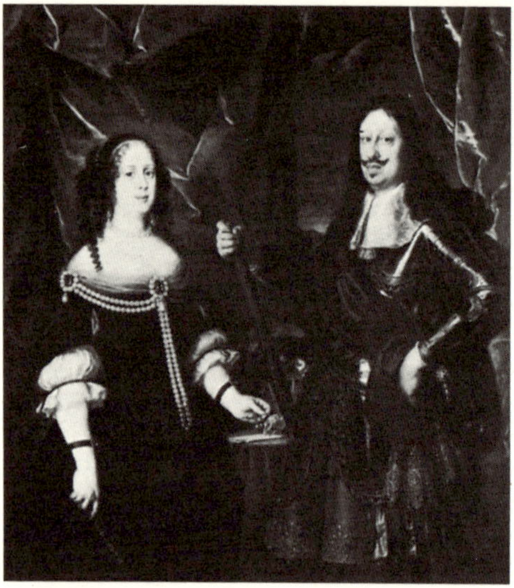

ФЕРДИНАНД II ТОСКАНСКИЙ И ВИКТОРИЯ ДЕЛЛА РОВЕРЕ.
СУСТЕРМАНС.
1597–1681

увиден и вблизи, и издалека. Можно провести аналогию с образцами, рассматриваемыми под микроскопом. Вот они перед нами, мы можем изучать их, но нельзя представить, чтобы они аналогичным образом рассматривали нас.

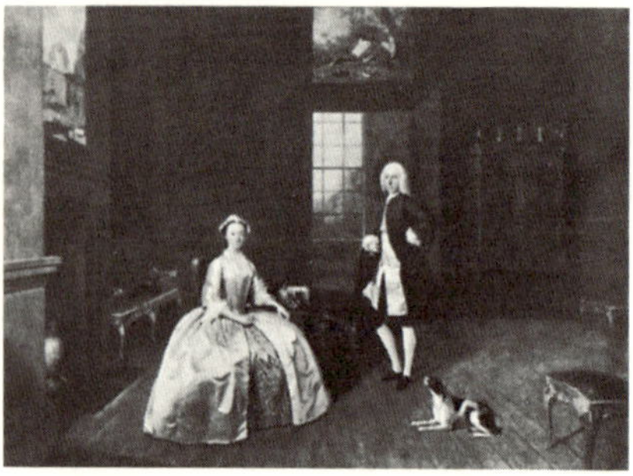

МИСТЕР И МИССИС УИЛЬЯМ АТЕРТОН.
ДЕВИС.
1711–1787

Официальный портрет (в противоположность автопортрету и неформальному дружескому портрету) так и не смог решить эту проблему. Однако по мере развития традиции манера изображения лица заказчика становилась все более обобщенной.

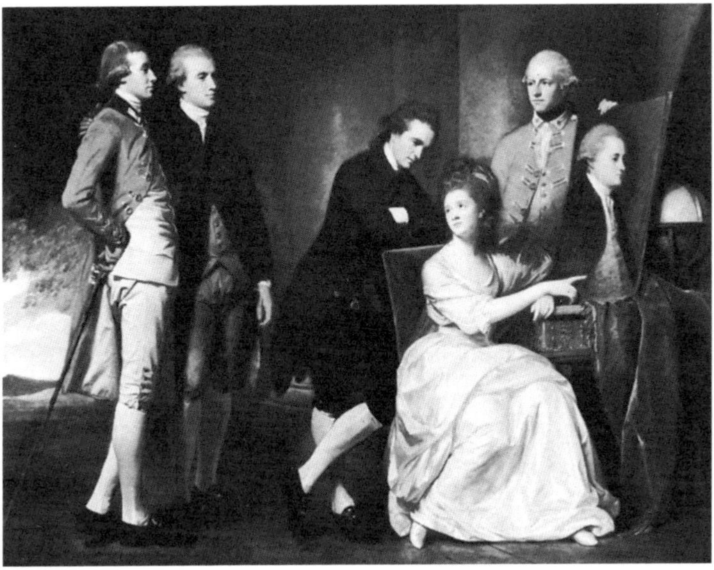

СЕМЬЯ БОМОНТ. РОМНИ. 1734–1802

Его черты превращались в маску, которая прилагалась к костюму. Итог развития этой традиции – телевизионные выступления современных политиков.

Рассмотрим вкратце некоторые жанры масляной живописи, бывшие частью этой живописной традиции – и ни в какой другой не существовавшие.

До эпохи масляной живописи средневековые художники использовали в своей работе сусальное золото. Позднее золото исчезает из живописи и используется только для оформления рам. Однако полотна сами зачастую были просто демонстрацией того, что можно купить за деньги и золото. Подлинной темой искусства стал товар.

Изображение пищи. Такая картина не только демонстрирует мастерство ее создателя. Она подтверждает богатство ее хозяина и привычный для него стиль жизни.

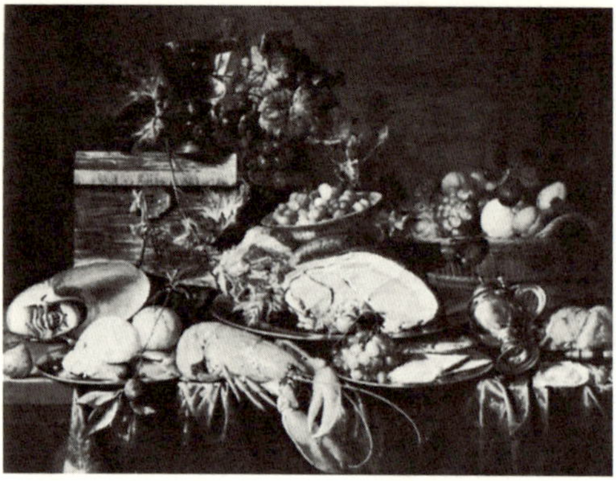

НАТЮРМОРТ С ОМАРОМ.
ДЕ ХЕМ.
1606–1684

Изображение животных. Не животных в их естественной среде обитания, а домашнего скота, родословная которого подчеркивается как доказательство его ценности – и сама подчеркивает социальный статус его владельцев. (Животные изображаются как мебель.)

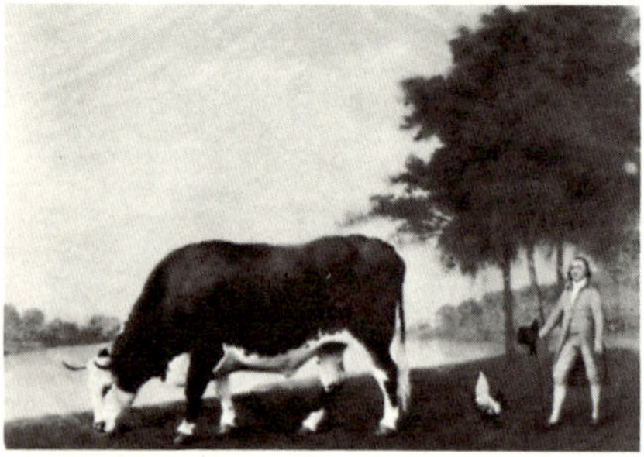

ЛИНКОЛЬНШИРСКИЙ БЫК.
СТАББС.
1724–1806

Изображение предметов – тех предметов, которые (что весьма примечательно) стали называться *предметами искусства.*

Изображение зданий. Здания рассматриваются не как совершенные произведения архитектуры (что можно увидеть в работах некоторых художников раннего Ренессанса), но как объект собственности.

Высшей категорией масляной живописи была историческая, или мифологическая, живопись. Изображе-

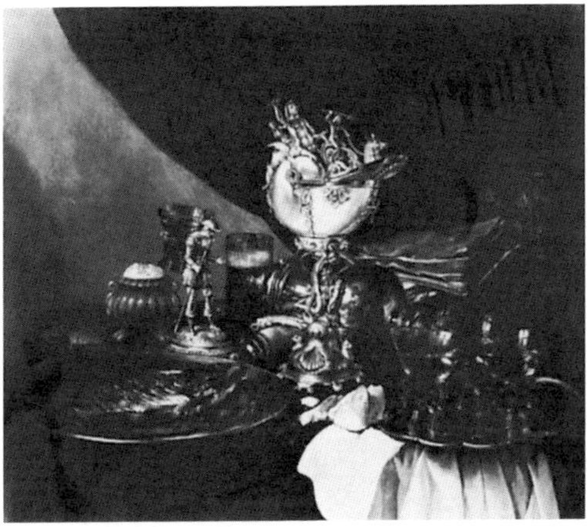

НАТЮРМОРТ.
ПРИПИСЫВАЕТСЯ КЛАСУ.
1596/7–1661

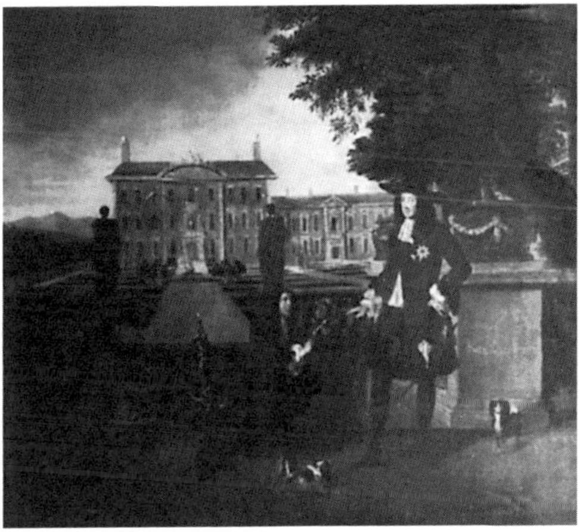

РОУЗ, КОРОЛЕВСКИЙ САДОВНИК, ПРЕПОДНОСИТ АНАНАС КАРЛУ ВТОРОМУ.
КОПИЯ ХЬЮАРТА С КАРТИНЫ ДАНКЕРТСА.
ОК. 1630–1678/9

ние героев древности по определению ценилось выше, чем натюрморт, портрет или пейзаж. За исключением нескольких *исключительных* работ, в которых художник смог выразить свое собственное лирическое чувство, именно эти мифологические полотна больше остальных поражают нас своей пустотой. Они похожи на дорогие, но уже поблекшие от времени сувениры. Однако их престиж и их пустота были самым непосредственным образом связаны.

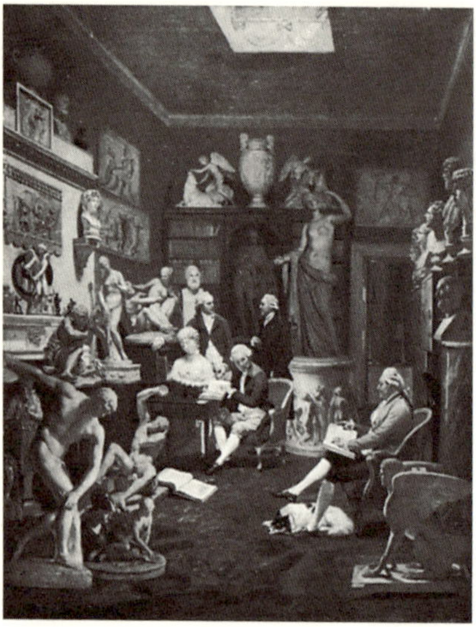

ЧАРЛЬЗ ТАУНЛИ И ЕГО ДРУЗЬЯ.
ЦОФФАНИ.
1734/5–1810

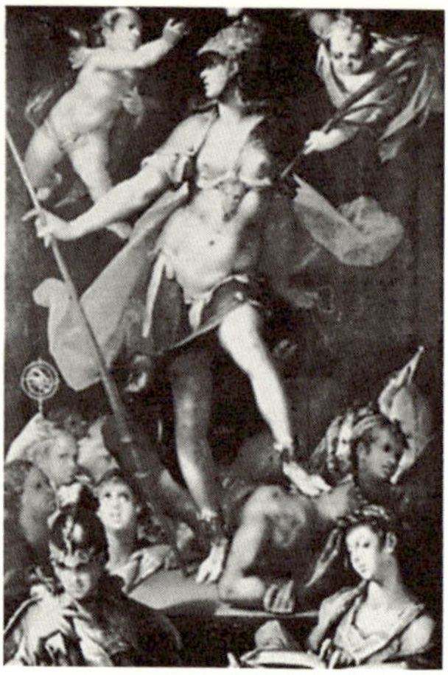

МИНЕРВА, ПОБЕЖДАЮЩАЯ
НЕВЕЖЕСТВО.
СПРАНГЕР.
1546–1627

До самого недавнего времени (а в определенных кругах даже сегодня) изучению античной классики приписывалось определенное нравственное значение. Дело в том, что классические античные тексты (вне зависимости от их внутренней ценности) предоставляли высшим слоям правящего класса систему прецедентных форм идеального поведения. Точно так же, как поэзия, логика и философия, античная литература предлагала систему этикета. Она предлагала примеры того, как возвышенные моменты жизни (которые обнаруживаются в героических поступках, благородных физических упражнениях, страсти, мужественной смерти, в благородном стремлении к наслаждению) должны проживаться или, по крайней мере, должны быть увидены.

Тогда почему изображение этих сцен, которые якобы должны воскреснуть перед нами, так пусто и поверхностно? Дело в том, что этим картинам вовсе не надо было будить воображение. В противном случае они не так эффективно достигали бы своей цели. А целью их было отнюдь не погрузить зрителя в новый для него опыт, а приукрасить тот опыт, который у него уже был. На этих холстах зритель-владелец рассчитывал увидеть классическое изображение собственной страсти, или горя, или великодушия. Идеализированные образы, которые он находил на этих картинах, поддерживали его представление о самом себе. Это был образец, глядя на который зритель-владелец создавал свой собственный (или своей жены, или дочерей) благородный облик.

Иногда это было простое заимствование классических образов (как на картине Рейнольдса, где дочери семейства представлены *Грациями, украшающими герму Гименея*).

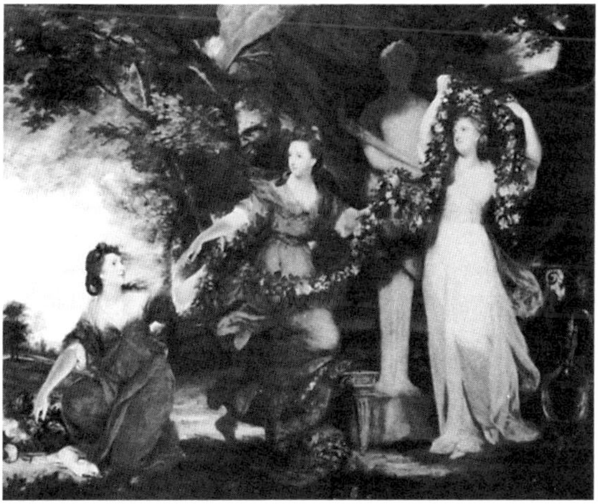

ТРИ ГРАЦИИ УКРАШАЮТ ГЕРМУ ГИМЕНЕЯ. РЕЙНОЛЬДС. 1723–1792

Иногда мифологическая сцена целиком представляет собой своего рода костюм, в который зрителю-владельцу предлагается облачиться. Тот факт, что эта сцена одновременно материальна и, тем не менее, за этой материальностью, пуста, облегчает «надевание» такого «костюма».

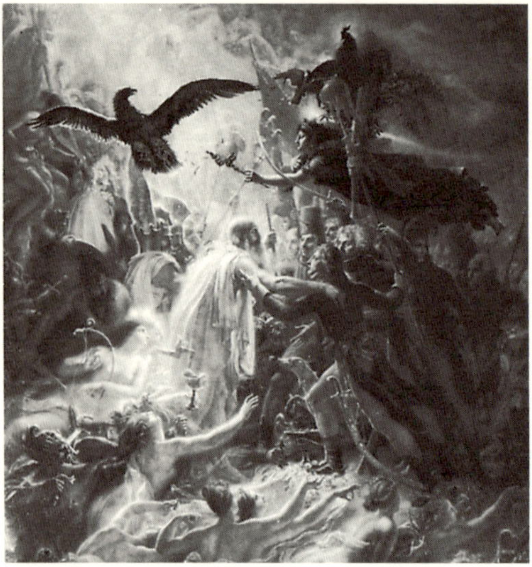

ТЕНИ ФРАНЦУЗСКИХ ГЕНЕРАЛОВ, ВСТРЕЧАЕМЫЕ В ЕЛИСЕЙСКИХ ПОЛЯХ ОССИАНОМ.
ЖИРОДЕ.
1767–1824

Так называемая «жанровая» живопись – изображение «низкой действительности» – мыслилась как противоположность живописи мифологической. В противовес благородству последней она изображала жизнь черни. Целью «жанровой» живописи было доказать (прямо или от противного), что добродетель в этом мире награждается социальным и финансовым благополучием. Таким образом те, кто мог позволить себе купить эти картины (как бы дешевы они ни были), получали подтверждение собственной добродетели. Эти картины были особенно популярны в среде новой буржуазии, идентифицировавшей себя не с изображенными на них людьми, а с той моралью, которую они иллюстрировали. Опять-таки, способность масляной краски создавать иллюзию материальности придавала убедительности сентиментальной лжи о том, что честные и работящие всегда преуспевают, а ничего не имеют (и заслужили это) лишь бездельники.

Адриан Браувер был единственным исключением из этого правила. Его картины, изображающие дешевые та-

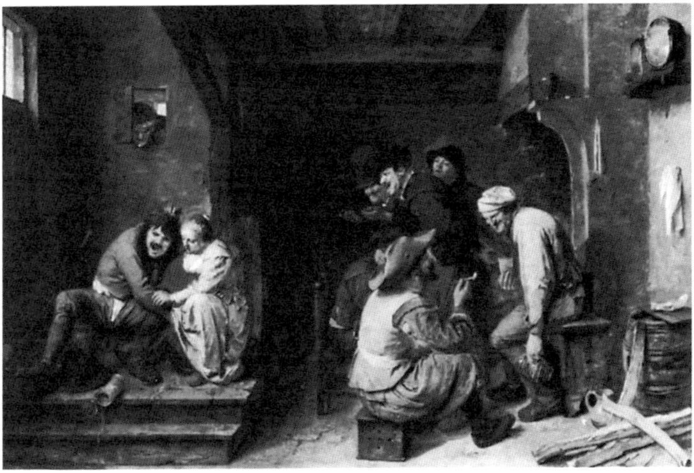

СЦЕНА В ТАВЕРНЕ. БРАУВЕР. 1605–1638

верны и их завсегдатаев, полны того горького и наивного реализма, который не оставляет места сентиментальному морализаторству. Как результат – его картины не покупал никто, за исключением нескольких других художников, таких как Рембрандт и Рубенс.

Среднестатистическая «жанровая» картина (даже написанная таким «мастером», как Хальс) представляла собой нечто совсем иное.

СМЕЮЩИЙСЯ МАЛЬЧИК. ХАЛЬС. 1580–1666

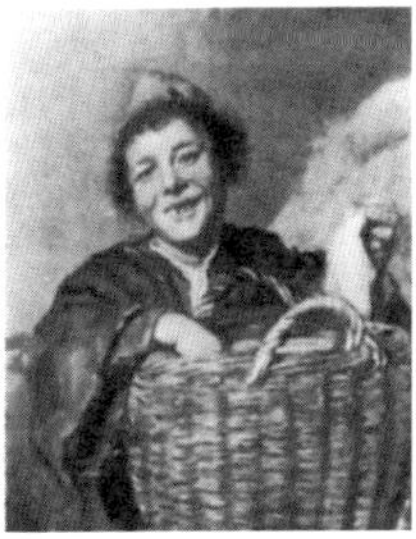

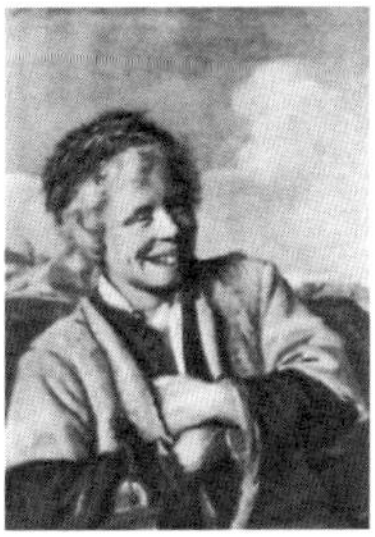

МАЛЕНЬКИЙ РЫБАК. ХАЛЬС. 1580–1666

Это бедняки. Бедняков можно увидеть на улице или в деревне. Однако изображения бедняков в доме выглядят жизнеутверждающе. Изображенные здесь бедняки улыбаются, предлагая то, что у них есть на продажу. (Они улыбаются, показывая зубы, чего богатые на картинах не делают никогда.) Они улыбаются богатым, заискивая перед ними и рассчитывая на работу или на то, что у них что-нибудь купят. Такие картины утверждают две вещи: что бедные люди счастливы и что богатые – источник надежды для окружающего мира.

В наименьшей степени наш главный тезис приложим к такой категории масляной живописи, как пейзаж.

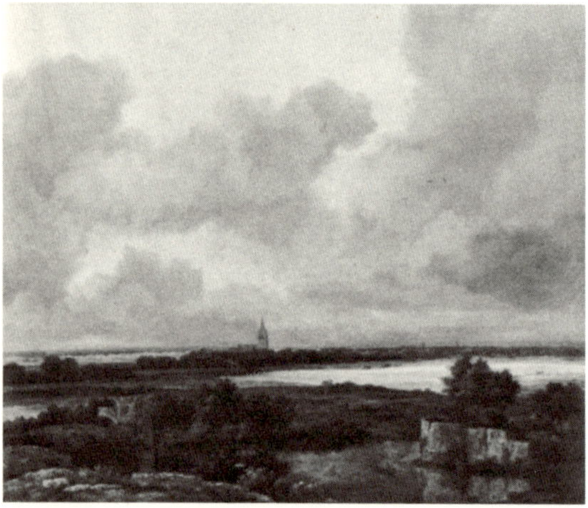

ПЕЙЗАЖ С РУИНАМИ.
РЁЙСДАЛ.
1628/9–1682

До недавнего всплеска интереса к экологии природа не рассматривалась как объект капиталистической деятельности; скорее она мыслилась как арена, на которой осуществляются и капитализм, и социальная жизнь вообще, и каждая отдельная человеческая жизнь в частности. Различные аспекты природы становились предметами научного исследования, но природа в целом отрицала идею собственности.

Можно сформулировать это еще проще. Небо – это не поверхность, его нельзя потрогать; небо нельзя превра-

РЕЧНОЙ ПЕЙЗАЖ С РЫБАКАМИ.
ГОЙЕН.
1596–1656

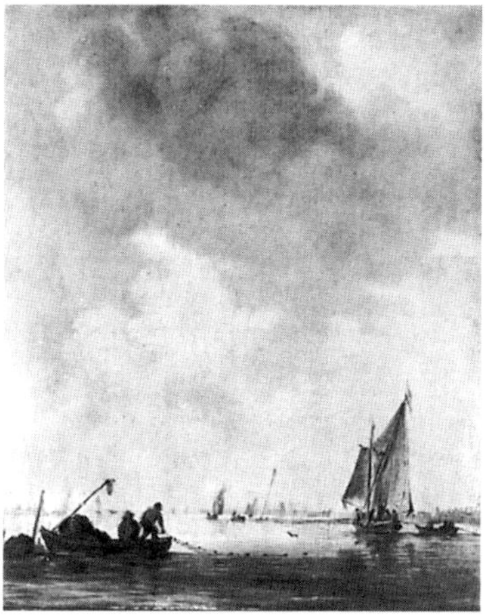

тить в вещь или измерить. Проблема изображения неба и расстояния – то, с чего начинается пейзаж.

Первые пейзажи, написанные в Голландии в XVII веке, не отвечали никакой непосредственной социальной потребности. (Как следствие, Рёйсдал голодал, а Хоббема вынужден был забросить живопись.) Пейзажная живопись с самого своего начала была деятельностью относительно независимой. Безусловно, будучи частью традиции, пейзажисты унаследовали ее нормы и методы и в целом их придерживались. Но всякий раз, когда традиция масляной живописи значительно модифицировалась, первый шаг к этому делался именно в живописи пейзажной. Начиная с XVII века выдающимися реформаторами способов видения, а значит, и техники, были Рёйсдал, Рембрандт (характер использования света в его поздних работах пришел из его пейзажных этюдов), Констебль (в своих набросках), Тёрнер и, в конце этого периода, Моне и импрессионисты. Более того, их нововведения постепенно вели от материального и осязаемого к неопределенному и неосязаемому.

Тем не менее специфические отношения между масляной живописью и собственностью сыграли свою роль и в развитии пейзажного жанра. Рассмотрим в качестве примера известную картину Гейнсборо *Портрет четы Эндрюс.*

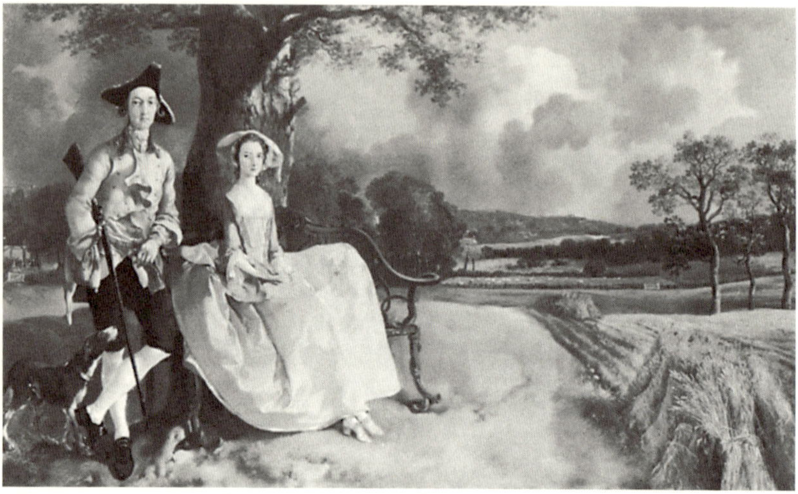
ПОРТРЕТ ЧЕТЫ ЭНДРЮС. ГЕЙНСБОРО. 1727–1788

Кеннет Кларк так пишет о Гейнсборо и этой его картине:

> «В самом начале карьеры радость от увиденного вдохновляла его на создание в картине фона, прописанного с тончайшей наблюдательностью, – как, например, хлебное поле, куда он поместил мистера и миссис Эндрюс. Это очаровательное произведение написано с такой любовью и мастерством, что следовало бы ожидать движения Гейнсборо в том же направлении, но он отказался от живописи с натуры и занялся написанием картин в том нежном стиле, каковым и прославился. Биографы Гейнсборо пришли к выводу, что работа над заказными портретами не оставляла ему времени на этюды с натуры, и в подтверждение того, что Гейнсборо, имей он возможность, был бы натуралистическим пейзажистом, цитировали его знаменитое

письмо, в котором говорится, что «его тошнит от портретов и ему хочется взять виолу да гамба и пешком отправиться в какую-нибудь прелестную деревушку, где можно заняться пейзажами». Однако письмо о виоле да гамба — не более чем проявление руссоизма Гейнсборо. Его истинное мнение на сей счет выражено в письме к одному из его покровителей, который оказался настолько простодушен, что обратился к художнику с просьбой изобразить на холсте его парк. «М-р Гейнсборо выражает нижайшее почтение лорду Хардвику и почтет за честь выполнить любое поручение его светлости; что же до подлинных видов с натуры, то он берет на себя смелость заметить, что не видел в этой стране ни одного места, которое давало бы тему, достойную самых жалких подражаний Дюге или Лоррену».[4]

Зачем лорду Хардвику нужна была картина с изображением его парка? Зачем мистер и миссис Эндрюс заказали своей портрет на фоне знакомого им пейзажа – своих владений?

Они отнюдь не пара на лоне Природы, как эту природу представлял себе Руссо. Они землевладельцы, и то, что окружающее принадлежит им, явно читается в их позах и выражении лиц.

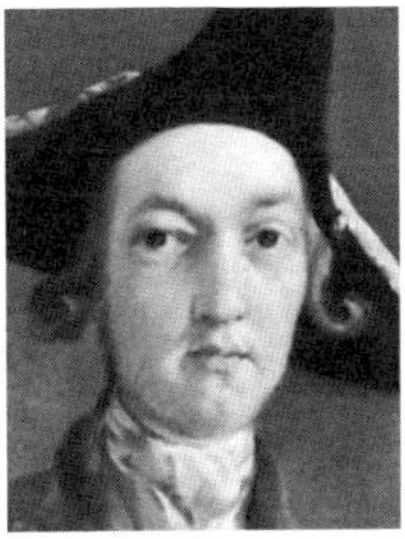

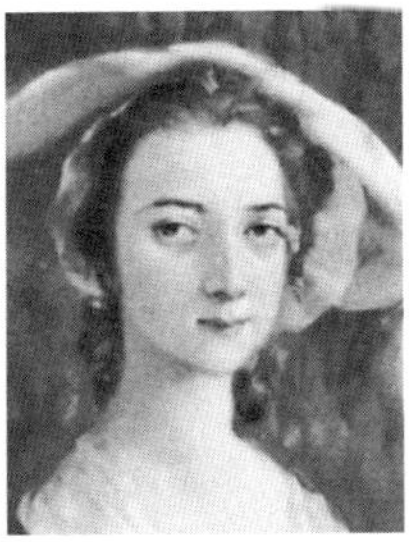

[4] Кеннет Кларк. Пейзаж в искусстве. Пер. Н. Н. Тихонова. – СПб.: Азбука-классика, 2004.

Профессор Лоуренс Гоуинг с негодованием отверг нашу мысль о том, что мистера и миссис Эндрюс интересует их собственность:

> «Прежде чем Джон Бергер снова встанет между нами и явным смыслом хорошей картины, я хотел бы отметить, что есть свидетельства, подтверждающие, что мистер и миссис Эндрюс у Гейнсборо не просто владеют своим кусочком земли. Прямое следование чрезвычайно похожей и известной Гейнсборо композиции, найти которую можно у его учителя Френсиса Хеймана, подразумевает, что люди на таких картинах погружены в наслаждение «высшим Законом... истинным светом неиспорченной и неискаженной Природы».

Аргументацию профессора стоит процитировать, поскольку она замечательно иллюстрирует то лицемерие, которым страдает история искусства. Разумеется, вполне возможно, что мистер и миссис Эндрюс наслаждаются неискаженной Природой. Но это никоим образом не мешает им быть одновременно и гордыми собой землевладельцами. В большинстве случаев владение землей было необходимым условием такого философского наслаждения – отнюдь не редкого среди поместного дворянства. Однако это наслаждение «неиспорченной и неискаженной природой» обычно не распространялось на природу человеческую. Наказанием за браконьерство была высылка. И если человек своровал картофелину, его могли публично высечь по приказу судьи, в роли которого выступал сам землевладелец. То, что считалось *природным*, имело, между тем, очень строгие границы как частная собственность.

Мысль, которую я тут провожу, заключается в том, что среди удовольствий, которые этот портрет доставлял чете Эндрюс, было удовольствие видеть себя в роли землевладельцев; удовольствие это усиливалось благодаря свойствам масляной живописи, позволяющим изобразить их землю во всей ее материальности. И данное наблюдение необходимо озвучить именно потому, что история культуры (как она обычно нам преподается) делает вид, будто оно не стоит внимания.

Наш обзор европейской масляной живописи был очень сжатым, а потому поверхностным. Это не более чем проект исследования, которое, возможно, найдет своего автора. Исходная же точка исследования должна быть видна уже сейчас. Благодаря своим особым качествам масляная живопись легла в основу особой системы правил воспроизведения видимого мира. Суммарный итог этих правил — способ видения, изобретенный в масляной живописи. Часто говорят, что написанная маслом картина в раме подобна окну, за которым открывается мир. Примерно так в общих чертах и видит саму себя эта художественная традиция, с поправкой на те стилистические изменения (маньеризм, барокко, неоклассицизм, реализм и т. д.), которые происходили с ней на протяжении четырех веков. Мы пытаемся доказать, что если изучать культуру европейской масляной живописи в целом и если оставить в стороне ее утверждения о себе самой, то ее ближайшей аналогией окажется не окно, открытое в мир, а сейф, встроенный в стену, сейф, в котором хранится то, что можно увидеть.

Меня обвиняют в том, что я помешался на собственности. Все совсем наоборот. На собственности помешались это общество и эта культура. Но для маньяка его навязчивая идея кажется чем-то, что в природе вещей, а потому и не осознается как навязчивая идея. Отношения между собственностью и искусством в европейской культуре кажутся этой культуре естественными, а потому, если кто-то в пределах данного культурного поля вы-ходит за рамки идеи собственности, то считается, что это *он* таким образом демонстрирует свою собственную манию. И это позволяет культурному истеблишменту еще какое-то время поддерживать собственный обманчивый образ.

Сущность масляной живописи была скрыта общим непониманием отношений между ее «традицией» и ее «мастерами». Исключительные художники в исключительных обстоятельствах освобождались от норм традиции и создавали произведения, прямо противоположные ее ценностям; и именно эти художники объявляются лучшими представителями традиции. Утверждать это тем легче, что после их смерти традиция смыкалась вокруг их произведений, вбирая второстепенные новшества технического характера и продолжаясь так, словно ничто принципиально не изменилось. Именно по этой причине ни Рембрандт, ни Вермеер, ни Пуссен, ни Шарден, ни Гойя, ни Тёрнер не имели последователей – лишь поверхностных подражателей.

В рамках традиции возник и стереотип о «великом художнике». Великий художник – это человек, вся жизнь которого тратится на борьбу: на борьбу с материальными условиями, на борьбу с непониманием, на борьбу с самим собой. Он как Иаков, борющийся с Ангелом. (Примеров тому множество – от Микеланджело до Ван Гога.) Ни одна другая культура так не мыслит своих художников. Почему же так происходит в этой? Мы ужс упоминали открытый художественный рынок и его требования. Однако борьба художника не сводилась к борьбе за выживание. Когда художник осознавал, что его не устраивает ограниченная роль живописи как инструмента прославления собственности и статуса ее владельца, он неизбежно обнаруживал, что вынужден бороться с самим языком своего творчества – с тем, как этот язык понимается той традицией, к которой мастер принадлежит.

Для нашей аргументации крайне существенны два понятия, а именно: исключительного и среднестатистического (типичного) произведения. Но эти категории не могут механистически применяться в качестве критерия для критики. Критик должен понимать обстоятельства этого антагонизма. Каждое выдающееся произведение было результатом долгой и успешной борьбы. Огромное количество картин было написано без борьбы. Случалась также и долгая, но безуспешная борьба.

Чтобы стать исключением, художник, чье видение было сформировано традицией (вероятно, в шестнадцать лет он уже поступил в подмастерья или в ученики), должен был понять, что представляет собой это видение, а затем отделить его от сферы творчества, в которой оно укоренилось. И так, в одиночку, он должен был бороться с нормами искусства, сформировавшими его. Он должен был видеть себя художником, отрицающим способ видения мира, присущий художникам. Это значит, что он видел себя делающим нечто такое, чего никто другой не мог предвидеть. Меру требуемых усилий можно оценить по двум автопортретам Рембрандта.

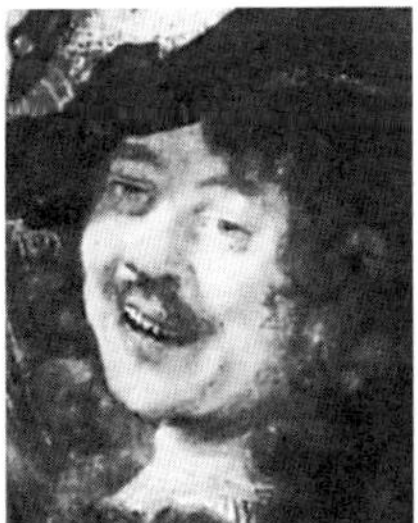

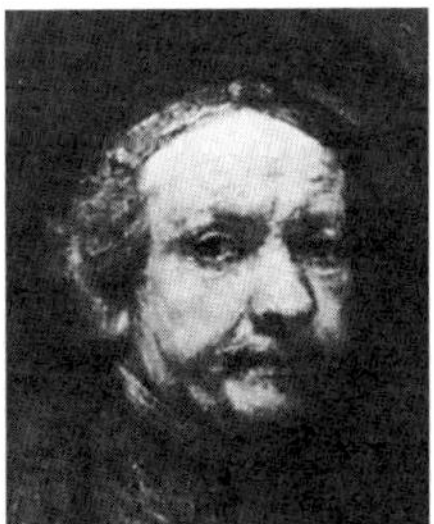

Первый был написан в 1634 году, когда Рембрандту было 28 лет; второй – 30 лет спустя. Но различие между ними не сводится к тому факту, что время изменило внешность и характер художника.

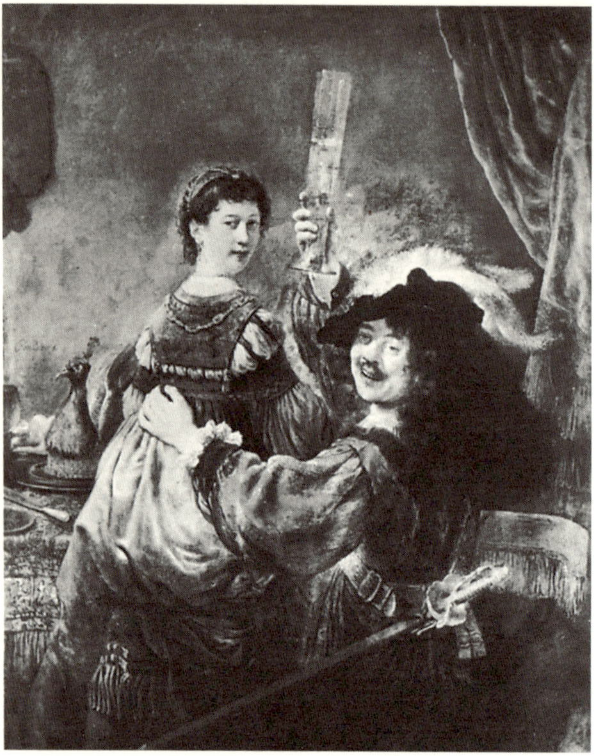

АВТОПОРТРЕТ С САСКИЕЙ НА КОЛЕНЯХ. РЕМБРАНДТ. 1606–1669

Первая картина занимает особенное место в повествовании о жизни Рембрандта. Он написал ее в год своей первой женитьбы. Здесь он похваляется Саскией, своей невестой. Через шесть лет она умрет. Считается, что эта картина воплощает в себе так называемый счастливый период жизни Рембрандта. Однако если рассмотреть ее сегодня без всякой сентиментальности, то можно увидеть, что изображенное на ней счастье – внешнее и неискреннее. Рембрандт использует здесь традиционные приемы в традиционных целях. Пожалуй, уже начинает узнаваться его индивидуальный стиль. Но это не более чем стиль новичка, исполняющего традиционную роль. Картина в целом остается ре-

АВТОПОРТРЕТ.
РЕМБРАНДТ.
1606–1669

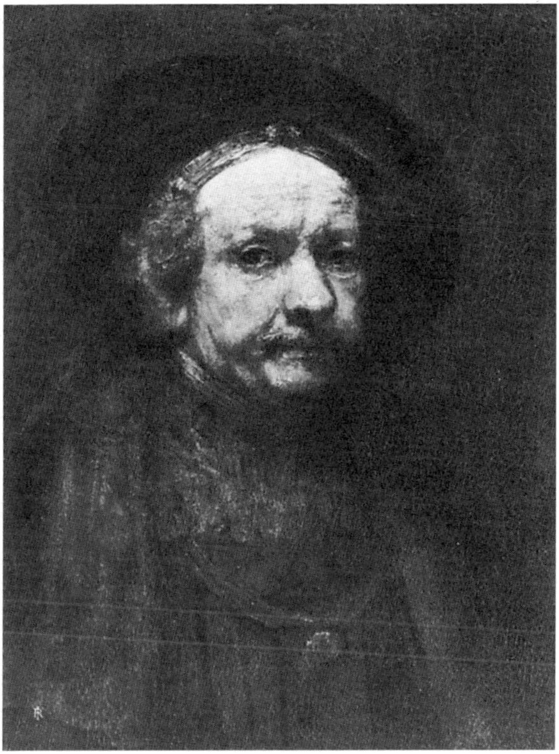

кламой счастья, авторитета и богатства изображенного на ней человека (в данном случае самого Рембрандта). И, как в любой такой рекламе, в ней нет настоящего чувства.

В поздней своей картине художник направил традицию против нее самой. Он отнял у нее ее язык. Он старик. Все ушло, осталось лишь переживание вопроса о существовании, переживание существования как вопроса. И живущий в старике художник (который одновременно и больше, и меньше, чем просто старик) нашел возможность выразить это и только это, используя изобразительные средства, исконно разработанные для того, чтобы исключить подобного рода вопросы.

6

ЕВРОПА, ПОДДЕРЖИВАЕМАЯ АФРИКОЙ И АМЕРИКОЙ

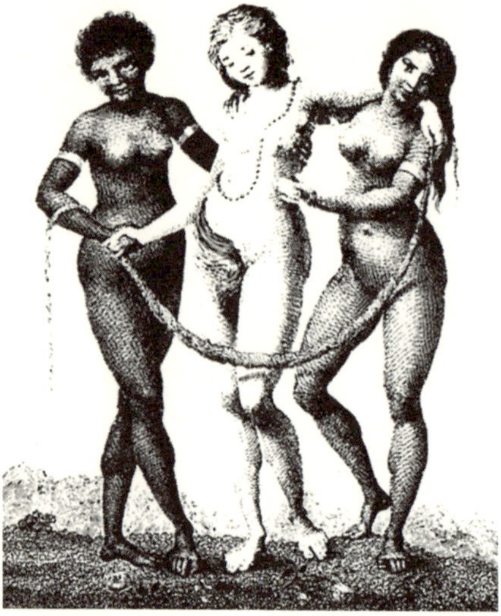

ПЬЕТА

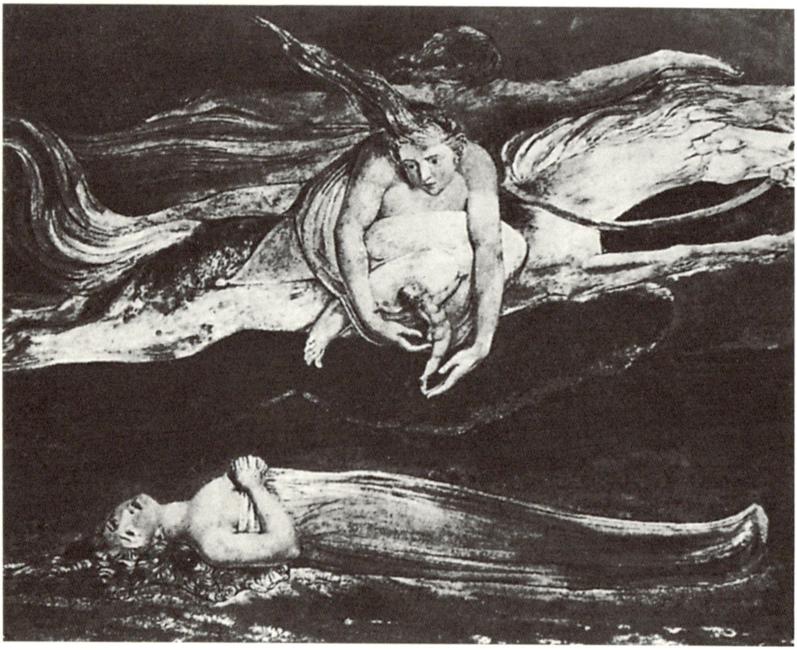

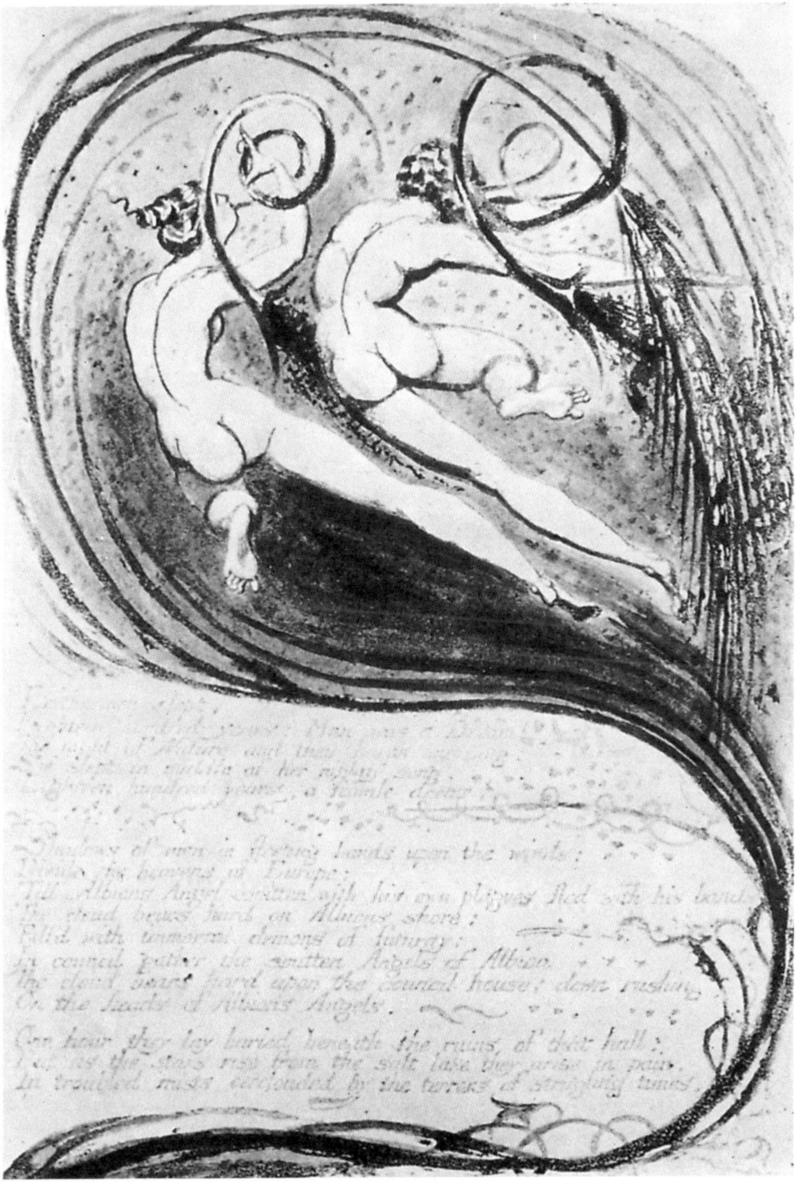
Shadows of men in fleeting bands upon the winds:
Divide the heavens of Europe:
Till Albions Angel smitten with his own plagues fled with his bands
The cloud bears hard on Albions shore:
Fill'd with immortal demons of futurity:
In council gather the smitten Angels of Albion
The cloud bears hard upon the council house; down rushing
On the heads of Albions Angels.
One hour they lay buried beneath the ruins of that hall;
But as the stars rise from the salt lake they arise in pain.
In troubled mists o'erclouded by the terrors of struggling times.

ЗЕРНО, ПОРАЖАЕМОЕ БОЛЕЗНЬЮ

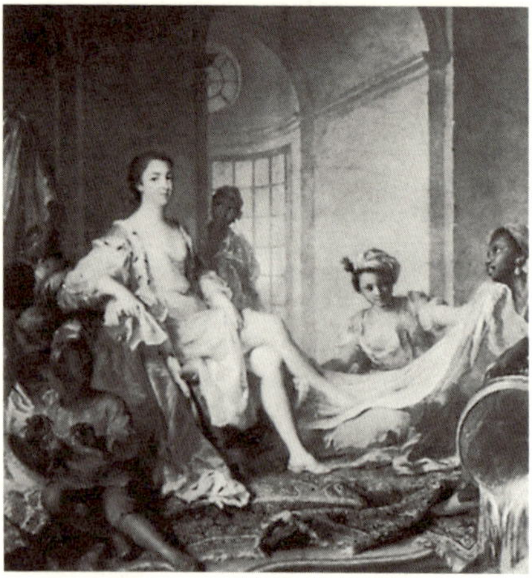

ПРОДАЖА КАРТИН И РАБОВ В РОТОНДЕ НОВОГО ОРЛЕАНА. 1842

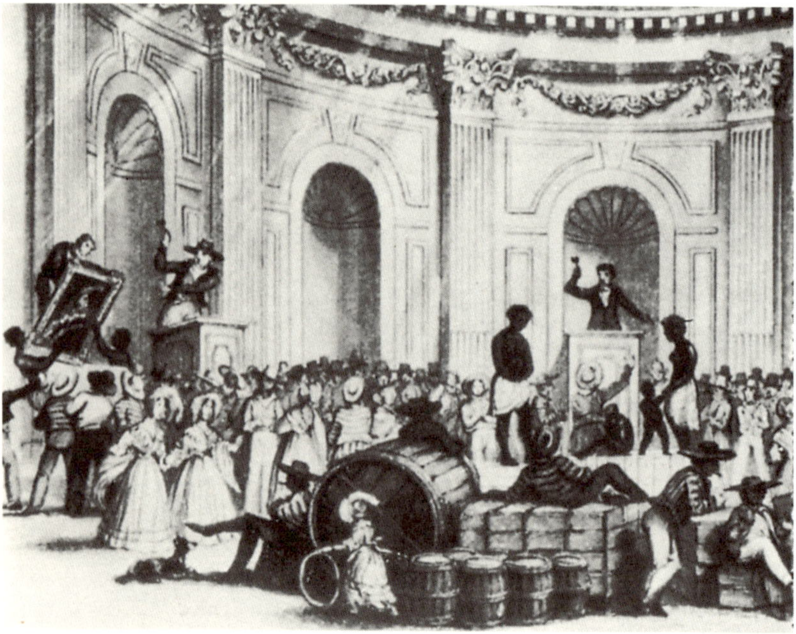

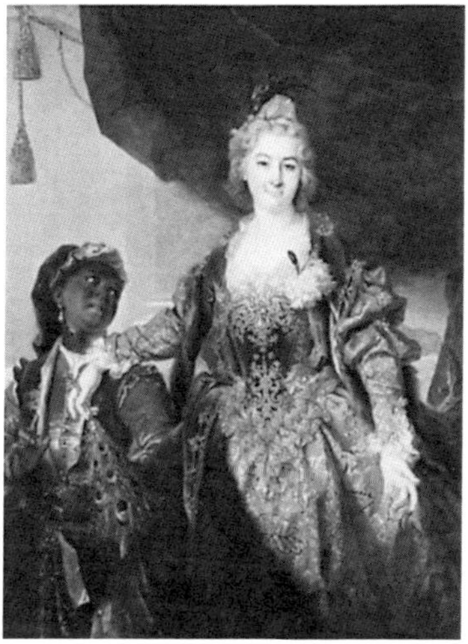

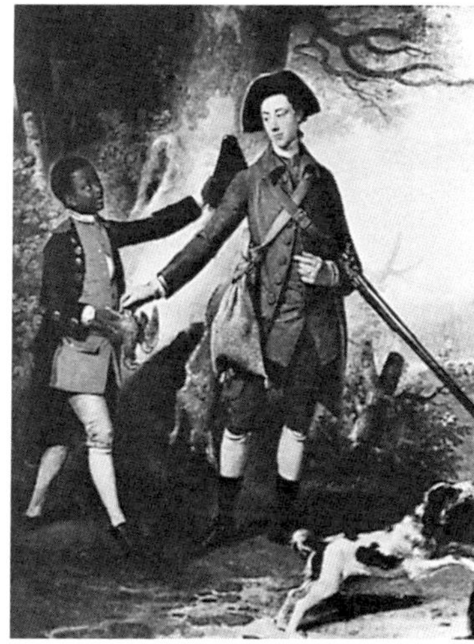

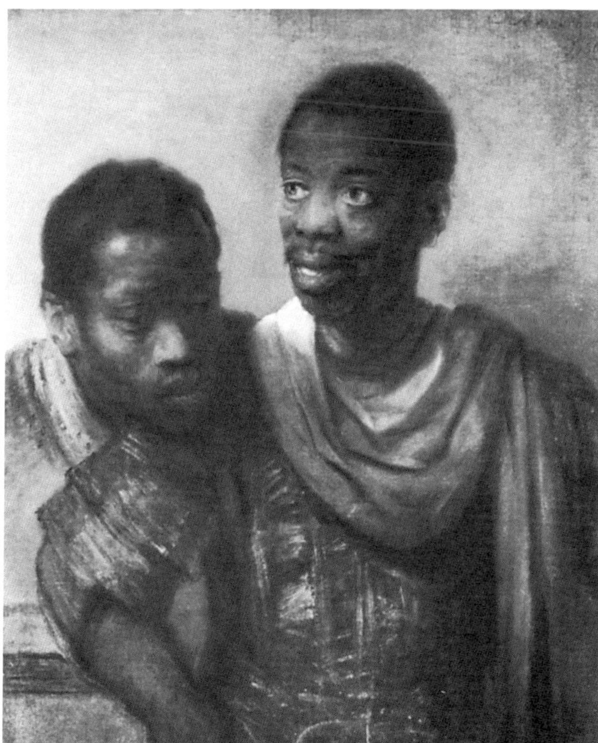

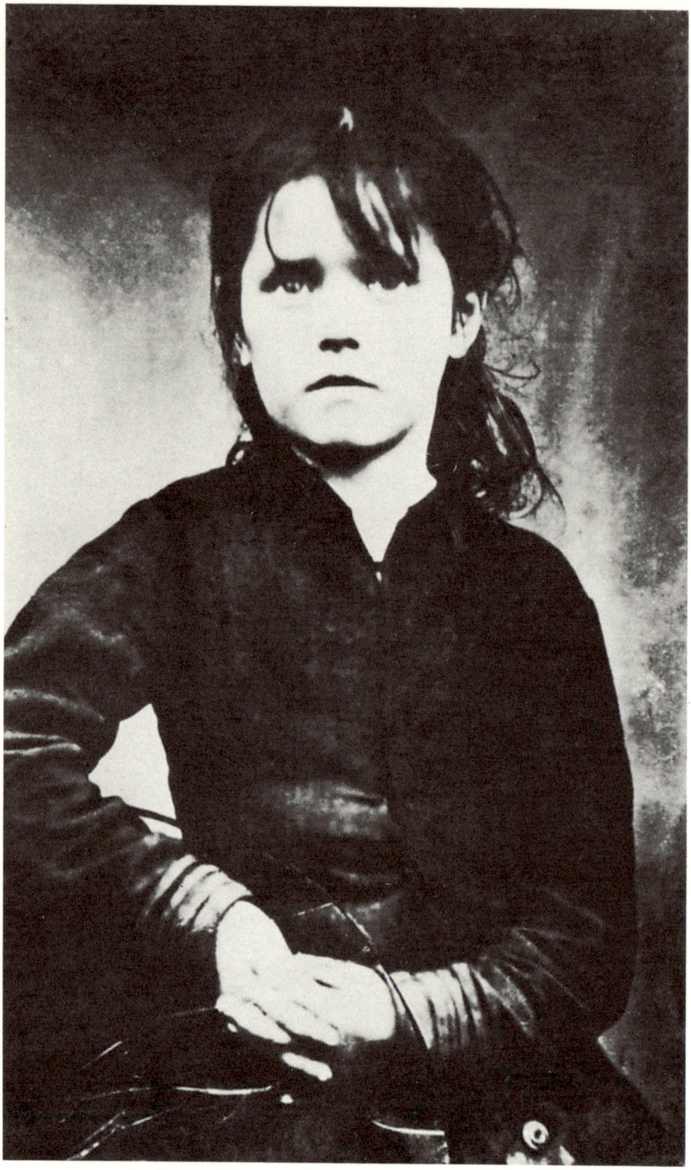

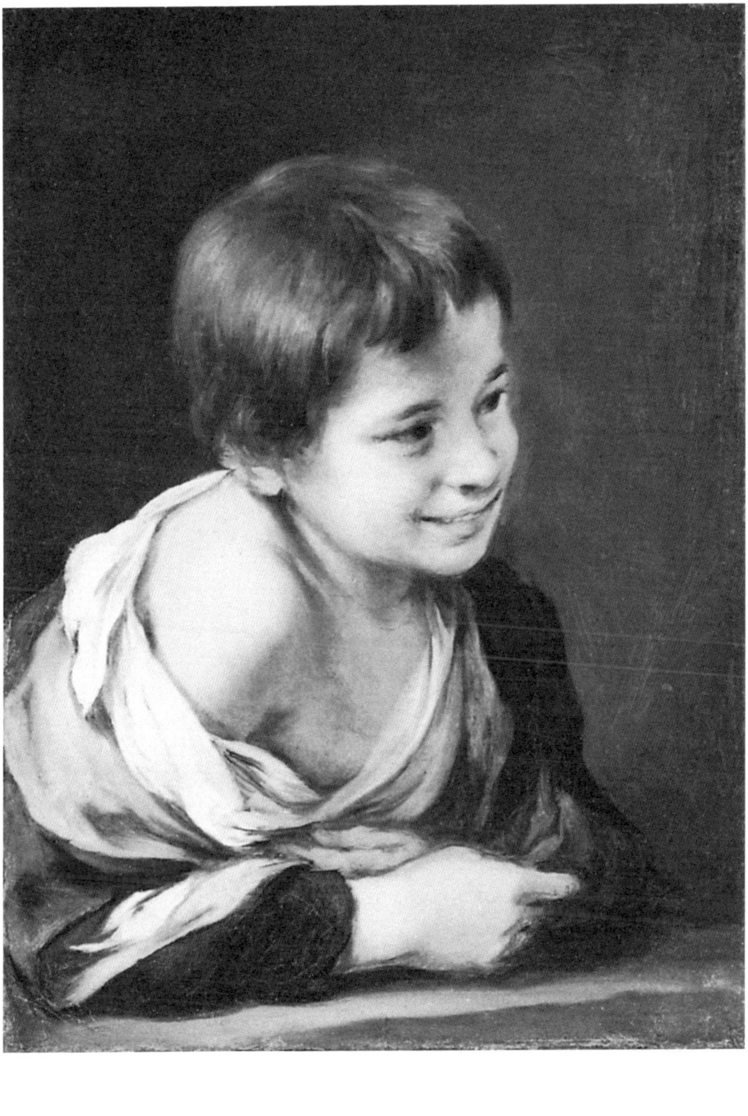

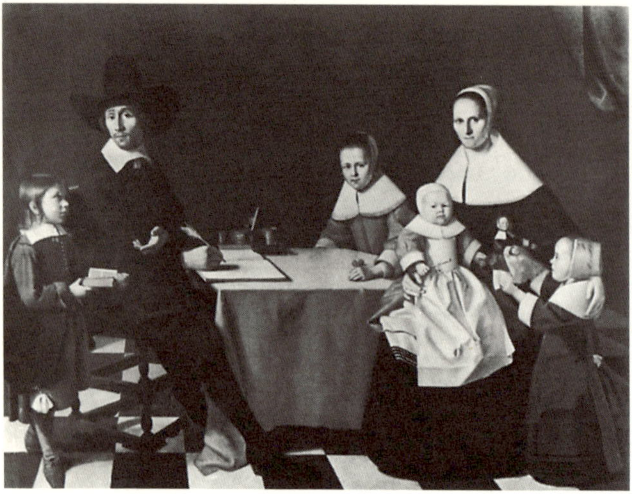

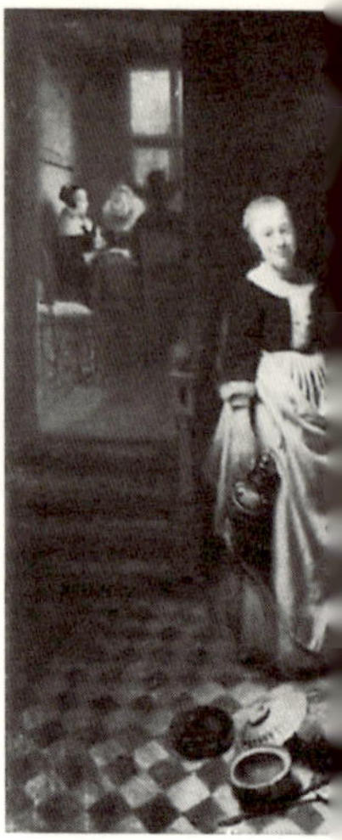

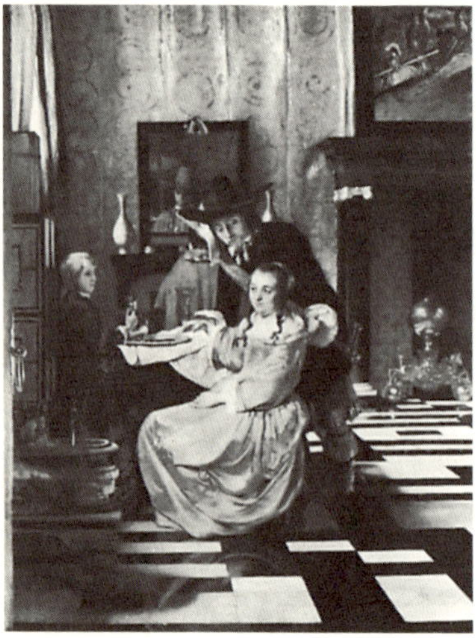

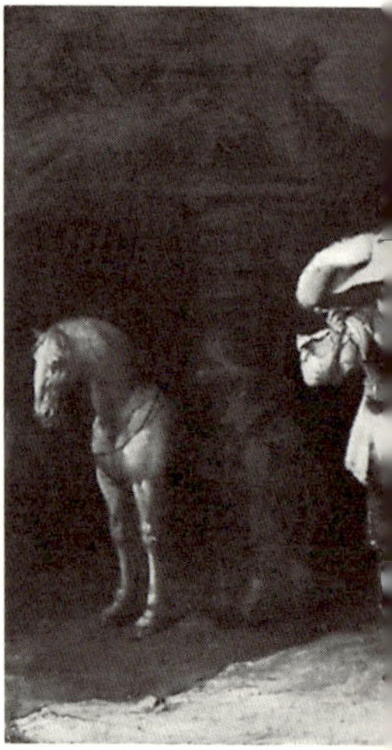

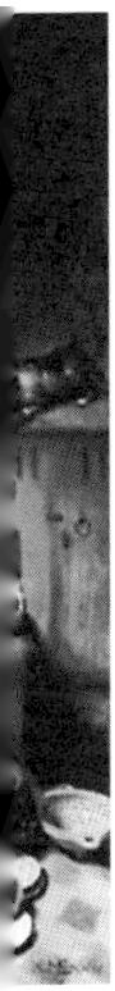

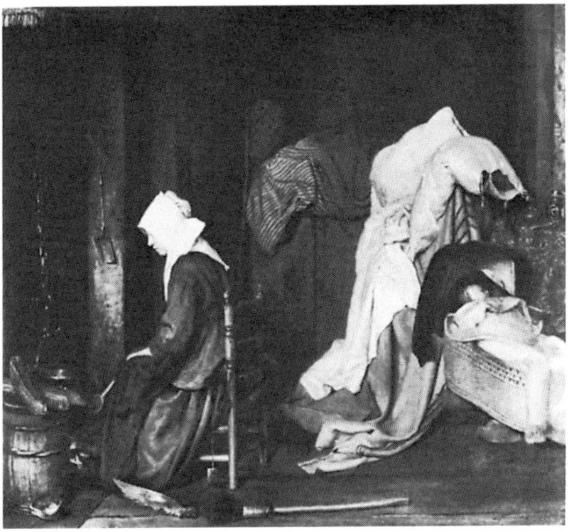

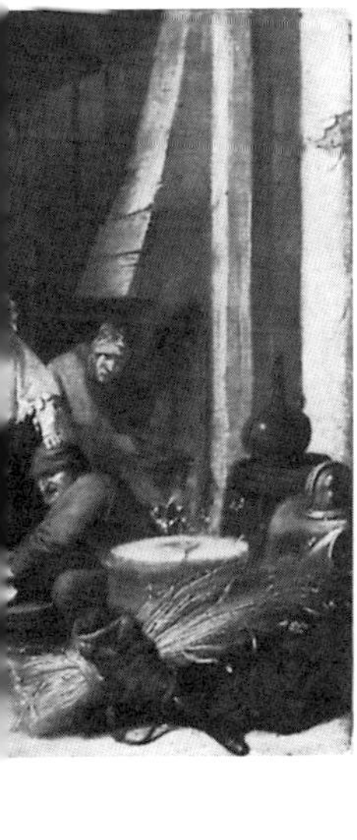

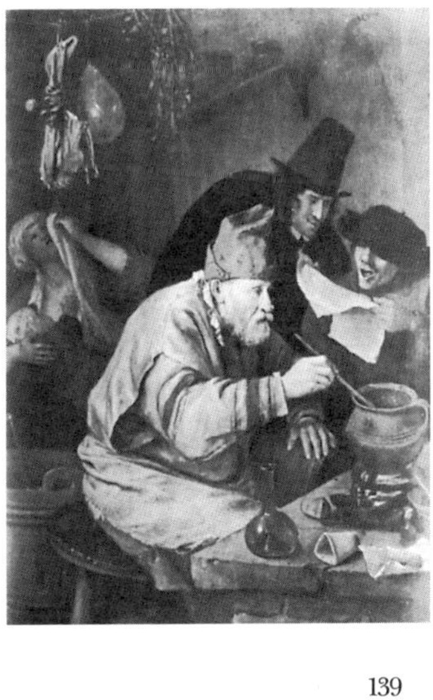

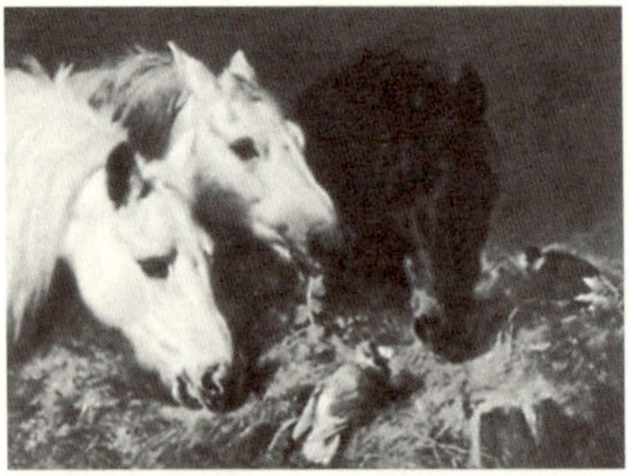
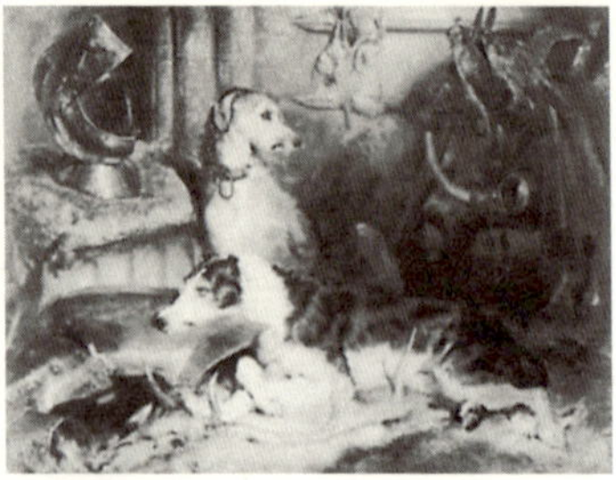
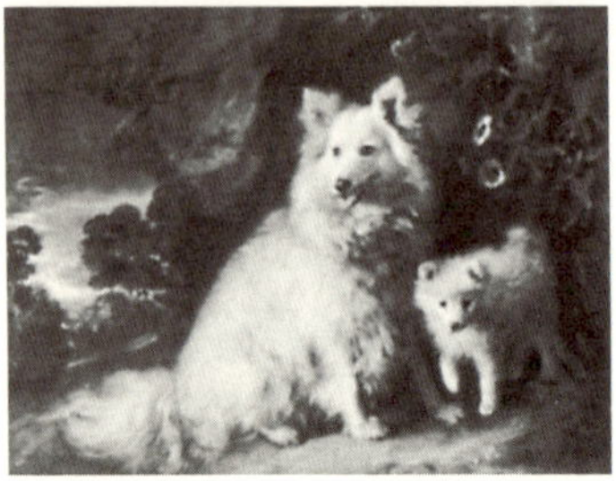
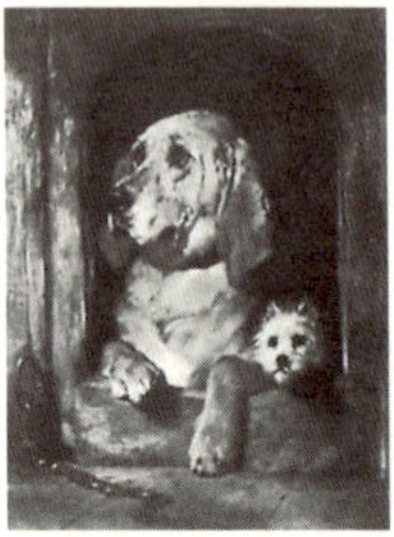
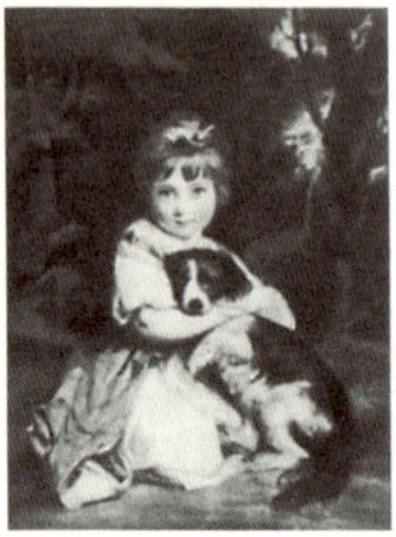
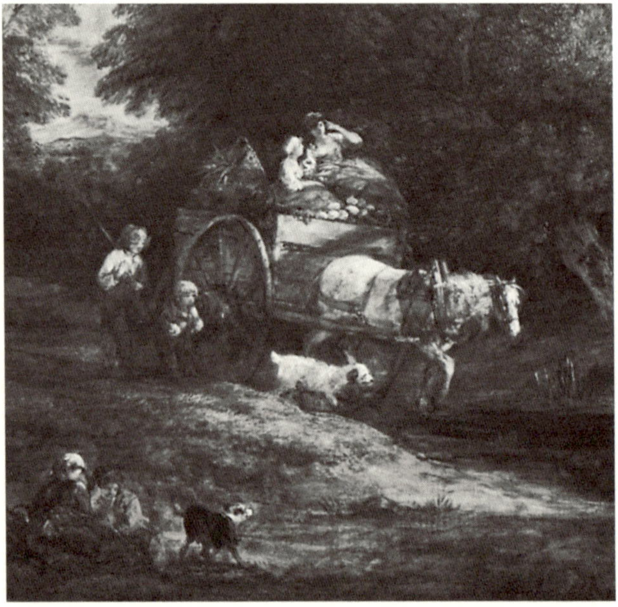

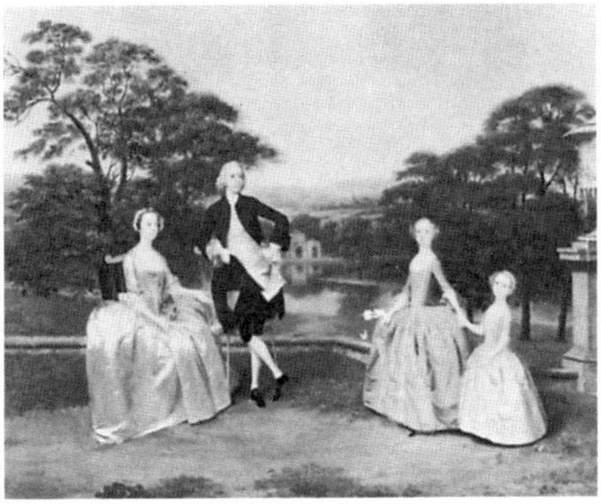

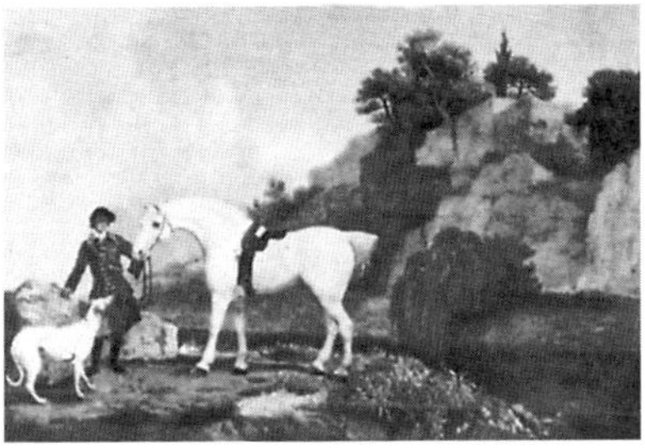

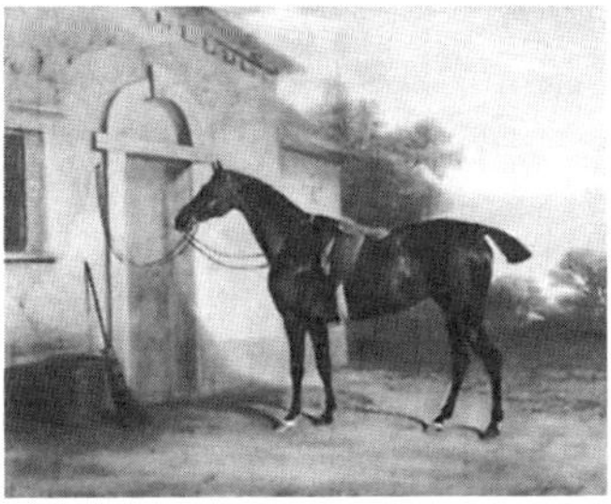

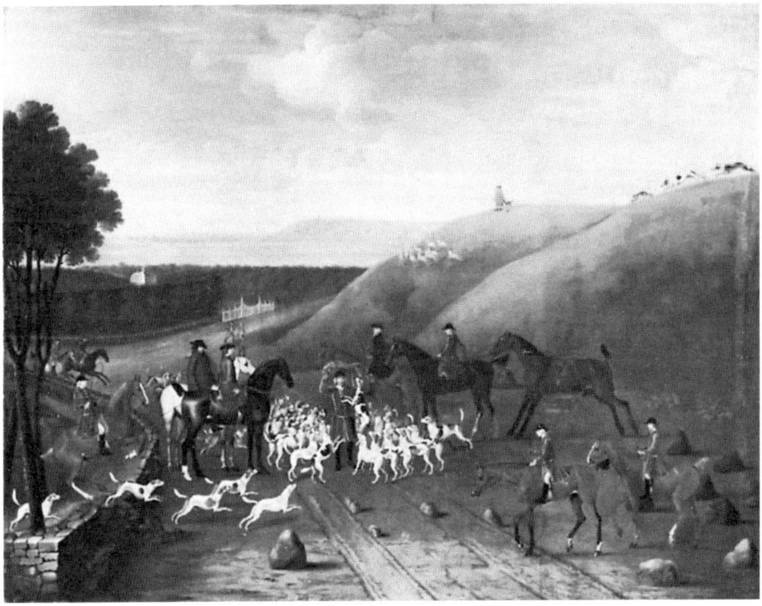

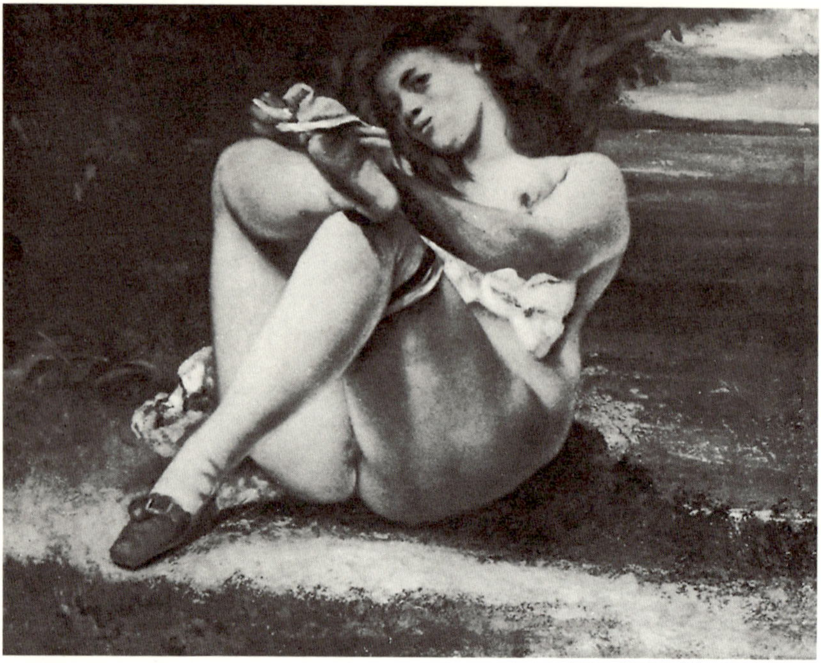

ЖЕНЩИНА С БЕЛЫМИ ЧУЛКАМИ

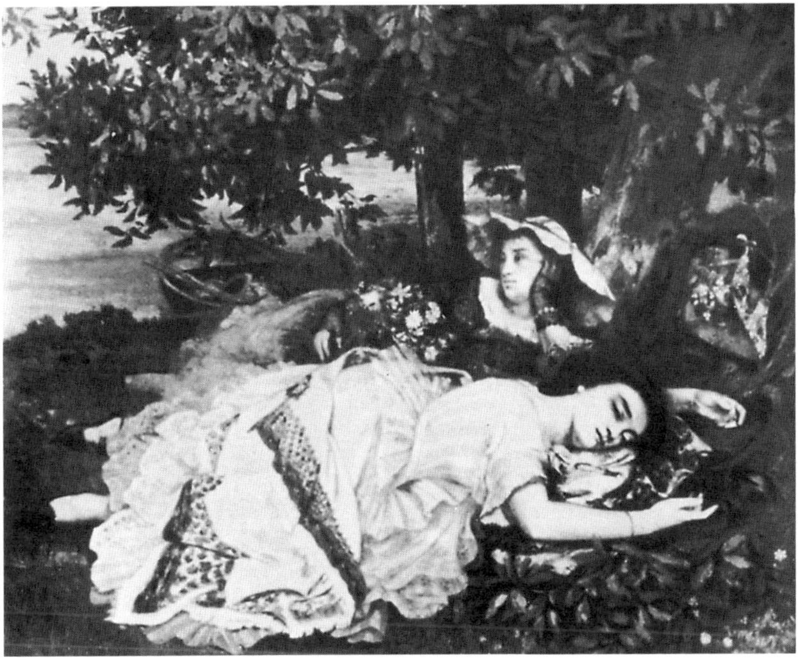

ДЕВУШКИ НА БЕРЕГУ СЕНЫ

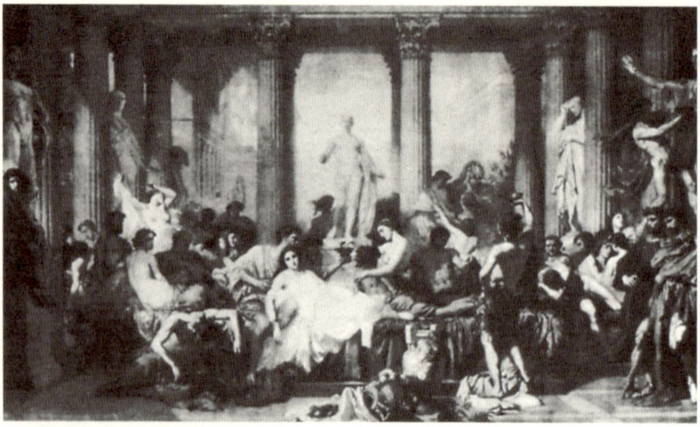

РИМЛЯНЕ
ЭПОХИ
УПАДКА

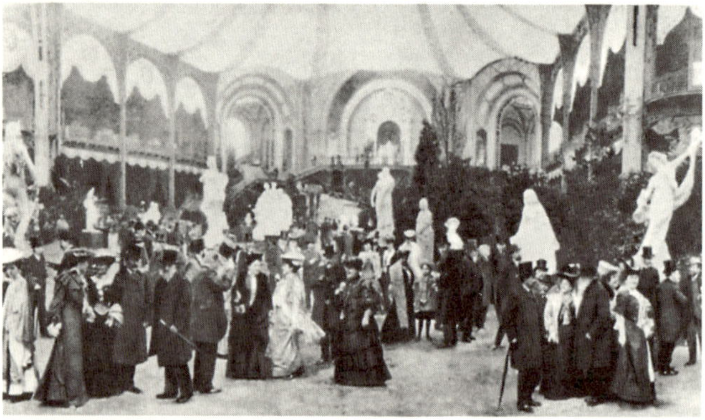

САЛОН

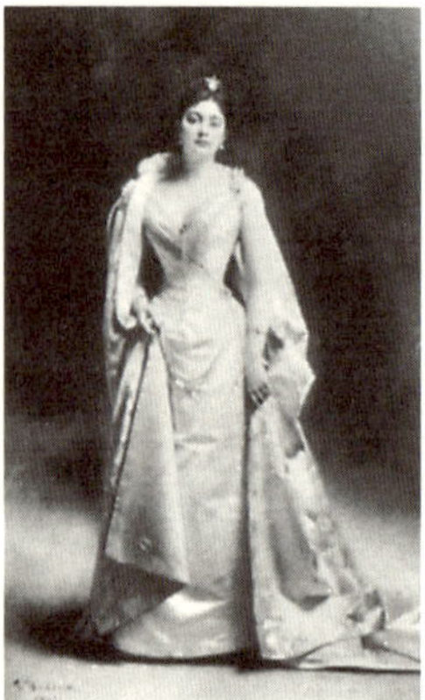

МАДАМ КАЭН Д’АНВЕР

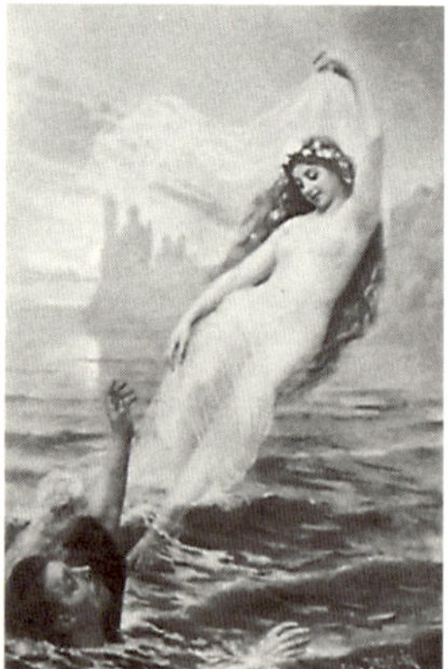

УНДИНА

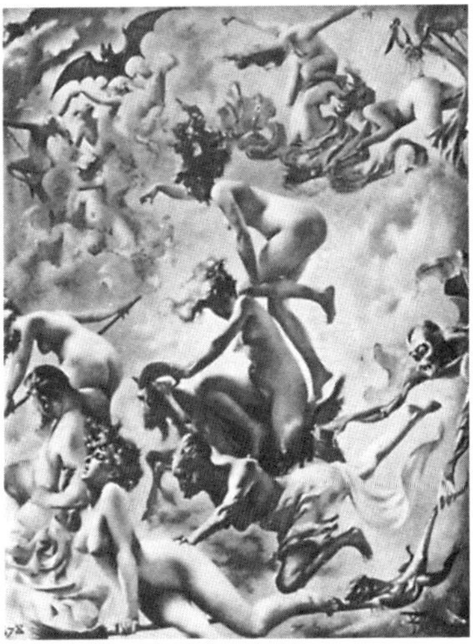

НА ШАБАШ

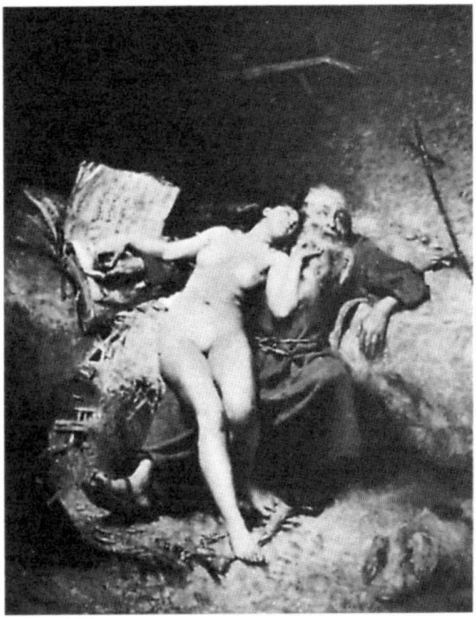

ИСКУШЕНИЕ СВЯТОГО АНТОНИЯ

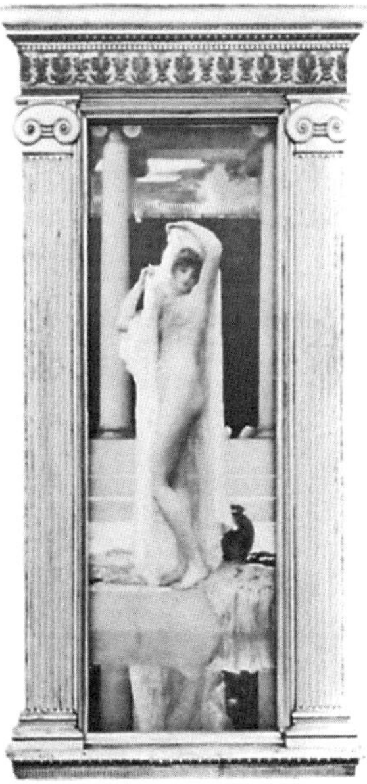

КУПАНИЕ ПСИХЕИ

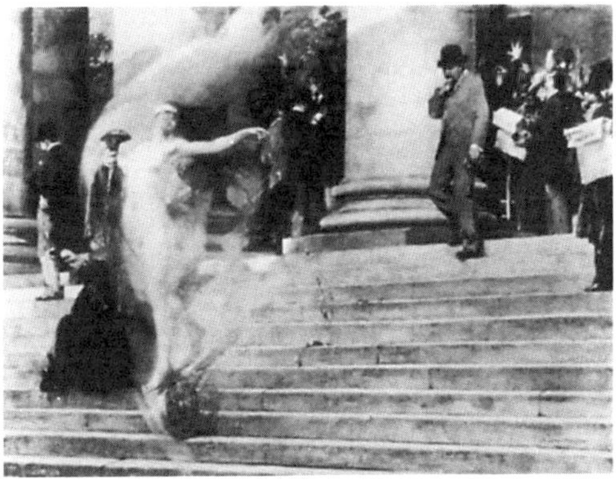

ФОРТУНА

7

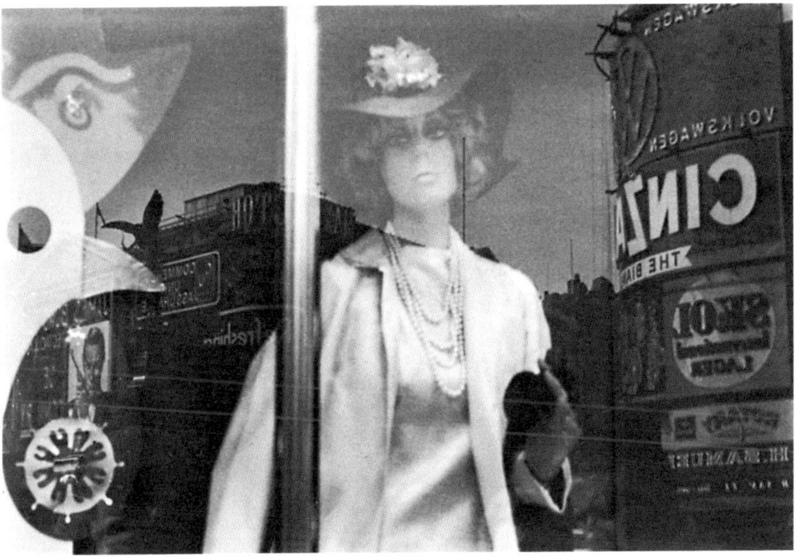

В городах, где мы живем, каждый день нашей жизни каждый из нас видит сотни рекламных изображений. Никакие другие образы не возникают перед нами так часто.

Ни в каком другом обществе в прошлом не существовало такой концентрации образов, такой плотности визуальной информации.

Человек может запомнить или забыть эту информацию, но какое-то мгновение он все-таки воспринимает ее, и она стимулирует его воображение при посредстве либо памяти, либо ожидания. Рекламный образ принадлежит мгновению. Мы замечаем его, переворачивая страницу, поворачивая за угол, глядя на проезжающий мимо автобус. Или видим его на экране телевизора, дожидаясь, когда же кончится рекламная пауза. Рекламные образы принадлежат мгновению также и в том смысле, что они все время должны обновляться, дабы оставаться актуальными. И, тем не менее, они никогда не говорят о настоящем. Они часто отсылают к прошлому и всегда говорят о будущем.

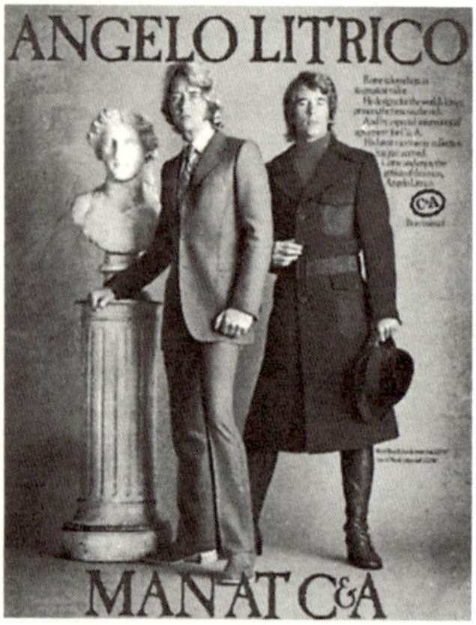

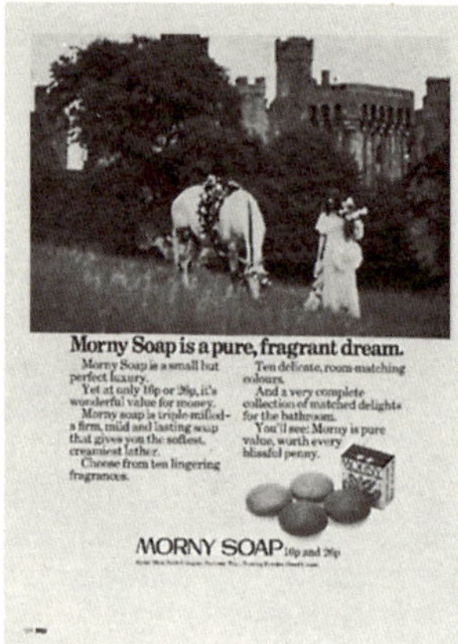

Мы сегодня совсем привыкли к тому, что эти образы обращаются к нам, и практически не замечаем их совокупного воздействия на нас. Человек может обратить внимание на отдельную картинку (и на ту информацию, которую она несет), поскольку она отвечает некоему его конкретному интересу. Но система рекламных образов в цслом воспринимается нами просто как постоянный фон. Например, тот факт, что эти образы принадлежат текущему мгновению, но говорят о будущем, создает странный эффект, ставший столь привычным, что мы почти не замечаем его. Обычно это мы проходим мимо изображения – идя пешком, проезжая на машине или переворачивая страницу книги; если перед нами экран телевизора, то дело обстоит несколько иначе, однако и тогда теоретически мы являемся активными участниками процесса – мы можем отвернуться, выключить звук, пойти сделать кофе. И, несмотря на это, у нас создается впечатление, что рекламные образы постоянно проносятся мимо нас, подобно скорым поездам, стремящимся к своему далекому пункту назначения. Мы стоим на месте, а они движутся, пока газета не выкидывается, телевизионная программа не заканчивается, а афиша не заклеивается новой.

О рекламе обычно говорят, объясняя ее значение и оправдывая ее существование, как о двигателе прогресса, в конечном счете работающем на общество (потребителя) и лучших из производителей – и, таким образом, на всю национальную экономику. Эта мысль тесно связана с некоторыми идеями относительно свободы – свободы выбора для покупателя, свободы предпринимательства для производителя. Огромные плакаты и неоновая реклама капиталистических городов – типичный «видимый» признак «Свободного Мира».

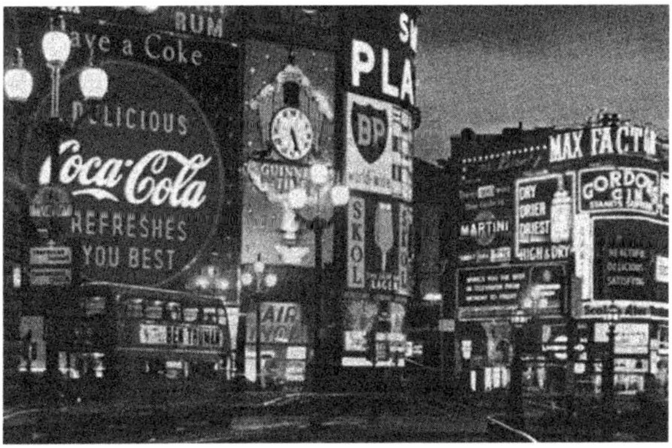

Для многих жителей Восточной Европы эти образы символизируют все то, чего им там, на Востоке, не хватает. Предполагается, что реклама создает возможность свободного выбора.

Действительно, благодаря рекламе одна торговая марка, одна фирма соперничает с другой; но вместе с тем эффект от каждого рекламного образа подкрепляет и усиливает воздействие всех остальных рекламных образов. Реклама – это не просто совокупность конкурирующих между собой сообщений, это самодостаточный язык, который используется для того, чтобы донести одно и то же главное сообщение. Внутри рекламного текста нам предлагается выбор между этими сливками и теми сливками, между той машиной и этой машиной, но реклама как система предлагает нам одну-единственную вещь.

Она предлагает каждому из нас изменить себя (или свою жизнь), купив что-нибудь еще.

Это что-то, как она утверждает, сделает нас неким образом богаче (хотя мы и станем беднее, потратив свои деньги).

Реклама убеждает нас в возможности такой трансформации, показывая нам людей, якобы прошедших через нее и теперь вызывающих у нас зависть. Стремление вызывать зависть – вот что лежит в основе гламура. И реклама – это производство гламура.

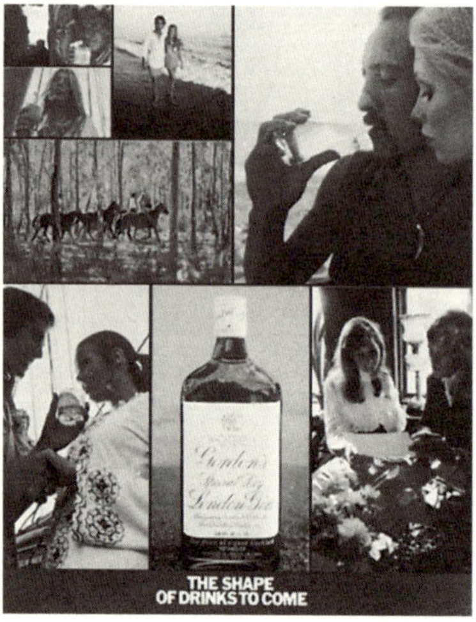

Тут важно разделить собственно рекламу и то удовольствие или пользу, которые можно получить от рекламируемых вещей. Реклама действенна постольку, поскольку она опирается на реальность. Одежда, еда, машины, косметика, море, солнце – все это вполне реальные вещи, которыми можно непосредственно наслаждаться. Реклама начинается с возбуждения естественной жажды удовольствий. Но она не может предоставить сам объект удовольствия и не предлагает никакой подходящей замены этому удовольствию. Чем убедительнее реклама изображает удовольствие от купания в теплом, далеком море, тем яснее становится зрителю-покупателю, что он в сотнях километров от этого моря, и тем менее реальной кажется ему возможность искупаться. Именно по этой причине реклама не может позволить себе говорить непосредственно о продукте или возможности, предлагаемых покупателю, который ими еще не наслаждается. Реклама никогда не прославляет удовольствие как таковое. Она всегда говорит о будущем покупателе. Она предлагает покупателю его собственный образ, но ставший гламурным под воздействием того продукта, который эта реклама пытается продать. То есть рекламный образ за-

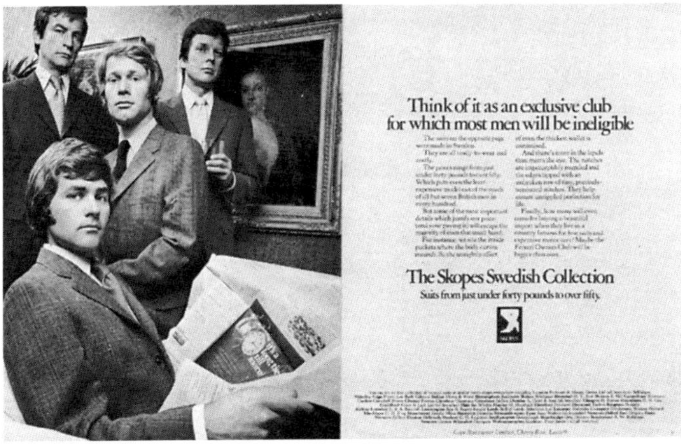

ставляет покупателя завидовать самому себе, каким он мог бы быть. Однако что же делает это возможное будущее достойным зависти? Зависть других. Реклама имеет отношение не столько к вещам, сколько к социальным отношениям. Она обещает не удовольствие, а счастье. А счастье быть предметом зависти – это гламур.

Чтобы самоутвердиться за счет зависти окружающих, необходимо дистанцироваться от них. Делиться опытом с теми, кто завидует, было бы неразумно. На тебя смотрят заинтересованно, но ты смотришь без интереса – в противном случае тебе будут меньше завидовать. В этом отношении те, кому завидуют, подобны чиновникам: чем более они безличны, тем убедительнее (для них самих и для окружающих) иллюзия их силы. Сила гламура коренится в приписываемом ему счастье; сила бюрократии – в приписываемой ей власти. Этим и объясняется пустой, расфокусированный взгляд, характерный для многих гламурных изображений. Они смотрят поверх завидующих взглядов, обеспечивающих их существование.

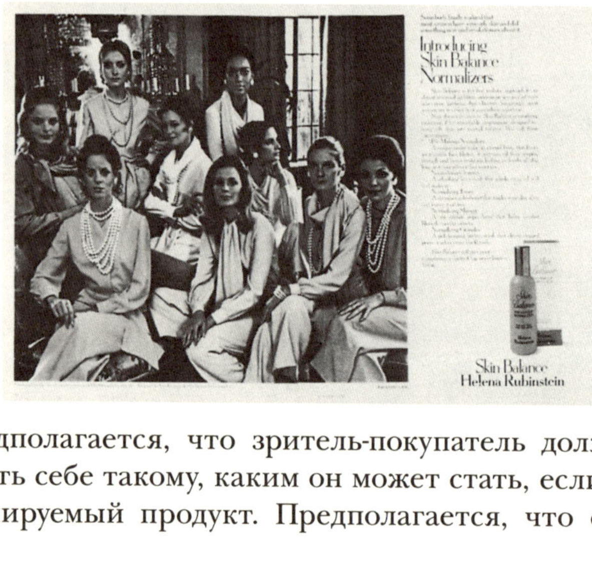

Предполагается, что зритель-покупатель должен завидовать себе такому, каким он может стать, если купит рекламируемый продукт. Предполагается, что он должен представить себя преображенным этим продуктом в объект чужой зависти – зависти, которая должна затем оправдать его любовь к самому себе. Можно сформулировать это иначе: рекламный образ крадет у потребителя его любовь к самому себе и предлагает получить ее обратно за цену продвигаемого продукта.

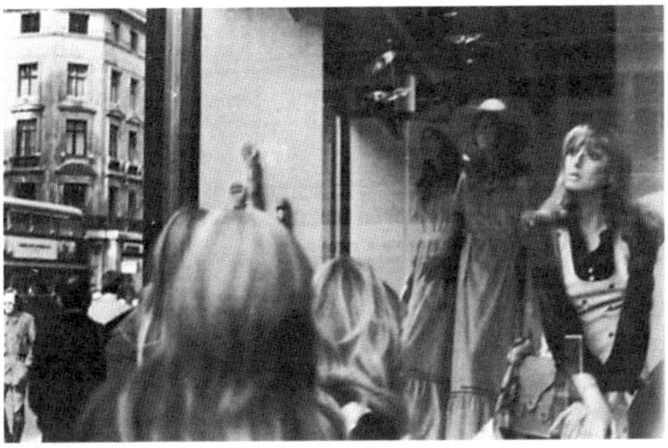

Имеет ли язык рекламы что-то общее с языком масляной живописи, который на протяжении четырех столетий, вплоть до изобретения фотоаппарата, доминировал в европейском видении мира?

Это один из тех вопросов, которые надо просто задать, для того чтобы ответ стал очевиден. Тут существует прямая преемственность. И только для сохранения авторитета культуры эта связь замалчивается. И, тем не менее, несмотря на эту преемственность, между ними существует принципиальное различие, которое не менее важно изучить.

В рекламе возникает масса отсылок к произведениям искусства минувших эпох. Иногда вся рекламная картинка представляет собой откровенную стилизацию под классическое полотно.

Рекламные образы нередко используют скульптуру и живопись, для того чтобы добавить себе обаяния и солидности. Картины в рамах часто висят в магазинных витринах вместе с другими товарами.

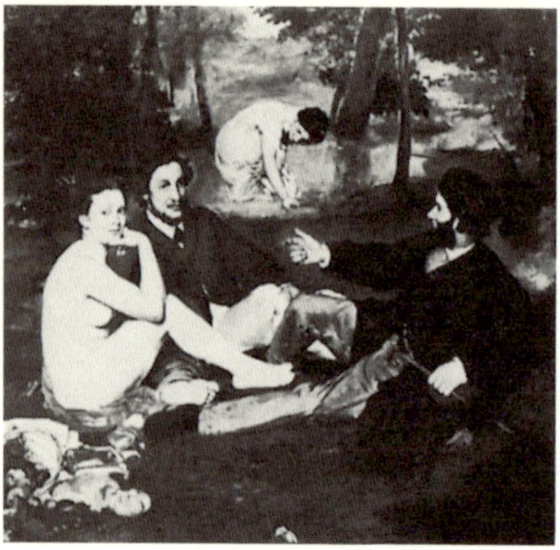

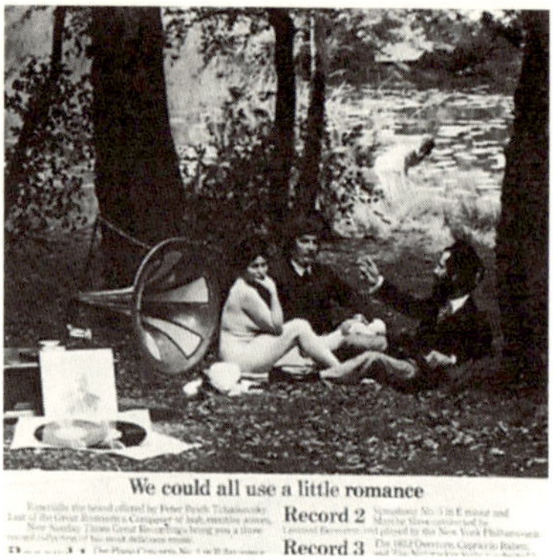

ЗАВТРАК НА ТРАВЕ. МАНЕ. 1832–1883

Любое произведение искусства, будучи «процитированным» рекламой, служит двум целям. Искусство – знак богатства, спутник хорошей жизни, это составляющая мира богатых и красивых.

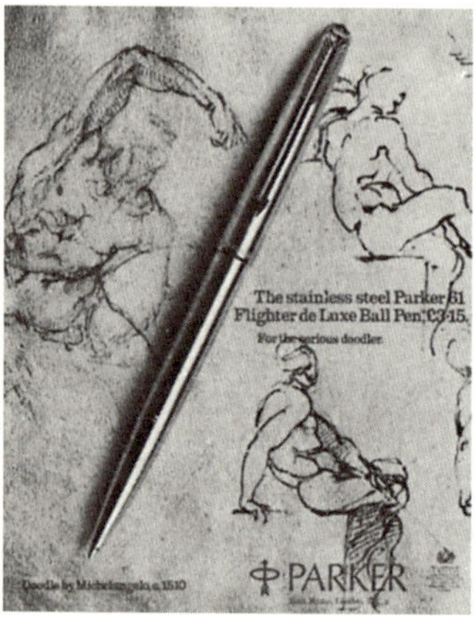

Но произведение искусства обладает еще и культурным авторитетом, своего рода величием или даже мудростью, что куда существеннее любого заурядного материального интереса. Масляная живопись принадлежит к культурному наследию: она напоминает нам, что значит быть цивилизованным европейцем. И, таким образом, произведение искусства, будучи процитированным, говорит две практически противоположные вещи (и этим-то оно полезно рекламе): оно символизирует одновременно богатство и духовность, оно утверждает, что покупка, которую предлагается сделать, – это и роскошь, и культурная ценность. На самом деле реклама поняла традицию масляной живописи лучше, чем большинство искусствоведов. Уловив подразумеваемые масляной живописью отношения между произведением искусства и его зрителем-владельцем, реклама при их посредстве пытается убедить зрителя-покупателя и польстить ему.

При этом связь между масляной живописью и рекламой лежит глубже простого «цитирования» того или иного произведения. Реклама в очень большой степени опирается на язык масляной живописи. Она тем же голосом говорит о тех же вещах. Порой визуальное сходство так велико, что можно играть в «мемори», используя вместо карточек эти совершенно одинаковые картинки или детали картинок.

Однако преемственность проявляется не только и не столько на уровне прямого образного сходства, сколько на уровне использованных знаков.

Сравните рекламные картинки и живописные полотна, приведенные в этой книге, или пройдитесь по оживленной торговой улице, заглядывая в витрины магазинов, а затем полистайте какой-нибудь иллюстрированный музейный каталог, – и вы увидите, сколь сходный смысл они транслируют. Это требует систематического исследования. Здесь мы можем лишь указать те сферы, в которых сходство приемов и целей особенно бросается в глаза.

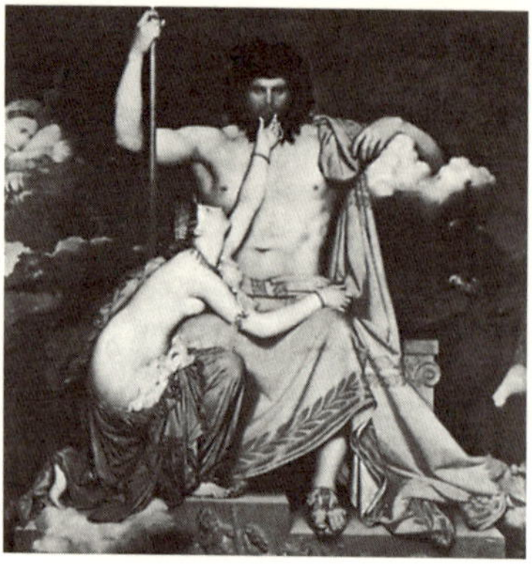

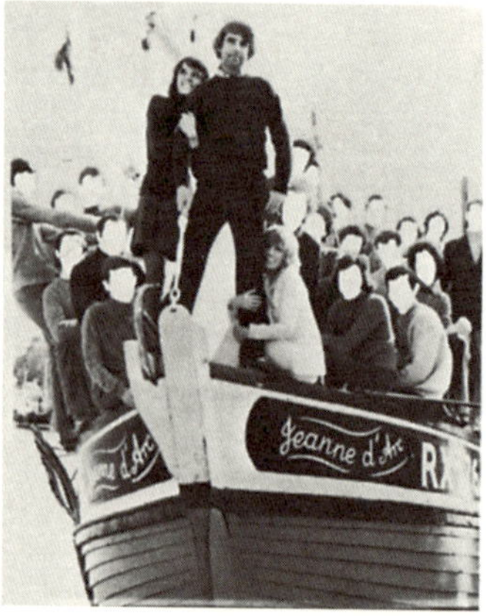
Jeanne d'Arc

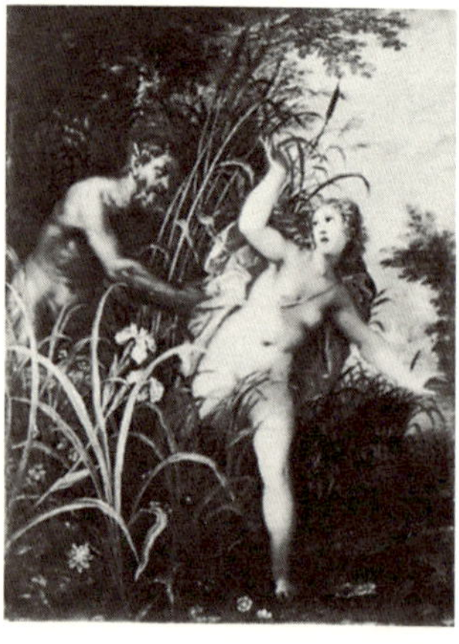

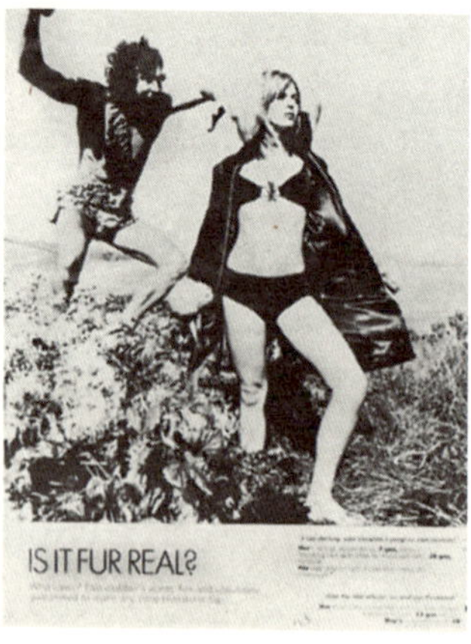
IS IT FUR REAL?

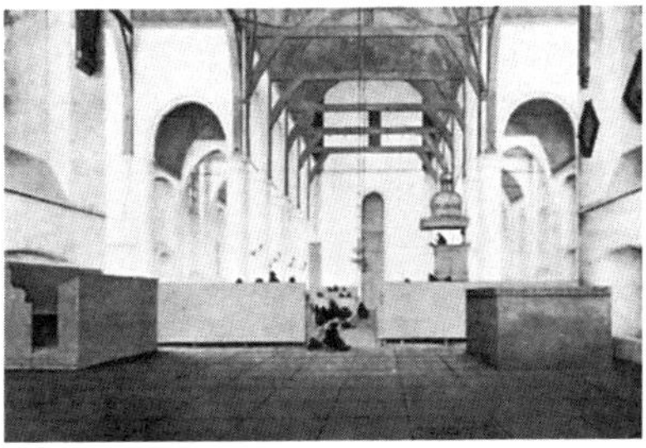

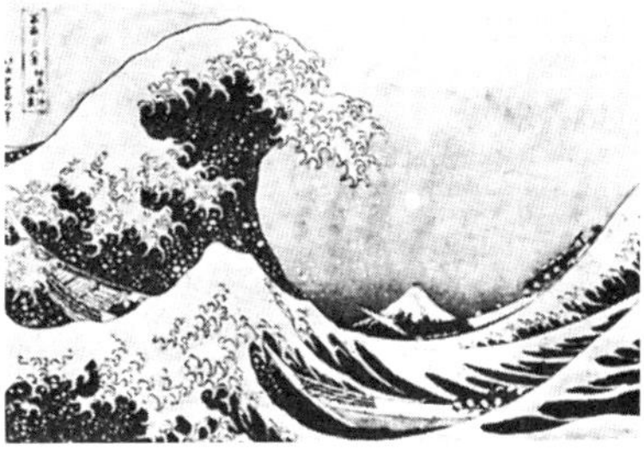

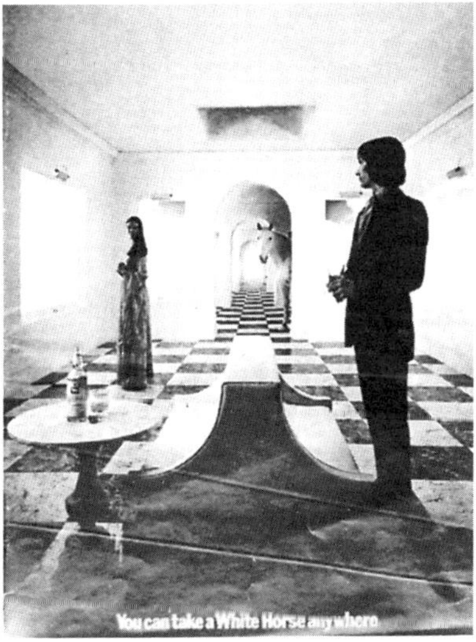
You can take a White Horse anywhere

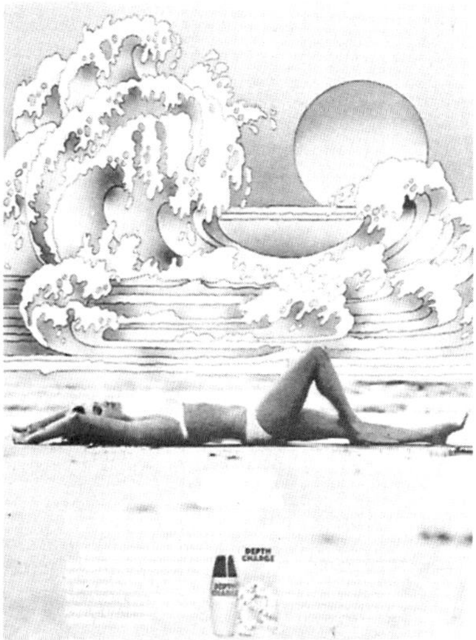
DEPTH CHARGE

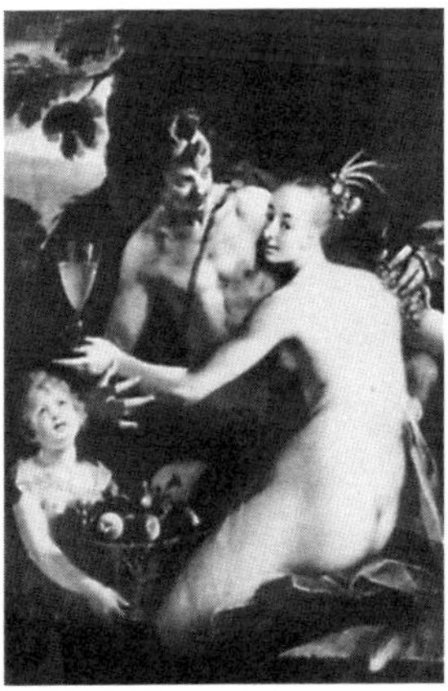

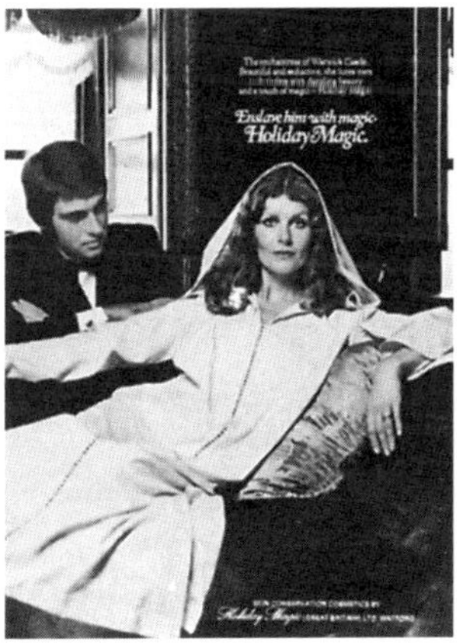
Enslave him with magic.
Holiday Magic.

Жесты моделей (манекенов) и мифологических персонажей.

Романтическое использование природы (листвы, деревьев, воды) с целью изображения места, где может быть вновь обретена невинность.

Экзотическое и ностальгическое влечение к Средиземноморью.

Позы, используемые для обозначения того или иного женского стереотипа: безмятежная мать (мадонна), фривольная секретарша (актриса, любовница короля), идеальная хозяйка (жена зрителя-владельца), объект сексуального желания (Венера, застигнутая врасплох нимфа) и т. д.

Особый сексуальный акцент на женских ногах.

Материалы, преимущественно используемые для обозначения роскоши: гравированный металл, меха, блестящая кожа и т. д.

Жесты и объятия любовников, показанные так, чтобы зритель мог их хорошо рассмотреть.

Море, сулящее новую жизнь.

Физическая форма мужчин, говорящая об их богатстве и мужественности.

Перспективные искажения пространства, создающие таинственность.

Спиртные напитки как показатель успешности.

Мужчина из рыцаря (всадника) превращается в мотоциклиста.

Почему же реклама так зависит от визуального языка масляной живописи?

Реклама – это культура общества потребления. Она посредством визуальных образов поддерживает веру этого общества в себя. Есть несколько причин тому, что для этого используется язык масляной живописи.

Масляная живопись, прежде всего остального, была прославлением частной собственности. Как форма искусства она выросла из убеждения: *ты – это то, чем ты владеешь.*

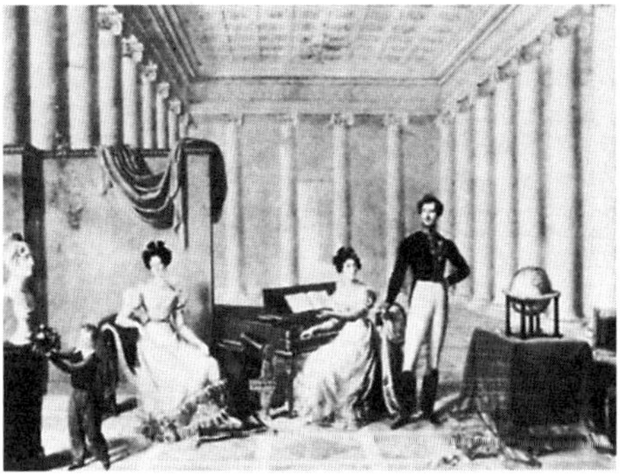

КАРЛ ЛЮДОВИК БУРБОН ПАРМСКИЙ С ЖЕНОЙ, СЕСТРОЙ И БУДУЩИМ КАРЛОМ III ПАРМСКИМ. НЕИЗВЕСТНЫЙ ХУДОЖНИК. XIX ВЕК

Будет ошибкой считать, что реклама заняла место искусства постренессансной Европы: она последняя, умирающая форма этого искусства.

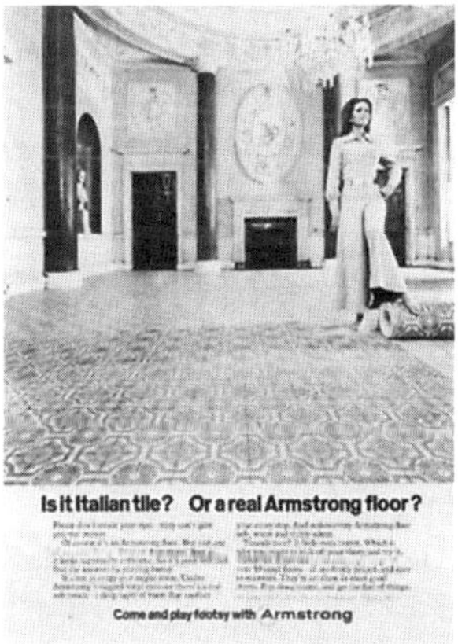

Реклама по сути своей ностальгична. Она призвана продать прошлое будущему. Она сама не в состоянии обеспечить собственные стандарты. Так что все ее указания на качество вынуждены быть ретроспективными и традиционными. Если она будет использовать только современный язык, то окажется неубедительной и не внушающей доверия.

Реклама вынуждена извлекать выгоду из традиционного образования среднего зрителя-покупателя. Все то, что он узнал в школе об истории, мифологии и поэзии, может быть использовано при производстве рекламы. Сигары могут продаваться именем короля, нижнее белье – при поддержке сфинкса, а новая машина – при помощи аллюзии на статусность загородного дома.

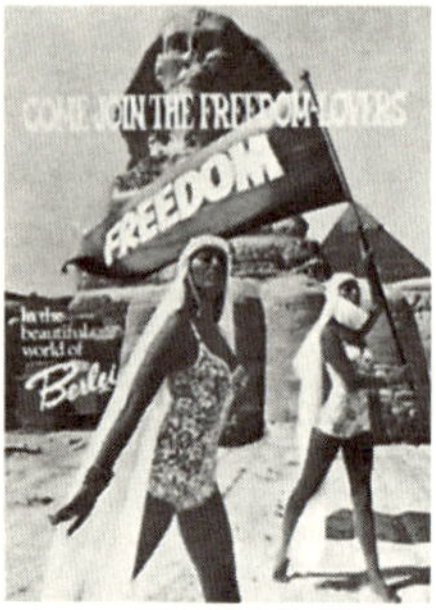

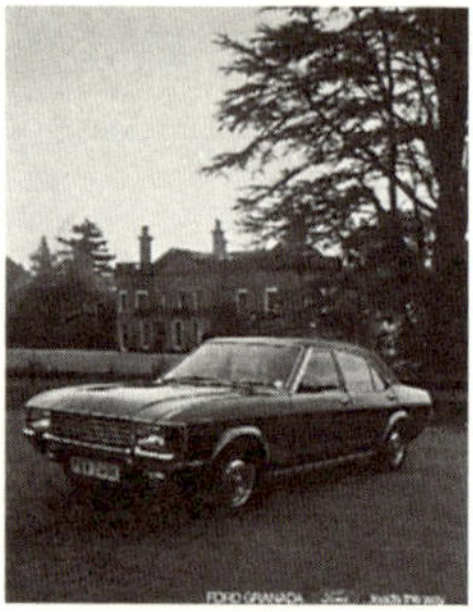

В языке масляной живописи эти смутные исторические, поэтические и нравоучительные отсылки всегда присутствуют. Тот факт, что они остаются неопределенными и, в конечном счете, бессмысленными, идет только на пользу: не нужно, чтобы их понимали, они должны быть просто отголоском некогда полученных знаний. Реклама всю историю превращает в мифологию, но чтобы это вполне получалось, ей нужен визуальный язык, обладающий историческим измерением.

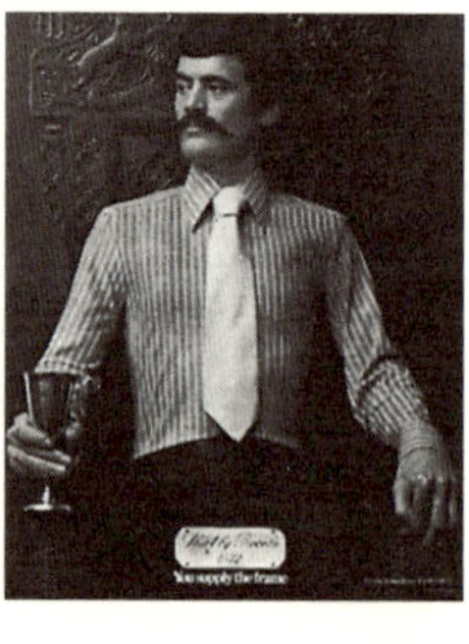

И наконец, технический прогресс очень облегчил перевод с языка масляной живописи на язык рекламных клише. Этому послужило изобретение в середине XX века дешевой цветной фотографии. Такая фотография способна воспроизводить цвет, текстуру и осязаемость вещей, как раньше могла только масляная живопись. Цветная фотография стала для зрителя-покупателя тем, чем была для зрителя-владельца масляная живопись. И то и другое использует одни и те же ориентированные на осязание приемы, для того чтобы вызвать у зрителя ощущение, будто он приобретает настоящую вещь, в действительности же лишь изображенную. В обоих случаях ощущение, будто он может прямо дотронуться до того, что изображено, напоминает ему о том, что он мог бы владеть или уже владеет этой вещью в реальности.

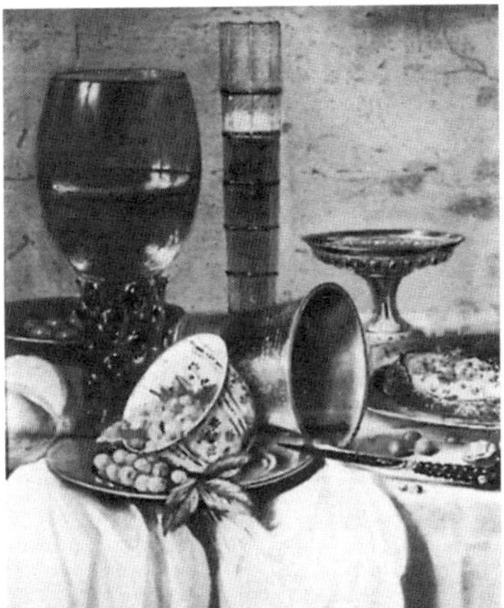

НАТЮРМОРТ С БОКАЛАМИ.
КЛАС. 1596/7–1661

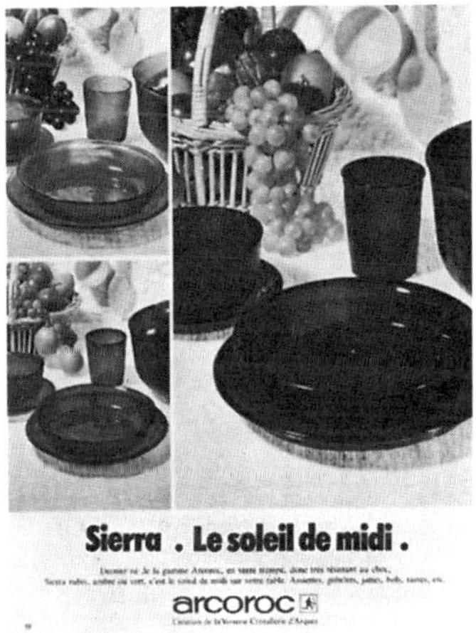

Однако, несмотря на преемственность языка, функция рекламы очень отличается от функции масляной живописи. Зритель-покупатель находится в иных отношениях с миром, чем зритель-владелец.

Масляная живопись показывала то, чем ее владелец уже обладает и что уже входит в его образ жизни. Она подкрепляла его сознание собственной значительности. Она поддерживала его уже существующее представление о самом себе. Она началась с фактов, с фактов его жизни. Картины украшали интерьеры, в которых их хозяин жил.

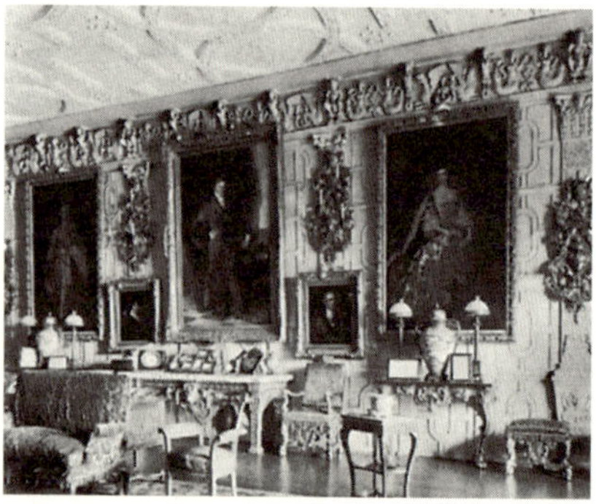

Цель рекламы – заставить зрителя испытать некоторое неудовлетворение от той жизни, которую он ведет. Не жизни общества в целом, но его собственной жизни. Реклама утверждает, что, если он купит предлагаемое, жизнь его станет лучше. Она предлагает ему усовершенствованный вариант его самого.

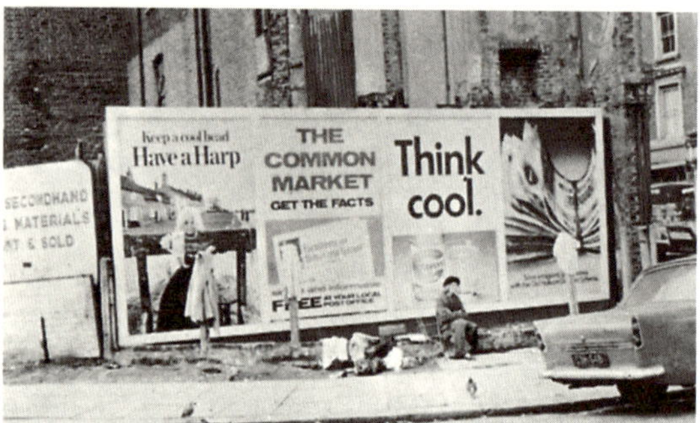

Масляная живопись обращалась к тем, кто извлекал прибыль из рынка. Реклама обращается к тем, кто, собственно, и представляет собой рынок, – к зрителю-покупателю, одновременно являющемуся потребителем-производителем; прибыль из него извлекается дважды – сперва как из работника, а потом как из покупателя. Единственное пространство, остающееся относительно свободным от рекламы, – это кварталы, где живут очень богатые люди; на их деньги никто не покушается.

Любая реклама играет на тревоге. Все в конечном счете сводится к деньгам; получить деньги – значит преодолеть тревогу.

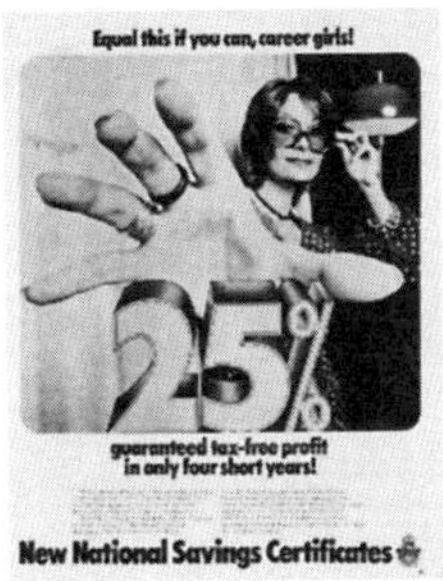

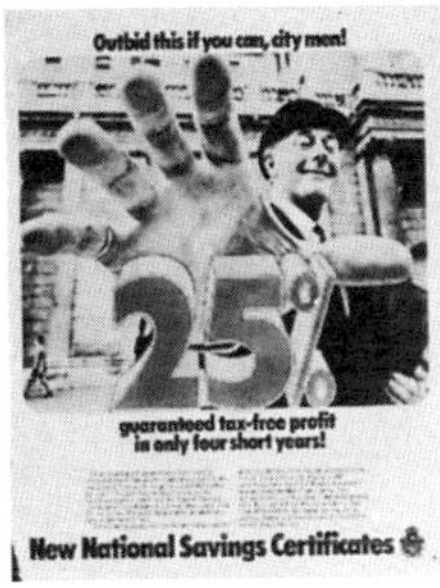

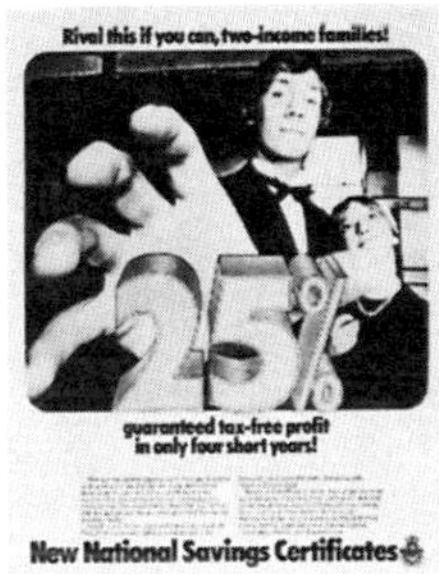

Другая тревога, на которой играет реклама, – это страх того, что, не имея ничего, ты останешься ничем.

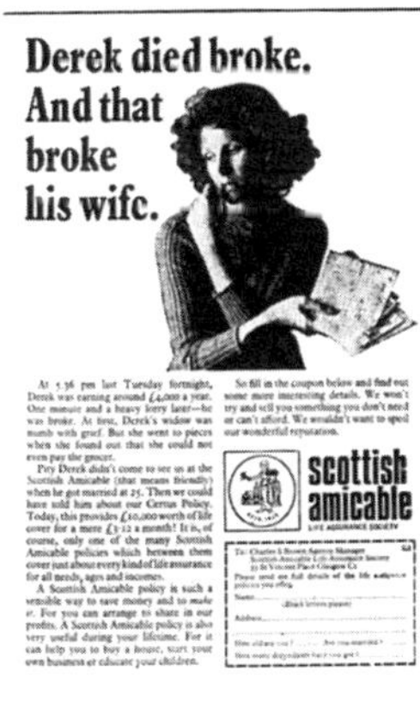

Деньги – это жизнь. Не в том смысле, что без денег тебе придется голодать. Не в том смысле, что капитал дает одному классу власть над жизнью другого класса. Но в том смысле, что деньги – это ключ ко всем человеческим возможностям и знак этих возможностей. Способность тратить деньги – это жизненная сила. Согласно рекламным максимам те, кому не хватает этой силы, становятся в буквальном смысле безликими. А те, кто ею наделен, привлекают к себе любовь окружающих.

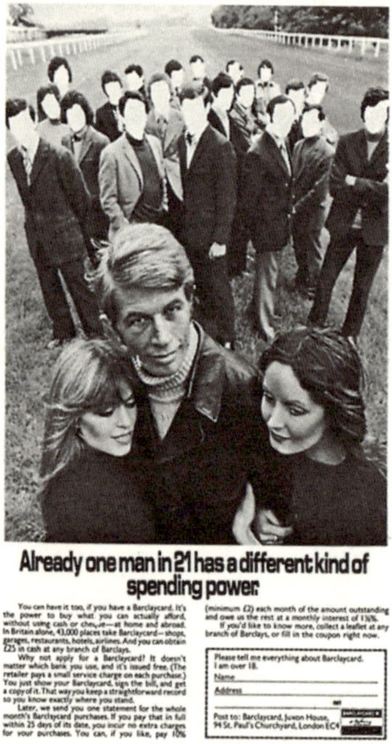

Реклама все больше и больше апеллирует к сексуальности, продавая любые продукты и услуги. Но это, в сущности, не сексуальность сама по себе, она является символом чего-то большего, чем она сама, – хорошей жизни, в которой ты можешь покупать все, что захочешь. Иметь возможность купить – все равно что обладать сексуальной привлекательностью; иногда этот смысл лежит на самой поверхности, как в приведенной выше рекламе кредитных карт. Обычно же этот посыл выражен не столь явно, но, тем не менее, он есть: если ты сможешь купить эту вещь, тебя будут любить. Если не сможешь – будут любить меньше.

Для рекламы то, что существует сейчас, по определению неудовлетворительно. Масляная живопись мыслилась как фиксация реальности навечно. Одним из наслаждений, которые живописное полотно доставляло своему владельцу, была мысль о том, что картина перенесет образ его настоящего в будущее его потомков. Таким образом, масляная живопись, естественно, говорила обо всем в настоящем времени. Художник рисовал то, что находилось перед ним, в реальности или в воображении. А эфемерный рекламный образ использует только будущее время. Получив это, ты станешь желанным. В этой обстановке твои отношения с людьми станут счастливыми и лучезарными.

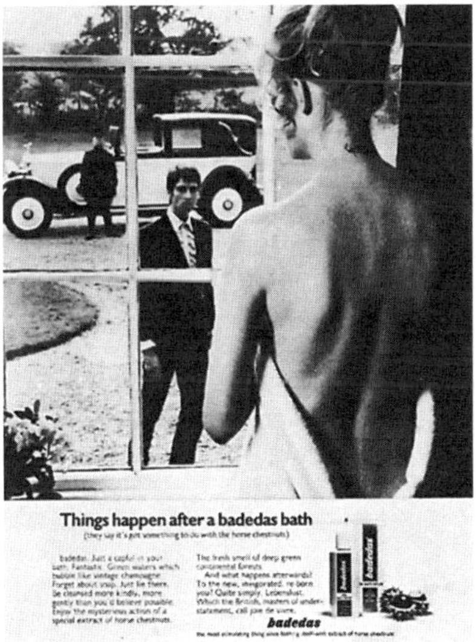

Реклама, адресованная рабочему классу, обычно обещает преображение за счет некой функции того продукта, который она продает (Золушка); реклама для среднего класса обещает преображение отношений за счет общей атмосферы, которую создает набор продуктов (Заколдованный дворец).

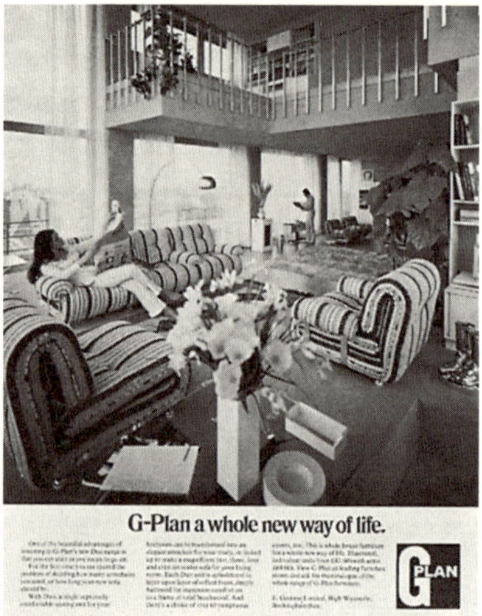

Реклама говорит в будущем времени, однако наступление этого будущего бесконечно откладывается. Как же рекламе удается по-прежнему вызывать доверие, по крайней мере, настолько, чтобы оказывать то влияние, которое она оказывает? Ей доверяют, поскольку ее правдивость доказана – не воплощением в реальность ее обещаний, а тем, насколько ее фантазии соответствуют фантазиям зрителя-покупателя. Она обращается не столько к реальности, сколько к мечтам.

Чтобы лучше с этим разобраться, нужно вернуться к понятию *гламура*.

Гламур – современное изобретение. В пору расцвета масляной живописи его не существовало. Представления об изяществе, элегантности, авторитете складывались во что-то с виду сходное, но в основе своей принципиально иное.

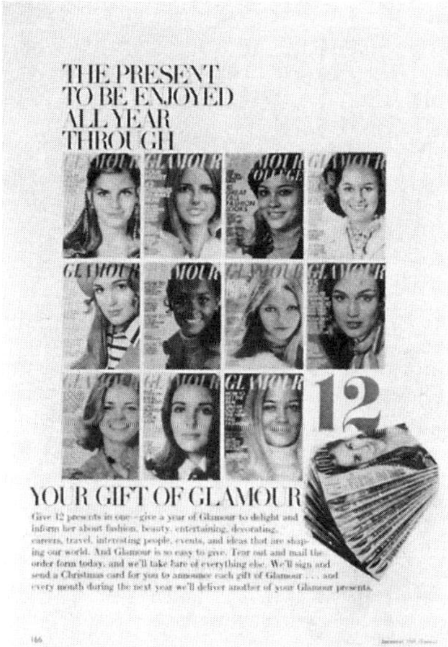

Портрет Сары Сиддонс кисти Гейнсборо – это не гламур, потому что она не представлена здесь как вызывающая зависть, а потому счастливая. Ее можно увидеть как

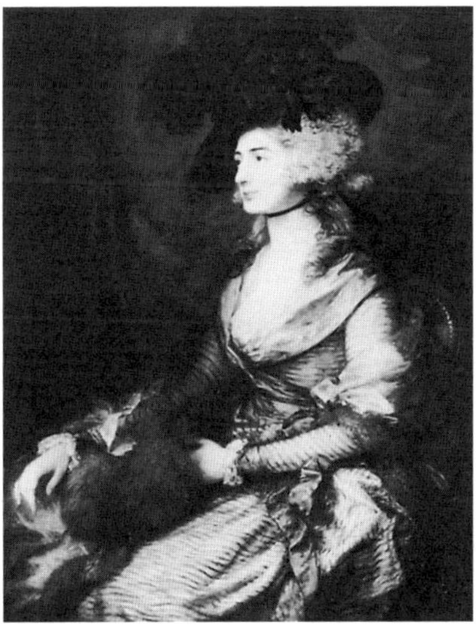

ПОРТРЕТ САРЫ СИДДОНС. ГЕЙНСБОРО. 1727–1788

богатую, красивую, талантливую, успешную женщину. Но это ее личные качества, и они именно так и понимаются. То, чем она является, не зависит полностью от других, жаждущих быть такой, как она. Она не является созданием чужой зависти, в отличие от, например, Мэрилин Монро, как она предстает у Энди Уорхола.

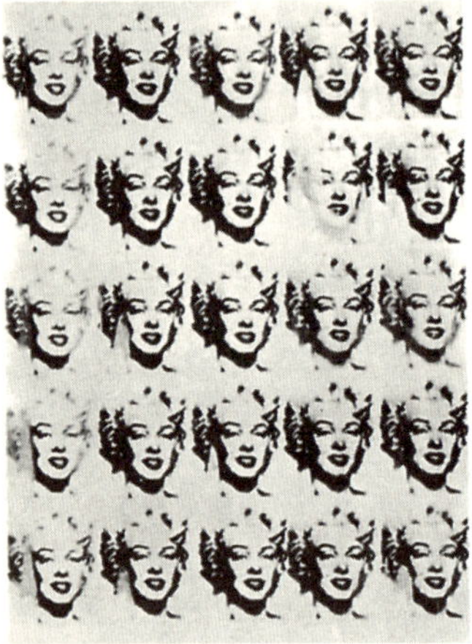

МЭРИЛИН МОНРО.
ЭНДИ УОРХОЛ

Гламур не может существовать без опоры на социальную зависть – эмоцию обычную и широко распространенную. Индустриальное общество, двигавшееся в сторону демократии, но остановившееся на полпути, – идеальная среда для выработки этой эмоции. Стремление к личному счастью было признано всеобщим правом. Но в существующих социальных условиях человек чувствует себя беспомощным. Его все время разрывает противоречие между тем, кем он является, и тем, кем он хотел бы быть. Либо он вполне осознает это противоречие и его причины и включается в борьбу за полную демократию, предполагающую, среди всего прочего, и свержение капитализма; либо он продолжает жить во власти зависти, которая, соединяясь с его ощущением беспомощности, преображается в порождаемых вновь и вновь фантазиях.

Это позволяет понять, почему люди до сих пор верят рекламе. Разрыв между тем, что реклама действительно предлагает, и тем будущим, которое она сулит, соответствует разрыву между тем, кем зритель-покупатель себя чувствует, и тем, кем он хотел бы быть. Два разрыва становятся одним; но вместо того чтобы преодолевать этот разрыв с помощью действия или проживаемого опыта, его заполняют гламурными фантазиями.

Этот процесс часто поддерживается условиями труда.

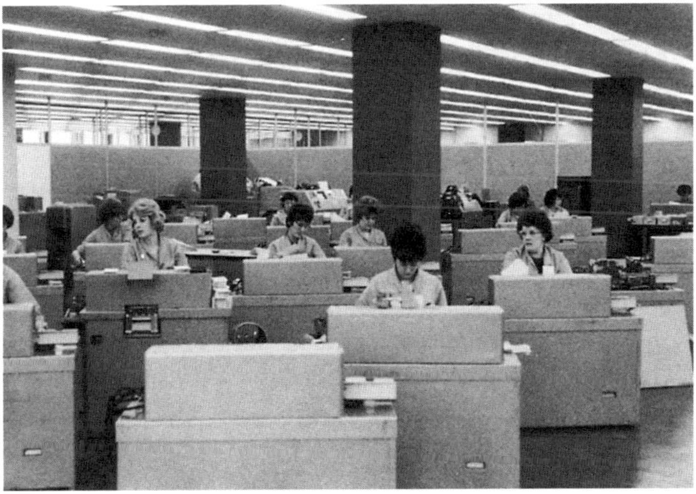

Бесконечное настоящее бессмысленных рабочих часов «сбалансировано» вымечтанным будущим, в котором воображаемая активность замещает имеющуюся пассивность. В своих фантазиях пассивный работник превращается в активного потребителя. Работающее «я» завидует потребляющему «я».

Все мечты разные. Одни краткие, а другие долгие. Мечты у каждого мечтателя свои. Реклама не производит меч-

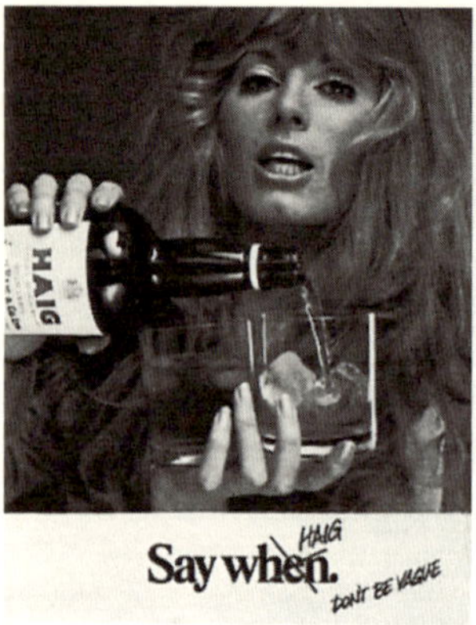

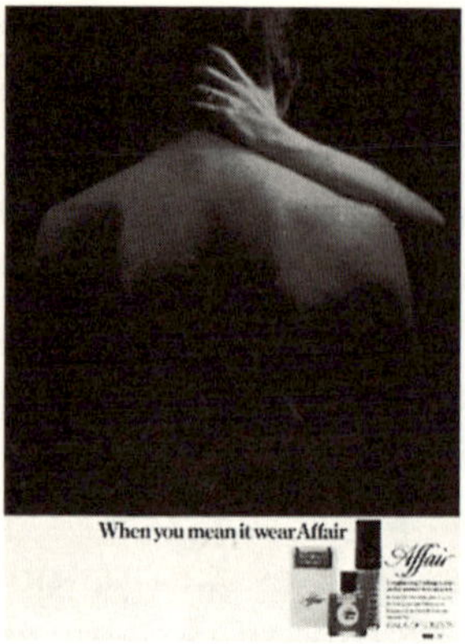

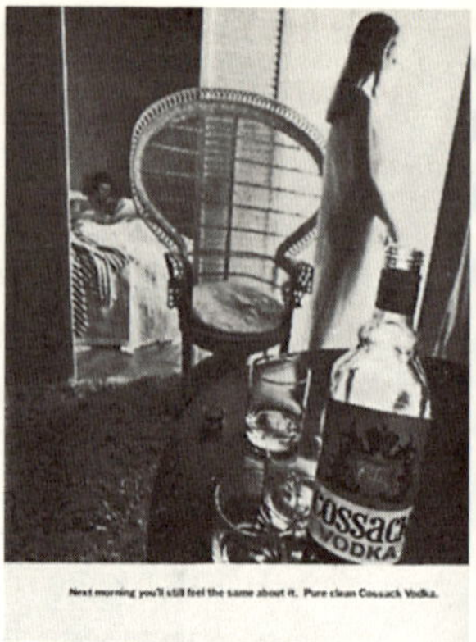

ты. Единственное, что она делает, – это говорит каждому из нас, что нам пока нельзя позавидовать, но что это можно изменить.

У рекламы есть и другая важная социальная функция. Тот факт, что появление этой функции никогда не было целью тех, кто создает и использует рекламу, нисколько не умаляет ее значения. Реклама превращает потребле-

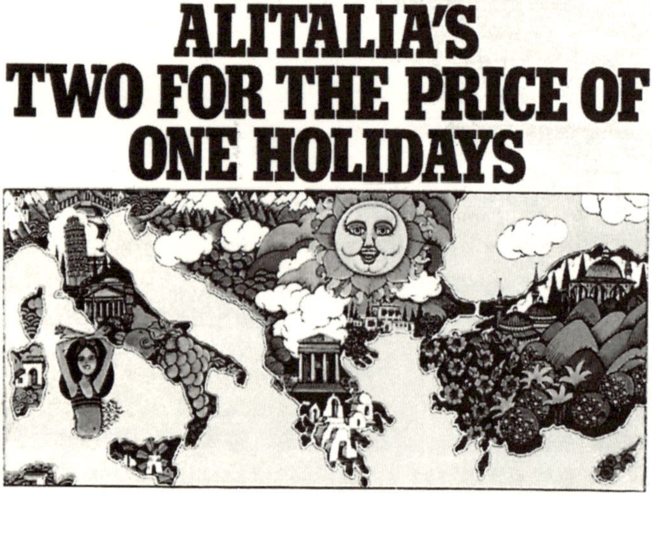

ние в субститут демократии. Возможность выбрать, что есть (или что носить, или на чем ездить), заменяет собой возможность значимого политического выбора. Реклама помогает замаскировать и компенсировать все, что есть недемократического в обществе. Кроме того, она скрывает то, что происходит во всем остальном мире.

Реклама складывается в своего рода философскую систему. Она объясняет все в своих собственных координатах. Она интерпретирует мир.

Весь мир превращается в декорации, в которых должно исполняться рекламное обещание лучшей жизни. Мир улыбается нам. Он предлагает нам себя. И поскольку весь мир воображается как предлагающий себя нам, то весь мир становится более или менее одинаковым.

Согласно рекламе, быть умным – значит обходить конфликты стороной.

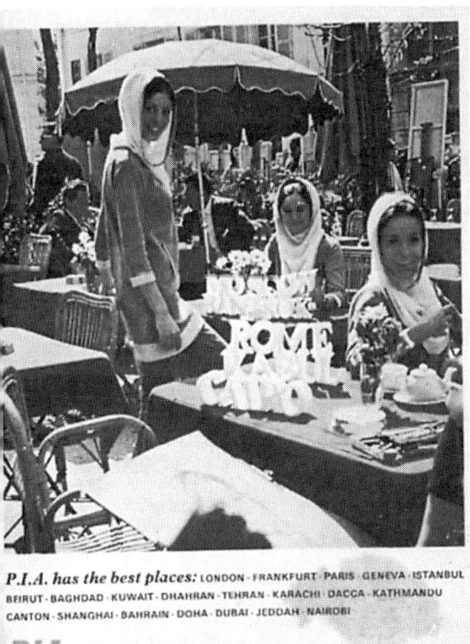

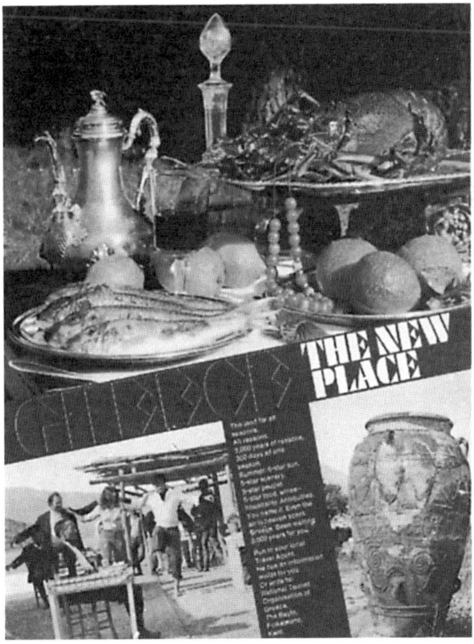

Реклама даже революцию может проинтерпретировать по-своему.

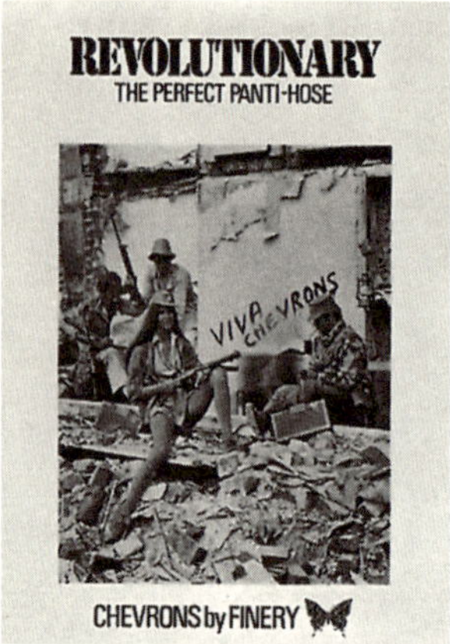
REVOLUTIONARY
THE PERFECT PANTI-HOSE
VIVA CHEVRONS
CHEVRONS by FINERY

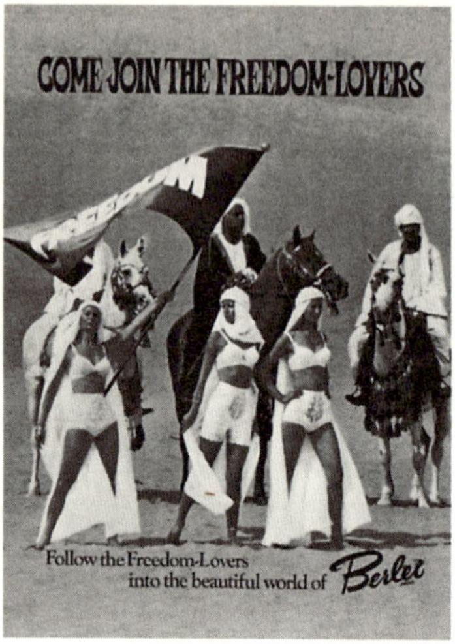
COME JOIN THE FREEDOM-LOVERS
Follow the Freedom-Lovers
into the beautiful world of Berlei

Контраст между предлагаемой рекламой интерпретацией мира и реальным его состоянием может быть разителен; иногда он становится очевидным в глянцевых журналах, говорящих о текущих событиях. Вот картинки с разворота подобного журнала.

Такого рода контрасты шокируют, причем не только сосуществованием двух показанных миров, но и цинизмом культуры, показывающей их на одной странице, друг над другом. Допустим, столь близкое соседство этих картинок не было запланировано. И, тем не менее, текст, фотографии, сделанные в Пакистане, фотографии, сделанные для рекламы, работа редактора, верстка рекламы, печать всего вместе, тот факт, что новости и реклама не могут быть скоординированы, – все это продукты одной и той же культуры.

Что следует особенно подчеркнуть, так это отнюдь не нравственный шок от такого рода контрастов. Рекламо-

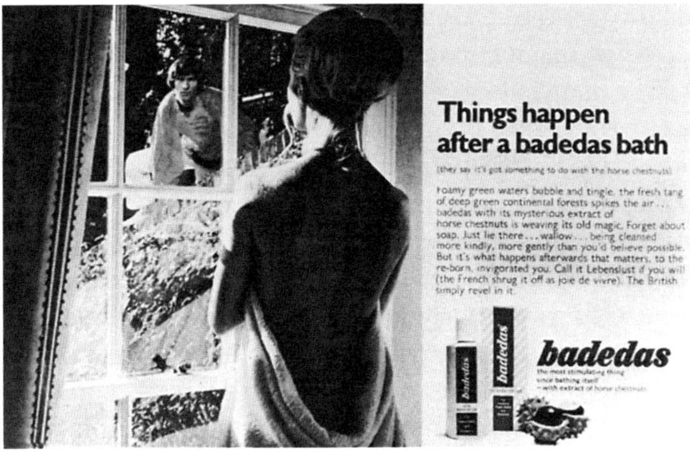

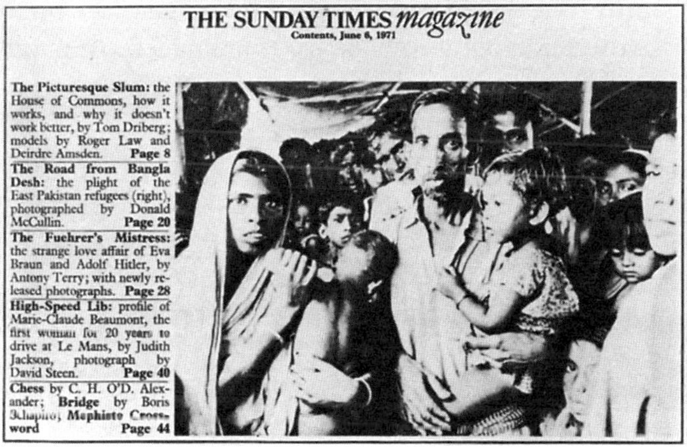

THE SUNDAY TIMES *magazine*

Contents, June 6, 1971

The Picturesque Slum: the House of Commons, how it works, and why it doesn't work better, by Tom Driberg; models by Roger Law and Deirdre Amsden. **Page 8**

The Road from Bangla Desh: the plight of the East Pakistan refugees (right), photographed by Donald McCullin. **Page 20**

The Fuehrer's Mistress: the strange love affair of Eva Braun and Adolf Hitler, by Antony Terry; with newly released photographs. **Page 28**

High-Speed Lib: profile of Marie-Claude Beaumont, the first woman for 20 years to drive at Le Mans, by Judith Jackson, photograph by David Steen. **Page 40**

Chess by C. H. O'D. Alexander; **Bridge** by Boris Schapiro; **Mephisto Crossword** **Page 44**

датели и сами осознают этот эффект. В Advertisers Weekly от 3 марта 1972 года писали, что некоторые рекламные агентства, осознавшие коммерческую опасность такого рода неудачных соположений в новостных журналах, решили использовать менее дерзкие, неяркие образы, часто черно-белые, а не цветные. Что нам нужно осознать, так это то, чтó такие контрасты говорят о природе рекламы.

Реклама по сути своей бессобытийна. Она длится, пока ничего другого не происходит. Для рекламы все события реальности – это исключения, происходящие только с чужаками. На фотографиях из Бангладеш показаны события трагические и очень далекие. Но контраст не был бы менее разительным, если бы это были события, произошедшие неподалеку. Более того, такой контраст создается не только событиями трагическими. Если они трагичны, то эта трагичность взывает к нашему нравственному чувству. Однако даже если это события веселые, но сняты непосредственно и не стереотипно, контраст все равно будет очень сильным.

Реклама, живущая в отложенном будущем, исключает все настоящее и, значит, все становящееся, все развивающееся. В ее рамках невозможен опыт. Все, что происходит, происходит за ее пределами.

То, что реклама бессобытийна, было бы тут же замечено, если бы она не использовала язык, который саму осязаемость делает событием. Все, что показывает реклама, ждет, когда же его приобретут. Приобретение как действие заняло место всех остальных действий; чувство обладания вытеснило все остальные чувства.

Реклама оказывает невероятное влияние и является политическим феноменом огромной важности. Но ее предложения столь же немногочисленны, сколь многообразны содержащиеся в ней ссылки на культурный опыт. Она не знает ничего, кроме возможности приобретать. Все другие человеческие способности и нужды оказываются второстепенными по отношению к этой возможности. Все мечты и надежды объединяются, делаются однородными, упрощаются – так, чтобы они совпали с тем сильным, но смутным, волшебным, но повторяющимся рекламным посулом. Никакие другие надежды, удовольствия и наслаждения уже не могут быть помыслены в рамках культуры капитализма.

Реклама – жизнь этой культуры (постольку, поскольку без рекламы капитализм не может существовать), и в то же время реклама – это ее мечта.

Капитализм выживает, заставляя эксплуатируемое большинство определять свои интересы как можно более узко. Раньше это достигалось за счет ущемления его прав. Сегодня в развитых странах это достигается путем навязывания ложных стандартов того, к чему следует, а к чему не следует стремиться.

НА ПОРОГЕ СВОБОДЫ.
РЕНЕ МАГРИТТ.
1898–1967

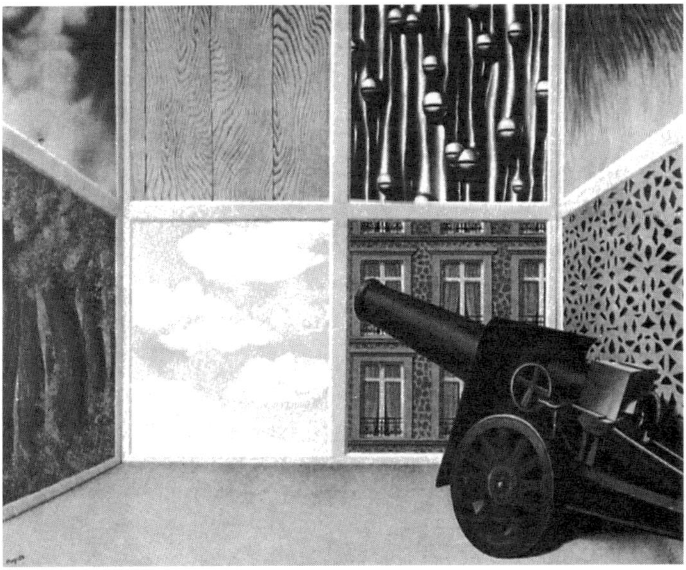

СПИСОК ИЛЛЮСТРАЦИЙ

С. 10. Ключ к грезам. Рене Магритт (1898–1967). Частная коллекция.
С. 15. Регенты приюта для престарелых. Франс Хальс (1580–1666). Музей Франса Хальса. Харлем.
С. 15. Регентши приюта для престарелых. Франс Хальс (1580–1666). Музей Франса Хальса. Харлем.
С. 23. Натюрморт с плетеным стулом. Пикассо (1881–1973).
С. 25. Мадонна в скалах. Леонардо да Винчи (1452–1519). Лондонская Национальная галерея.
С. 27. Мадонна в скалах. Леонардо да Винчи (1452–1519). Лувр, Париж.
С. 31. Венера и Марс. Сандро Боттичелли (1445–1510). Лондонская Национальная галерея.
С. 33. Шествие на Голгофу. Питер Брейгель-старший (1525–1569). Музей истории искусства, Вена.
С. 33. Пшеничное поле с воронами. Винсент Ван Гог (1853–1890). Городской музей (Стеделек-музей) Амстердама.
С. 37. Служанка с кувшином молока. Ян Вермеер (1632–1675). Государственный музей (Рейксмюзеум), Амстердам.
С. 46. *(вверху слева)* Обнаженная. Пикассо (1881–1973).
С. 46. *(вверху справа)* Обнаженная. Модильяни (1884–1920). Галерея Института Курто, Лондон.
С. 46. *(внизу слева)* Больше никогда. Гоген (1848–1903). Галерея Института Курто, Лондон.
С. 46. *(внизу справа)* Стоящая обнаженная. Джакометти. Галерея Тейт, Лондон.
С. 47. Вирсавия. Рембрандт ван Рейн (1606–1669). Лувр, Париж.
С. 51. Суд Париса. Питер Пауль Рубенс (1577–1640). Лондонская Национальная галерея.
С. 53. Обнаженная на шкуре пантеры. Феликс Трюта (1824–1848). Музей изящных искусств, Дижон.
С. 57. Райский сад; Искушение; Грехопадение и изгнание из рая. Миниатюры из «Великолепного часослова герцога Беррийского». Поль де Лимбург и братья (до 1416). Музее Конде, Шантийи.
С. 57. Адам и Ева. Ян Госсарт по прозванию Мабюз (умер ок. 1533). Коллекция Ее Величества королевы Елизаветы II.

С. 58. Пара. Макс Слефогт (1868–1932).
С. 58. Сусанна и старцы. Якопо Тинторетто (1518–1594). Лувр, Париж.
С. 59. Сусанна и старцы. Якопо Тинторетто (1518–1594). Музей истории искусства, Вена.
С. 59. Земное тщеславие и божественное искупление. Ханс Мемлинг (1435–1494). Страсбургский музей.
С. 60. Суд Париса. Лукас Кранах-старший (1472–1553). Краеведческий музей города Гота.
С. 61. Суд Париса. Питер Пауль Рубенс (1577–1640). Лондонская Национальная галерея.
С. 61. Нелль Гвин. Сэр Питер Лели (1618–1680).
С. 62. Керамика Моче, изображающая сексуальные отношения. Фотография Шипи-Джонсона, Лима, Перу.
С. 62. Раджастан (XVIII век). Аджит Мукерджи, Нью-Дели.
С. 62. Вишну и Лакшми (XI век). Храм Парсваната, Каджурахо.
С. 64. Венера, Купидон, Безрассудство и Время. Аньоло Бронзино (1503–72). Лондонская Национальная галерея.
С. 65. Большая одалиска (фрагмент). Ж.-О.-Д. Энгр (1780–1867). Лувр, Париж.
С. 65. Вакх, Церера и Купидон. Ханс фон Аахен (1552–1615). Музей истории искусства, Вена.
С. 66. Ореады. Вильям Бугро (1825–1905). Частная коллекция.
С. 68. Даная (деталь). Рембрандт ван Рейн (1606–1669). Эрмитаж, Санкт-Петербург.
С. 71. Шубка. Портрет Елены Фоурмен. Питер Пауль Рубенс (1577–1640). Музей истории искусства, Вена.
С. 73. Художник, рисующий лежащую женщину. Альбрехт Дюрер (1471–1528).
С. 73. Гравюра на дереве из «Четырех книг о пропорциях». Альбрехт Дюрер (1471–1528).
С. 74. Венера Урбинская. Тициан (1487/90–1576). Галерея Уффици, Флоренция.
С. 74. Олимпия. Эдуард Мане (1832–1883). Лувр, Париж.
С. 78. *(сверху слева)* Мадонна на троне. Чимабуэ (ок. 1240–1302(?)), Лувр, Париж.
С. 78. *(сверху справа)* Мадонна с младенцем и четырьмя ангелами. Пьеро делла Франческа (1410/20–1492). Уильямстоун, Художественный институт Кларк.
С. 78. *(внизу слева)* Мадонна с младенцем. Фра Филиппо Липпи (1457/8–1504).
С. 78. *(внизу справа)* Отдых на пути в Египет. Герард Давид (ум. 1523). Вашингтонская Национальная картинная галерея, коллекция Меллона.
С. 79. *(вверху слева)* Сикстинская Мадонна. Рафаэль (1483–1520). Галерея Уффици, Флоренция.

С. 79. *(вверху справа)* Мадонна с младенцем. Мурильо (1617–1682). Палаццо Питти, Флоренция.
С. 79. *(внизу)* Симпатичные барашки. Форд Мэдокс Браун (1821–1893). Музей города Бирмингем.
С. 80. *(вверху)* Смерть святого Франциска. Джотто (1266/7–1337). Санта-Кроче, Флоренция.
С. 80. *(внизу)* Триумф смерти. Питер Брейгель (1525/30–1569). Музей истории искусств, Вена.
С. 81. *(вверху слева)* Головы казненных. Теодор Жерико (1791–1824). Национальный музей, Стокгольм.
С. 81. *(вверху справа)* Три возраста женщины и Смерть. Ханс Бальдунг Грин (1483–1545). Прадо, Мадрид.
С. 81. *(внизу)* Мертвый тореадор. Эдуард Мане (1832–1883).
С. 82. *(вверху)* Натюрморт. Жан Батист Симеон Шарден (1699–1779). Лондонская Национальная галерея.
С. 82. *(внизу)* Натюрморт. Франсиско Гойя (1746–1828). Лувр, Париж.
С. 83. *(вверху)* Натюрморт. Жан Батист Удри (1686–1755). Коллекция Уоллеса, Лондон.
С. 83. *(внизу)* Натюрморт. Ян Фейт. Коллекция Уоллеса, Лондон.
С. 84. Дафнис и Хлоя. Бьянки-Феррари. Коллекция Уоллеса, Лондон.
С. 85. *(вверху)* Венера и Марс. Пьеро ди Козимо (1462–1521). Картинная галерея, Берлин-Далем.
С. 85. *(внизу)* Пан. Лука Синьорелли (ок. 1441/50–1523). Оригинал утрачен, хранился в Музее кайзера Фридриха, Берлин.
С. 86. *(вверху)* Руджеро, спасающий Анжелику. Ж.-О.-Д. Энгр (1780–1867). Лондонская Национальная галерея.
С. 86. *(внизу)* Римский пир. Тома Кутюр (1815–1879). Коллекция Уоллеса, Лондон.
С. 87. *(вверху)* Пан и Сиринга. Буше (1703–1770). Лондонская Национальная галерея.
С. 87. *(внизу)* Любовь соблазняет Невинность, Удовольствие завлекает, а Раскаяние преследует. Пьер Поль Прюдон (1758–1823). Коллекция Уоллеса, Лондон.
С. 88. Зал в Ноул-Хаус.
С. 89. *(вверху слева)* Портрет Эммануила Филиберта, герцога Савойского. Антонис ван Дейк (1599–1641). Дулвич.
С. 89. *(внизу слева)* Портрет Эндимиона Портера. Уильям Добсон (1610–1646). Галерея Тейт, Лондон.
С. 89. *(справа)* Норман, 22-й глава клана Маклаудов. Аллан Рэмзи (1713–1784). Замок Данвеган.
С. 90. *(вверху)* Портрет Декарта. Франс Хальс (1580/5–1666). Копенгаген.
С. 90. *(внизу)* Портрет придворного шута Себастьяна де Морра. Диего Веласкес (1599–1660). Прадо, Мадрид.
С. 91. *(вверху слева)* Портрет доньи Тадеа Ариас де Энрикес. Франсиско Гойя (1746–1828). Прадо, Мадрид.

С. 91. *(вверху справа)* Возвращение с рынка. Жан Батист Симеон Шарден (1699–1779).
С. 91. *(внизу)* Похититель детей. Теодор Жерико (1791–1824). Спрингфилд, Массачусетс.
С. 92. *(вверху)* Автопортрет. Альбрехт Дюрер (1471–1528).
С. 92. *(внизу)* Автопортрет. Рембрандт ван Рейн (1606–1669).
С. 93. *(вверху)* Автопортрет. Франсиско Гойя (1746–1828). Музей Кастра.
С. 93. *(внизу)* Воспроизведение запрещено. Рене Магритт (1898–1967). Коллекция Э.-Ф.-У. Джеймса, Сассекс.
С. 95. Сокровища Пастонов в Окснид-холл. Фламандская школа (ок. 1665). Музей города Норидж.
С. 97. Эрцгерцог Леопольд-Вильгельм в своей картинной галерее. Давид Тенирс-старший (1582–1649). Музей истории искусства, Вена.
С. 99. Картинная галерея кардинала Валенти Гонзаги. Г.-П. Панини (1692–1765/8). Уодсворт Атенеум, Хартфорд, Коннектикут.
С. 99. Картинная галерея. Фландрия (XVII век). Лондонская Национальная галерея.
С. 102. Послы. Ханс Гольбейн-младший (1497/8–1543). Лондонская Национальная галерея.
С. 105. Vanitas. Виллем де Портер (1608–1648). Коллекция Башенгера, Женева.
С. 105. Читающая Магдалина. Мастерская Амвросия Бенсона (действовала в 1519–1550). Лондонская Национальная галерея.
С. 105. Мария Магдалина. Адриан ван дер Верф (1659–1722). Дрезден.
С. 106. Кающаяся Магдалина. Бодри (Салон 1859 г.). Музей изящных искусств, Нант.
С. 107. Акварельная иллюстрация к «Божественной комедии» Данте: Надпись на Дверях Ада. Уильям Блейк (1757–1827). Галерея Тейт, Лондон.
С. 109. Адмирал де Рюйтер в крепости Эльмина. Эмануэль де Витте (1617–1692). Коллекция вдовствующей Леди Харлек, Лондон.
С. 110. Индия приносит свои жемчуга Британии. Картина создана для Ост-Индской компании в конце XVIII века. Министерство иностранных дел и по делам Содружества.
С. 112. Фердинанд II Тосканский и Виктория делла Ровере. Юстус Сустерманс (1597–1681). Лондонская Национальная галерея.
С. 112. Мистер и миссис Уильям Атертон. Артур Девис (1711–1787). Художественная галерея Уокера, Ливерпуль.
С. 113. Семья Бомонт. Джордж Ромни (1734–1802). Галерея Тейт, Лондон.
С. 114. Натюрморт с омаром. Ян де Хем (1606–1684). Собрание Уоллеса, Лондон.
С. 114. Линкольнширский бык. Джордж Стаббс (1724–1806). Художественная галерея Уокера, Ливерпуль.

С. 115. Натюрморт. Приписывается Питеру Класу (1596/7–1661). Лондонская Национальная галерея.
С. 115. Роуз, королевский садовник, преподносит ананас Карлу Второму. Копия с картины Данкертса (ок. 1630–1678/9). Хэм-Хаус, Ричмонд.
С. 116. Чарльз Таунли и его друзья. Иоганн Цоффани (1734/5–1810). Картинная галерея Таунли-Холл, Бернли, Ланкашир.
С. 116. Минерва, побеждающая Невежество. Бартоломеус Спрангер (1546–1627). Венская галерея.
С. 117. Три грации, украшающие герму Гименея. Сэр Джошуа Рейнольдс (1723–1792). Галерея Тейт, Лондон.
С. 118. Тени французских генералов, встречаемые в Елисейских полях Оссианом. А.-Л. Жироде де Руси Триозон (1767–1824). Мальмезон.
С. 119. Сцена в таверне. Адриан Браувер (1605–1638). Лондонская Национальная галерея.
С. 119. Смеющийся мальчик. Франс Хальс (1580–1666). Бургштайнфурт, Вестфалия (коллекция князя Бентхайм-Штайнфурта).
С. 119. Мальчик-рыбак. Франс Хальс (1580–1666). Национальная галерея Ирландии, Дублин.
С. 120. Пейзаж с руинами. Рёйсдал (1628/9–1682). Лондонская Национальная галерея.
С. 121. Речной пейзаж с рыбаками. Ян ван Гойен (1596–1656). Лондонская Национальная галерея.
С. 122. Портрет четы Эндрюс. Томас Гейнсборо (1727–1788). Лондонская Национальная галерея.
С. 128. Автопортрет с Саскией на коленях. Рембрандт ван Рейн (1606–1669). Пинакотека, Дрезден.
С. 129. Автопортрет. Рембрандт ван Рейн (1606–1669). Галерея Уффици, Флоренция.
С. 132. *(вверху)* Европа, поддерживаемая Африкой и Америкой. Уильям Блейк (1757–1827).
С. 132. *(внизу)* Пьета. Уильям Блейк (1757–1827).
С. 133. Зерно, поражаемое болезнью. Уильям Блейк (1757–1827).
С. 134. *(вверху)* Мадмуазель де Клермон. Жан-Марк Наттье (1685–1766). Коллекция Уоллеса, Лондон.
С. 134. *(внизу)* Продажа картин и рабов в Ротонде Нового Орлеана. 1842.
С. 135. *(вверху слева)* Княгиня Ракоци. Никола Ларжильер (1656–1746). Лондонская Национальная галерея.
С. 135. *(вверху справа)* Чарльз, третий герцог Ричмондский. Иоганн Цоффани (1734/5–1810). Частная коллекция.
С. 135. *(внизу)* Два негра. Рембрандт ван Рейн (1606–1669). Гаага, галерея Маурицхёйс.
С. 136. Сара Бурдж, 1883. Приют Барнардо, неизвестный фотограф.

С. 137. Крестьянский мальчик у окна. Бартоломе Мурильо (1617–1682). Лондонская Национальная галерея.
С. 138. *(вверху слева)* Семейный портрет. Майкл Нутс (1656(?)). Лондонская Национальная галерея.
С. 138. *(вверху в центре)* Ленивая служанка. Николас Мас (1634–1693). Лондонская Национальная галерея.
С. 138. *(внизу слева)* Интерьер. Дельфтская школа (ок. 1650–1655(?)). Лондонская Национальная галерея.
С. 138. *(внизу в центре)* Мужчина и женщина на конюшне. Питер Кваст (1605/6–1647). Лондонская Национальная галерея.
С. 139. *(вверху справа)* Интерьер с готовящей женщиной. Исайя Боурсе. Коллекция Уоллеса, Лондон.
С. 139. *(внизу справа)* Сцена в таверне. Ян Стен (1626–1679). Коллекция Уоллеса, Лондон.
С. 140. *(вверху слева)* Скудная пища. Джон Фредерик Херринг (1795–1865). Галерея Тейт, Лондон.
С. 140. *(вверху справа)* Сцена в Абботсфорде. Сэр Эдвин Ландсир (1802–1873). Галерея Тейт, Лондон.
С. 140. *(в центре слева)* Две собаки (Бич и Паппи). Томас Гейнсборо (1727–1788). Лондонская Национальная галерея.
С. 140. *(в центре посередине)* Достоинство и Наглость. Сэр Эдвин Ландсир (1802–1873). Галерея Тейт, Лондон.
С. 140. *(в центре справа)* Портрет мисс Боулз с собакой. Сэр Джошуа Рейнольдс (1723–1792). Коллекция Уоллеса, Лондон.
С. 140. *(внизу)* Повозка, едущая на ярмарку (деталь). Томас Гейнсборо (1727–1788). Галерея Тейт, Лондон.
С. 141. *(вверху)* Семья Джеймс. Артур Девис (1711–1787). Галерея Тейт, Лондон.
С. 141. *(в центре слева)* Серая лошадь с собакой и грумом. Джордж Стаббс (1724–1806). Галерея Тейт, Лондон.
С. 141. *(в центре справа)* Гнедой. Джон Фернели (1782–1860). Галерея Тейт, Лондон.
С. 141. *(внизу)* Охота в Эшдаун-парк. Джеймс Сеймур. Галерея Тейт, Лондон.
С. 142. Женщина с белыми чулками. Гюстав Курбе (1819–1877).
С. 143. Девушки на берегу Сены. Гюстав Курбе (1819–1877). Музей Малого дворца, Париж.
С. 144. *(сверху)* Римляне эпохи упадка. Тома Кутюр (1815–1879).
С. 144. *(в центре)* Салон (фотография).
С. 144. *(внизу слева)* Мадам Каэн Д'Анвер. Л. Бонна.
С. 144. *(внизу справа)* Ундина. Э. Дёрстлинг.
С. 145. *(вверху слева)* На шабаш. Луи Фалеро.
С. 145. *(вверху справа)* Искушение Святого Антония. А. Моро.
С. 145. *(внизу слева)* Купание Психеи. Лейтон.
С. 145. *(внизу справа)* Фортуна. А. Меньян.

С. 147. Фотография Свена Бломберга.
С. 154. Завтрак на траве. Эдуард Мане (1832–1883). Лувр, Париж.
С. 156. *(сверху)* Юпитер и Фетида. Ж.-О.-Д. Энгр (1780–1867). Музей Гране, Экс-ан-Прованс.
С. 156. *(внизу слева)* Пан преследует Сирингу. Хендрик ван Бален-старший и ученик Яна Брейгеля-старшего, XVII век. Лондонская Национальная галерея.
С. 157. *(вверху слева)* Интерьер церкви святого Одульфа в Ассендельфте (1649). Питер Санредам (1547–1665).
С. 157. *(вверху справа)* Большая волна в Канагаве. Хокусай (1760–1849).
С. 157. (внизу слева) Вакх, Церера и Купидон. Ханс фон Аахен (1552–1615). Музей истории искусства, Вена.
С. 159. Карл Людовик Бурбон Пармский с женой, сестрой и будущим Карлом III Пармским. Неизвестный художник (XIX век). Собственность великого герцога Виареджо.
С. 161. Натюрморт с бокалами. Питер Клас (1596/7–1661). Лондонская Национальная галерея.
С. 167. Портрет Сары Сиддонс. Томас Гейнсборо (1727–1788). Лондонская Национальная галерея.
С. 168. Мэрилин Монро. Энди Уорхол.
С. 175. На пороге свободы. Рене Магритт (1898–1967).

РЕПРОДУКЦИИ В ЭТОЙ КНИГЕ ПЕЧАТАЮТСЯ
С ЛЮБЕЗНОГО РАЗРЕШЕНИЯ
СЛЕДУЮЩИХ ЛИЦ И ОРГАНИЗАЦИЙ:

Свен Бломберг; город Бирмингем; музей города Нориджа; замок Чидингстоун; Юэн Дафф; Evening Standard; Музей Франса Хальса; агентство «Жиродон»; Венский Музей истории искусства; Мэнселл; Жан Мор; Британский Национальный киноархив; Лондонская Национальная галерея; Британский Национальный трест (Country Life); Государственный музей (Рейксмюзеум) Амстердама; Галерея Тейт; Уодсворт Атенеум, Хартфорд; Коллекция Уоллеса; Художественная галерея Уокера.

Джон Бергер
ИСКУССТВО ВИДЕТЬ

Переводчик *Евгения Шрага*
Редакторы *Александр Гузман, Ольга Троицкая*
Выпускающий редактор *Мария-Анна Гущина*
Художественный редактор *Александр Веселов*
Верстка *Александра Веселова*
Корректор *Галина Година*
Издатель *Александр Троицкий*

Подписано в печать 01. 02. 2020.
Формат 60x88/16. Заказ № 0649/20.
Печать офсетная. Усл. печ. л. 11,5.
Отпечатано в соответствии с предоставленными материалами в ООО "ИПК Парето-Принт". 170546, Тверская область, Промышленная зона Боровлево-1, комплекс № 3А, www.pareto-print.ru

ООО «Морошка»
Издательство «Клаудберри»
www.klaudberri.ru